Oxygen Regulation of Ion Channels and Gene Expression

Oxygen Regulation of Ion Channels and Gene Expression

Edited by

José López-Barneo, MD, PhD

Professor of Physiology and Chairman
Department of Medical Physiology and Biophysics
Medical School, University of Seville
Seville, Spain

E. Kenneth Weir, MD

Professor of Medicine
University of Minnesota
School of Medicine
Department of Veterans Affairs Medical Center
Minneapolis, Minnesota

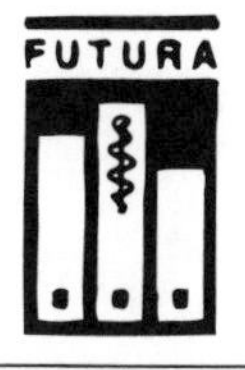

Futura Publishing Company, Inc.

Armonk, NY

Library of Congress Cataloging-in-Publication Data

Oxygen regulation of ion channels and gene expression / edited by José López-Barneo, E. Kenneth Weir.
p. cm.
Includes bibliographical references and index.
ISBN 0-87993-694-0
1. Tissue respiration. 2. Ion channels. 3. Genetic regulation.
4. Oxygen—Metabolism. I. López-Barneo, J. (Jóse)
II. Weir, E. Kenneth.
QP177.0956 1998
572′.47—dc21 97-50337
CIP

Published by
Futura Publishing Company, Inc.
135 Bedford Road
Armonk, New York 10504

LC#: 97-50337
ISBN#: 0-87993-694-0

Printed in the United States of America.

Printed on acid-free paper.

Contributors

Helmut Acker, MD [2]
Max Planck Institute for Molecular Physiology, Dortmund, Germany
Stephen L. Archer, MD [16,18]
Veterans Affairs Medical Center and University of Minnesota, Minneapolis, Minnesota
Pierre Boistard [4]
Laboratoire de Biologie Moléculaire des Relations Plantes-Microorganismes, Castanet Tolosan, France
Karlis Briviba, MD [1]
Institute for Physiologische Chemie I, Heinrich-Heine-Universitat Dusseldorf, Dusseldorf, Germany
Keith J. Buckler, PhD [12]
University Laboratory of Physiology, Parks Road, Oxford, England
H. Franklin Bunn, MD [9]
Hematology-Oncology Division, Brigham and Women's Hospital, Harvard Medical School, Boston, Massachusettes
Jaime Caro, MD [8]
Cardeza Foundation for Hematologic Research, Philadelphia, Pennsylvania
Emilio Cervantes [6]
Department of Biology, Biology Faculty, University of Salamanca, Salamanca, Spain
Dennis Choi, MD, PhD [22]
Center for the Study of the Nervous System Injury, Washington University in St. Louis, Department of Neurology, St. Louis, Missouri
David N. Cornfield, MD [16]
University of Minnesota and Veterans Affairs Medical Center, Minneapolis, Minnesota
Laura Conforti, PhD [15]
Department of Molecular and Cellular Physiology, College of Medicine, University of Cincinnati, Cincinnati, Ohio
Maria F. Czyzyk-Krzeska, MD, PhD [10]
Department of Molecular and Cellular Physiology, University of Cincinnati, Cincinnati, Ohio

---

Numbers in brackets indicate chapter(s) written or cowritten by the contributor.

Caroline Dart, PhD [20]
Ion Channel Group, Department of Cell Physiology and Pharmacology, University of Leicester, Leicester, United Kingdom
Christina S. Davie, BSc [20]
Ion Channel Group, Department of Cell Physiology and Pharmacology, University of Leicester, Leicester, United Kingdom
Laura L. Dugan, MD [22]
Center for the Study of the Nervous System Injury, Washington University in St. Louis, Department of Neurology, St. Louis, Missouri
Alfredo Franco-Obregón, PhD [19]
Department of Physiology and Biophysics, Medical Faculty, University of Seville, Seville, Spain
Jonathan M. Gleadle [7]
Institute of Molecular Medicine, John Radcliffe Hospital, Oxford, England
Constancio González, MD, PhD [24]
Department of Biochemistry and Molecular Biology and Physiology, Medical Faculty, University of Valladolid, Valladolid, Spain
Gabriel G. Haddad, MD [21]
Department of Pediatrics and Cellular and Molecular Physiology, Section of Respiratory Medicine, Yale University School of Medicine, New Haven, Connecticut
Chung Y. Hsu, MD, PhD [22]
Center for the Study of the Nervous System Injury,
Washington University in St. Louis,
Department of Neurology, St. Louis, Missouri
James Huang, PhD [18]
Veterans Affairs Medical Center and University of Minnesota, Minneapolis, Minnesota
L. Eric Huang, MD, PhD [9]
Hematology-Oncology Division, Brigham and Women's Hospital, Harvard Medical School, Boston, Massachusettes
Satoru Iwabuchi, MD, PhD [19]
Department of Physiology and Biophysics, Medical Faculty, University of Seville, Seville, Spain
Adele Jackson, PhD [14]
Department of Biology, McMaster University, Hamilton, Ontario, Canada
Shuichi Kobayashi, MD, PhD [15]
Department of Molecular and Cellular Physiology, College of Medicine, University of Cincinnati, Cincinnati, Ohio

Sandra L. Kroll, BS [10]
Department of Molecular and Cellular Physiology, University of Cincinnati, Cincinnati, Ohio
Prem Kumar, DPhil [23]
Department of Physiology, Medical School, University of Birmingham, Birmingham, United Kingdom
José López-Barneo, MD, PhD [11,19]
Department of Physiology and Biophysics, Medical Faculty, University of Seville, Seville, Spain
Patrick H. Maxwell [7]
Institute of Molecular Medicine, John Radcliffe Hospital, Oxford, England
Evangelos Michelakis, MD [18]
Veterans Affairs Medical Center and University of Minnesota, Minneapolis, Minnesota
David E. Millhorn, PhD [15]
Department of Molecular and Cellular Physiology, College of Medicine, University of Cincinnati, Cincinnati, Ohio
Rafael Montoro, MD, PhD [11]
Department of Physiology and Biophysics, Medical Faculty, University of Seville, Seville, Spain
Daniel P. Nelson, BS [16,18]
Veterans Affairs Medical Center and University of Minnesota, Minneapolis, Minnesota
Colin A. Nurse, PhD [14]
Department of Biology, McMaster University, Hamilton, Ontario, Canada
John F. O'Rourke [7]
Institute of Molecular Medicine, John Radcliffe Hospital, Oxford, England
Patricia Ortegá-Sáenz, PhD [11]
Department of Physiology and Biophysics, Medical Faculty, University of Seville, Seville, Spain
Waltke R. Paulding, PhD [10]
Department of Molecular and Cellular Physiology, University of Cincinnati, Cincinnati, Ohio
Chris Peers, PhD [13]
Institute for Cardiovascular Research, Leeds University, Leeds, England
David R. Pepper, PhD [23]
Department of Physiology, Medical School, University of Birmingham, Birmingham, United Kingdom

Olaf Pongs [3]
Institut für Neurale Signalverarbeitung, Center for Molecular Neurobiology, University of Hamburg, Hamburg, Germany
Christopher W. Pugh [7]
Institute of Molecular Medicine, John Radcliffe Hospital, Oxford, England
John M. Quayle, PhD [20]
Ion Channel Group, Department of Cell Physiology and Pharmacology, University of Leicester, Leicester, United Kingdom
Peter J. Ratcliffe [7]
Institute of Molecular Medicine, John Radcliffe Hospital, Oxford, United Kingdom
Helen L. Reeve, PhD [16,18]
Veterans Affairs Medical Center and University of Minnesota, Minneapolis, Minnesota
Susana Salceda, PhD [8]
Cardeza Foundation for Hematologic Research, Philadelphia, Pennsylvania
Helmut Sies, MD, PhD [1]
Institut für Physiologische Chemie I, Heinrich-Heine-Universitüt Düsselddorf, Düsseldorf, Germany
Tarik Smani [19]
Department of Physiology and Biophysics, Medical Faculty, University of Seville, Seville, Spain
Eric Soupène, PhD [4]
Laboratoire de Biologie Moléculaire des Relations Plantes-Microorganismes, Castanet Tolosan, France
Nicholas B. Standen, PhD [20]
Ion Channel Group, Department of Cell Physiology and Pharmacology, University of Leicester, United Kingdom
Barry L. Taylor, PhD [5]
Department of Microbiology and Molecular Genetics, Center for Molecular Biology and Gene Therapy, Loma Linda University, Loma Linda, California
Roger J. Thompson, BScH [14]
Department of Biology, McMaster University, Hamilton, Ontario, Canada
Simona Tolarova, MD [16,18]
Veterans Affairs Medical Center and University of Minnesota, Minneapolis, Minnesota
Dorothy M. Turetsky [22]
Center for the Study of the Nervous System Injury, Washington University in St. Louis, Department of Neurology, St. Louis, Missouri

Juan Ureña, PhD [11,19]
Department of Physiology and Biophysics, Medical Faculty, University of Seville, Seville, Spain
E. Kenneth Weir, MD [16,18]
University of Minnesota and Veterans Affairs Medical Center, Mineapolis, Minnesota
George C. Wellman, PhD [20]
Ion Channel Group, Department of Cell Physiology and Pharmacology, University of Leicester, Leicester, United Kingdom
S. Morwenna Wood [7]
Institute of Molecular Medicine, John Radcliffe Hospital, Oxford, England
Xiao-Jian Yuan, MD, PhD [17]
Department of Medicine, Division of Pulmonary and Critical Care Medicine, Department of Physiology, University of Maryland School of Medicine, Baltimore, Maryland
H. Zhong, PhD [14]
Department of Biology, McMaster University, Hamilton, Ontario, Canada
Wylie H. Zhu, MD, PhD [15]
Department of Molecular and Cellular Physiology, College of Medicine, University of Cincinnati, Cincinnati, Ohio

Preface

Why grass is green, or why our blood is red
Are mysteries which none have reach'd unto
John Donne
(1571–1631)

The observation that exposure to air in the lungs caused the color to change from dark venous blood to bright arterial blood was first reported in 1669 by Richard Lower, an Oxford physician. We now know why blood is red and why hemoglobin changes color when it combines with oxygen. However, there is much about the way in which oxygen is sensed in the body that we have not "reach'd unto." This book presents a summary of current views of the mechanisms whereby oxygen interacts with living cells, giving special emphasis to the biochemical and physiologic adaptations to hypoxia, and stressing the relevance of these phenomena in biology and medicine. The understanding of cellular responses to a lack of oxygen is an emerging topic of broad and well-recognized biological importance, but also with direct medical implications. Transient oxygen deficiency in the most labile organs, such as the heart or the brain, causes irreversible damage and considerable mortality and morbidity in humans. Moreover, advances in the knowledge of this field are also of interest in the conservation and protection of organs and tissues before transplantation and during reperfusion.

At the time of its discovery by Priestly (1733–1804), oxygen was recognized as the critical element of air necessary for the survival of living organisms. John Mayow (1643–1679), a physician working in Oxford at the same time as Richard Lower, had previously found that the same part of air was consumed in respiration and combustion. Lavoisier (1743–1794) coined the term "animal combustion" for the similarity found between the chemical reactions resulting from the combination of oxygen with inert compounds and its interaction with animal tissue. It is interesting to note that, when measured by weight, we consume as much oxygen each day as we consume food (approximately 0.7 kg oxygen and 0.64 kg food, dry weight, in a moderately active person).[1]

It is now well known that oxygen has a pivotal biological role as acceptor of electrons in the mitochondrial oxidation-reduction reactions necessary to generate metabolic energy. Oxygen also participates in numerous secondary cellular functions, which include the degradation of heme, the synthesis of steroid hormones, and the generation of reactive oxygen species in macrophages. Given the crucial importance of oxygen to the survival of most life forms, the provision of sufficient oxygen to the tissues and the protection of cells against damage due to oxygen deficiency are fundamental physiologic challenges. Hypoxia is known to alter cellular functions, such as the expression of genes encoding enzymes, hormones, and growth factors, but it also modifies excitability, contractility, and secretory activity. These changes constitute a widely operating system that, from bacteria to mammals, regulates, with a time course ranging from seconds to hours or days, the availability and utilization of oxygen in the immediate environment of cells and, thus, helps to minimize the deleterious effects of oxygen deficiency.

Modern research on the cellular mechanisms of oxygen sensing has developed following two main paths, without much intercommunication. On one side, there are studies focusing on oxygen dependent gene expression. This research, introduced by the pioneering work on erythropoietin, has lead to the discovery of numerous oxygen-sensitive enzymes and growth factors, such as vascular endothelial growth factor (VEGF), which mediates hypoxia-stimulated angiogenesis, and to important advances in the elucidation of the oxygen-sensitive signaling pathways that regulate gene transcription. On the other side, there are the recent advances in the characterization of the cellular mechanisms underlying the cardiovascular and respiratory reflexes evoked by low oxygen partial pressure (Po_2). It has become established that these fast functional adjustments to hypoxia depend on changes in membrane ionic permeability mediated by ion channels which are regulated by oxygen tension. Oxygen-sensitive channels have been discovered in the classic arterial chemoreceptors, such as the carotid body and pulmonary smooth muscle cells, as well as the neuroepithelial cells of the lung, systemic arterial myocytes, chromaffin cells, and central neurons. It is likely that the interaction between oxygen and ion channels was one of the most primitive accommodations made by living organisms. Free oxygen appeared in the atmosphere about 2 billion years ago,[2] while simple ion channels developed in prokaryotes more than 1.4 billion years ago.[3] This book aims to fill the gap that exists between molecular biology and biophysics, and to provide a common space where different ideas, concepts, and experimental methodologies can be evaluated. We are convinced that this interdisciplinary approach will help to elaborate a comprehensive view of the field of oxygen sensing.

The chapters of the book are organized in six sections. Section 1 introduces some general principles of oxygen sensing, such as the cellular metabolism of oxygen, as well as the possible role of reactive oxygen intermediates in the regulation of gene expression and ion channel gating. In Section 2, selected data are presented on recently identified oxygen sensors in bacteria, followed by a brief discussion on the mechanisms of oxygen sensing in plants. Section 3 summarizes the major field of oxygen dependent eukaryotic gene expression. Studies of the erythropoietin gene have shed light on general principles widely used in many cell types to adapt to low Po_2. Some important components of the signaling pathway linking oxygen tension and transcription are also presented, paying special attention to the hypoxia-inducible factor and the mechanisms of post-transcriptional stabilization. Section 4 deals with the numerous recent studies where oxygen-sensitive ion channels have been characterized. Some representative examples of oxygen-dependent neurosecretory systems are, besides the classic chemoreceptor cells of the carotid body, the adrenomedullary chromaffin cells of newborn animals and the related PC12 cell line. The second part of this section focuses on the role of oxygen-sensitive ion channels as mediators of the vasomotor responses to hypoxia both in systemic and pulmonary arterial myocytes. Section 5 contains two chapters which describe how hypoxia or redox alterations can produce fast changes in the excitability of some central neurones and, in a longer time range, regulate the expression of glutamate receptors. Finally, in Section 6, the relevance of studies at the cellular level is discussed when compared with the manifestations of hypoxia in animals and humans. To facilitate the reading of the book, we have introduced, when appropriate, cross references among the chapters, and have maintained a similar chapter format in all the sections.

This book was conceived during an international workshop in Madrid in December, 1996, and planned on the basis of a limited number of contributors. Nevertheless, the book has the "critical mass" necessary not only to provide a view of the present status of the field but, more importantly, to discern the fundamental questions. It seems to us that the field will reach complete maturity with the characterization of the oxygen sensor molecule(s). This molecular information will surely help to understand why there are cells (like neurons or cardiac muscle) so sensitive to the lack of oxygen while others can resist low Po_2 levels for hours without deleterious consequences. It will be also possible to elucidate whether the oxygen sensitivity of the various tissues depends on the differential distribution of one of various types of oxygen sensors, or on organ-dependent characteristics such as the geometry of blood distribution. It can be expected that, in the near future, oxygen-regulated channels and gene expression will appear as separate manifestations of common molecular mechanisms sensitive to oxygen tension.

This book owes all of its merit to the generosity of the authors of the different chapters. Their eager and enthusiastic attitude toward the project has made this final outcome possible. We would like also to express our gratitude to the March Foundation and Futura Publishing Company for their steady and unreserved support of international scientific communication and cooperation.

References

1. Engelberg J: How many pounds of oxygen do we ''eat'' each day? *Am J Physiol* 271 (*Adv Physiol Educ* 16):S43–S44, 1996.
2. Katz AM: Cardiac ion channels. *N Engl J Med* 328:1244–1251, 1993.
3. Halliwell B, Gutteridge JMC: *Free Radicials in Biology and Medicine.* Oxford: Clarendon Press; 1989.

José Lopez-Barneo, MD, PhD
E. Kenneth Weir, MD

Contents

SECTION 4

ION CHANNELS AND FUNCTIONAL RESPONSES TO HYPOXIA

Part 1
Neurosecretory Mechanisms

Part 2
Vascular Smooth Muscle

SECTION 5

OXYGEN SENSING IN NERVE CELLS

SECTION 6

SENSITIVITY TO HYPOXIA

Section 1

GENERAL PRINCIPLES OF OXYGEN SENSING

Chapter 1

Cellular Metabolism of Oxygen: Brief Overview and Current Aspects on Peroxynitrite and Singlet Oxygen

Karlis Briviba
Helmut Sies

Introduction

The bulk of cellular oxygen uptake is utilized for energy production in the form of adenosine triphosphate (ATP) by cytochrome oxidase in the mitochondrial respiratory chain. The net 4-electron reduction of molecular oxygen to water occurs without release of intermediate radical species. This means that far more than 95% of total oxygen uptake occurs without the formation of reactive oxygen species. The metabolism of hydroperoxides in mammalian systems has been a topic of long-standing interest, and the foundations of this field of research have been presented by Chance et al.[1] The mitochondrial respiratory chain may generate superoxide anion radicals at the level of ubisemiquinone, a process potentially related to long-term damage to mitochondria. Mitochondrial deoxyribonucleic acid (DNA) is afflicted by oxidation to an extent about tenfold higher than nuclear DNA.[2] Metabolism of hydrogen peroxide (H_2O_2) is, in part, compartmentalized in the subcellular organelle, the peroxisome.[3]

From: López-Barneo, J and Weir, EK: *Oxygen Regulation of Ion Channels and Gene Expression*. Armonk, NY: Futura Publishing Company, Inc., ©1998.

Sources of Reactive Oxygen Species

There are several enzymatic reaction sites in the cell where intermediate steps of oxygen reduction occur.[4] As shown in the Figure, major sites of generation of superoxide and of H_2O_2 can be found in the cytosol, in the mitochondria, in the peroxisome, and at membranes. The membranes of the endoplasmic reticulum are indicated, but other membranes, such as the plasma membrane, are also known to be sites of generation of reactive oxygen species. The 1-electron step, i.e., the formation of the superoxide anion radical, occurs enzymatically, and the process of redox cycling is driven by reductases utilizing nicotinamide adenine dinucleotide phosphate (NADPH). This process is of interest in toxicology, being the basis of the toxicity of quinones and nitroaromatics.[5] Various enzymes, such as xanthine oxidase, dopamine-β-hydroxylase, and D-amino acid oxidase, can oxidize endogenous or exogenous substrates and produce reactive oxygen species. Tissue ischemia leads to the degradation of ATP into hypoxanthine, a substrate for xanthine oxidase that has been proposed to be an important source of superoxide, H_2O_2, and species derived from them in reperfused tissue.[6]

Stimulation of phagocytes is associated with a burst of oxygen consumption[7] which is not due to enhanced mitochondrial respiration. In stimulated neutrophils after initiation of the respiratory burst, more than 90% of the consumed oxygen can be accounted for the generation of superoxide anion radical. This reaction is catalyzed by a plasma membrane-bound NADPH oxidase. H_2O_2 formed during the stimulation of phagocytic cells appears to be produced from the superoxide dismutase (SOD)-catalyzed dismutation of superoxide. Neither superoxide nor H_2O_2 are strong oxidants. The transition metal-catalyzed Haber-Weiss reaction leads to the formation of the more reactive hydroxyl radical. In addition, the strong oxidant peroxynitrite is formed by the reaction of superoxide anion and nitric oxide (NO) at a near diffusion-controlled rate.[8] Furthermore, the hypochlorite ion generated by myeloperoxidase can interact with H_2O_2 to produce singlet oxygen ($^1O_2$), another strong oxidant. Thus, the stimulation of phagocytic cells leads to the uptake of oxygen by the production of relatively mild oxidants like superoxide and H_2O_2, which then are modified into stronger damaging agents, depending on the respective biological environment.

Peroxynitrite

As characterized in assays employing several repair enzymes with defined substrate specificities, peroxynitrite formed by inflammatory cells leads to DNA damage by oxidizing guanine[9] and causing single strand breaks.[10,11] In proteins, peroxynitrite can lead to tyrosine nitration, potentially interfering with phosphorylation/dephosphorylation signaling pathways.[12] So far, there is no known enzymatic defense against peroxynitrite. Low-molecular-mass compounds such as ascorbate, cysteine, and methionine have been shown to react with peroxynitrite.

Our recent work shows that peroxynitrite appears to react preferentially with selenium compounds. Ebselen, an anti-inflammatory selenoorganic compound, reacts with peroxynitrite, forming the corresponding selenoxide[13] at a second order rate constant of $2 \times 10^6 M^{-1}s^{-1}$[14], which is about one hundredfold higher than the rate constant observed with ascorbate or methionine. Selenocompounds, such as selenomethionine, selenocysteine, or ebselen, protected dihydrorhodamine 123 from oxidation more effectively than their sulfur analogs or glutathione (GSH).[15] The selenoxide can be reduced back to the parent compound at the expense of GSH or other thiols, so that a steady state line of defense can be established.

Selenium-containing compounds protect plasmid DNA from single strand breaks better than the corresponding sulfur-containing analogs; e.g., selenomethionine protected DNA from peroxynitrite-induced damage more efficiently than methionine.[16] Likewise, nitration reactions were suppressed efficiently by selenocompounds.[15] We postulated, based on preliminary evidence, that defense against peroxynitrite is a novel function of selenoproteins such as GSH peroxidase.[17] (Evidence for GSH peroxidase as functioning as "peroxynitrite reductase" has been provided.[17A])

Singlet Molecular Oxygen

$^1O_2$ is an electronically excited and mutagenic form of oxygen that can be generated in biological systems by photoexcitation or by chemiexcitation (dark reactions), e.g., during the respiratory burst of phagocytes.[18] $^1O_2$ selectively reacts with the deoxyguanosine moiety and causes strand breaks in DNA.[19] $^1O_2$ generated by both photoexcitation and chemiexcitation inactivates herpes simplex virus type I in human plasma[20] and is involved in ultraviolet A light (UVA)-induced cytotoxicity.[21] At nontoxic concentrations, $^1O_2$ participates in signal transduction pathways that lead to the expression of various genes, such as heme oxygenase[22], collagenase,[23,24] and intercellular adhesion molecule (ICAM-1).[25]

The biological effects of UVA irradiation can be mediated by electron transfer or by a pathway involving $^1O_2$. UVA irradiation or $^1O_2$, generated in a dark reaction by thermal decomposition of the endoperoxide of

3,3′-(1,4-naphthylidene) dipropionate ($NDPO_2$), induced collagenase in human skin fibroblasts[23,24] and ICAM-1 in human keratinocytes[25], respectively. The effect of $NDPO_2$ or UVA irradiation in oxygen delivery (D_2O)-based buffer was more pronounced than that in normal buffer, attributable to the larger half-life of $^1O_2$ in D_2O. Sodium azide, a potent quencher of $^1O_2$, abrogated the induction of both collagenase and ICAM-1 after exposure to $NDPO_2$-generated $^1O_2$ and to UVA irradiation, respectively.

In human keratinocytes transfected with ICAM-1-based luciferase reporter gene constructs, it was shown that $^1O_2$-or UVA-mediated activation of the ICAM-1 promoter was completely abolished by deletion of the AP-2 binding site.[25] In contrast, deletion of AP-1 or NFkB binding sites did not affect the ICAM-1 promoter activation. This identifies the AP-2 site as the UVA as well as a $^1O_2$ responsive element of the human ICAM-1 gene.[25]

Antioxidants and Oxidative Stress

The pattern of oxidants is matched by an array of antioxidants. The nature of the diverse antioxidants encompasses enzymes and small molecules, including vitamins such as ascorbate or vitamin E[26] and micronutrients such as carotenoids.[27] An imbalance in the oxidant/antioxidant equilibrium in favor of the oxidants, leading to potential damage, is termed *oxidative stress*.'[28,29] Antioxidants may act at different levels in the oxidative process by 1) scavenging initiating radicals; 2) binding metal ions; 3) scavenging peroxyl radicals; or 4) removing oxidatively damaged molecules. Various antioxidants of low molecular weight, such as ascorbate, GSH, α-tocopherol, flavonoids, and antioxidant micronutrients, such as carotenoids and selenium, in conjunction with antioxidant enzymes, such as SOD, catalase, and GSH peroxidases, constitute a network of interlinked water-soluble or lipid-soluble antioxidant systems which protect the body from oxidative damage.[30]

The scheme shown in the Figure presents part of the GSH-linked defense line. The system is much more complex, even for GSH as such: post-translational modification of proteins by GSH, i.e., the formation of mixed disulfides between GSH and protein sulfhydryls, known as glutathionylation, has become of interest. We recently demonstrated the redox control of microsomal glutathione transferase.[31] Oxidants are involved in disease mechanisms, and there is interest in employing antioxidants in therapeutic strategies.[32]

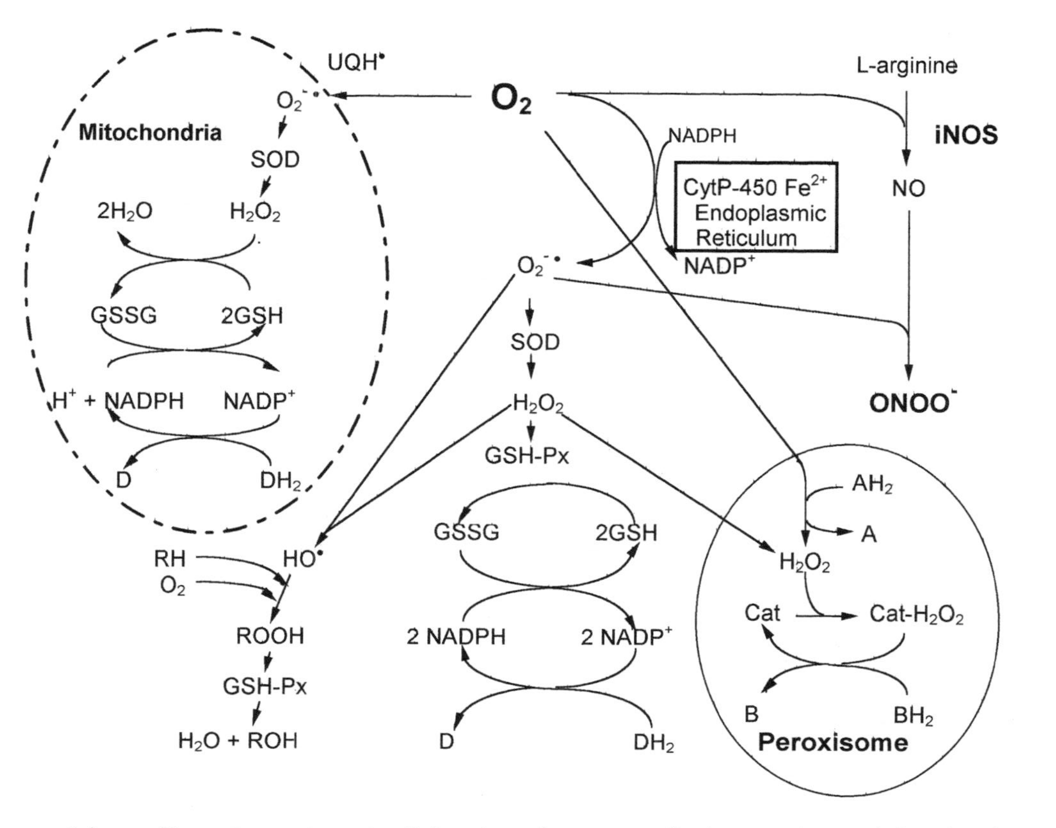

Figure. Scheme illustrating major subcellular sites of oxygen radical generation and the glutathione peroxidase/GSSG reductase defense line in hydroperoxide metabolism. (Modified with permission from References 1 and 5.)

Oxygen Sensing

Regarding oxygen sensing mechanisms during hypoxic transitions, the theme of this volume, it may be of interest to look back 20 years when it was stated:

> . . .that of the biochemical reactions intervening in O_2 sensing mechanisms, it is well possible that H_2O_2 may play a role in some yet unspecified peroxidative reaction. Catalase as a regulator of H_2O_2 concentration would have a role in such mechanism. One suitable peroxidatic reaction could be that of GSH peroxidase. This nonperoxisomal enzyme catalyzes the reduction of H_2O_2 and other hydroperoxides by GSH. The formation of glutathione disulfide in a steady state of hydroperoxide reduction leads to a transition of the thiol redox state in the cell which, in turn, has profound effects on active and passive cation permeability, as well as on the chemical stimulation of excitable cells.[33]

The fascinating advances in the regulation of ion channel activity by thiol/disulfide interchange, comprising much of the substance in this volume, provide a sound basis for a molecular understanding of oxygen sensing mechanisms.

Acknowledgments

The studies from the author's laboratory have been generously supported by the National Foundation for Cancer Research, Bethesda, Maryland, and by the Deutsche Forschungsgemeinschaft, Bonn, Germany.

References

1. Chance B, Sies H, Boveris A: Hydroperoxide metabolism in mammalian organs. *Physiol Revs* 59:527–605, 1979.
2. Richter C, Park JW, Ames BN: Normal oxidative damage to mitochondrial and nuclear DNA is extensive. *Proc Natl Acad Sci USA* 85:6465–6467, 1988.
3. Sies H: Biochemistry of the peroxysome in the liver cell. *Angew Chem Int Ed Engl* 13:706–718, 1974.
4. Sies H: Biochemistry of oxidative stress. *Angew Chem Int Ed Engl* 25:1058–1071, 1986.

5. Kappus H, Sies H: Toxic drug effects associated with oxygen metabolism. Redox cycling and lipid peroxidation. *Experientia* 37:1233–1241, 1981.
6. Omar B, McCord J, Downey J: Ischaemia-reperfusion. In: Sies H (ed). *Oxidative Stress: Oxidants and Antioxidants.* London: Academic Press; 493–527, 1991.
7. Babior BM: Oxygen-dependent microbial killing by phagocytes. *N Engl J Med* 298:659–668, 1978.
8. Huie RE, Padmaja S: The reaction of NO with superoxide. *Free Radical Res Commun* 18:195–199, 1993.
9. Douki T, Cadet J, Ames, NB: An adduct between peroxynitrite and 2′-deoxyguanosine: 4,5-dihydro-5-hydroxy-4-(nitrosooxy)-2′-deoxyguanosine. *Chem Res Toxicol* 9:3–7, 1996.
10. Salgo MG, Bermudez E, Squadrito GL, et al: DNA damage and oxidation of thiols peroxynitrite causes in rat thymocytes. *Arch Biochem Biophys* 322: 500–505, 1995.
11. Epe B, Ballmaier D, Roussyn I, et al: DNA damage by peroxynitrite characterized with DNA repair enzymes. *Nucleic Acid Res* 24:4105–4110, 1996.
12. Beckman JS, Ye YZ, Anderson P, et al: Extensive nitration of protein tyrosines observed in human atherosclerosis detected by immunohistochemistry. *Biol Chem Hoppe-Seyler* 375:81–88, 1994.
13. Masumoto H, Sies H: The reaction of ebselen with peroxynitrite. *Chem Res Toxicol* 9:262–267, 1996.
14. Masumoto H, Kissner R, Koppenol WH, et al: Kinetic study of the reaction of ebselen with peroxynitrite. *FEBS Lett* 398:179–182, 1996.
15. Briviba K, Roussyn I, Sharov VS, et al: Attenuation of oxidation and nitration reactions of peroxynitrite by selenomethionine, selenocystine and ebselen. *Biochem J* 319:13–15, 1996.
16. Roussyn I, Briviba K, Masumoto H, et al: Selenium containing compounds protect DNA from single-strand breaks caused by peroxynitrite. *Arch Biochem Biophys* 330:216–218, 1996.
17. Sies H, Masumoto H: Ebselen as a glutathione peroxidase mimic and as a reactant with peroxynitrite. *Adv Pharmacol* 38:229–246, 1997.
17A.Sies H, Sharov VS, Klotz L-O, Briviba K: Glutathione peroxidase protects against peroxynitrite-mediated oxidations. *J Biol Chem* 272:27812–27817, 1997.
18. Steinbeck MJ, Khan AU, Karnovsky MJ: Extracellular production of singlet oxygen by stimulated macrophages quantified using 9,10-diphenylanthracene and perylene in a polystyrene film. *J Biol Chem* 268:15649–15654, 1993.
19. Sies H: Damage to plasmid DNA by singlet oxygen and its protection. *Mutation Res* 299:183–191, 1993.
20. Müller-Breitkreutz K, Mohr H, Briviba K, et al: Inactivation of viruses by chemically and photochemically generated singlet molecular oxygen. *Photochem Photobiol* 30:63–70, 1995.
21. Tyrrell RM, Pidoux M: Singlet oxygen involvement in the inactivation of human skin fibroblasts by UVA (334 nm, 365 nm) and near-visible (405 nm) radiations. *Photochem Photobiol* 49:407–412, 1989.
22. Basu-Modak S, Tyrrell RM: A primary effector in the ultraviolet A near visible light induction of the human oxygenase gene. *Cancer Res* 53:4505–4510, 1993.
23. Scharffetter-Kochanek K, Wlaschek M, Briviba K, et al: Singlet oxygen induces collagenase expression in human skin fibroblasts. *FEBS Lett* 331:304–306, 1993.
24. Wlaschek M, Briviba K, Stricklin GP, et al: Singlet oxygen may mediate the

ultraviolet A-induced synthesis of interstitial collagenase. *J Invest Dermatol* 104: 194–198, 1995.
25. Grether-Beck S, Olaizola-Horn S, et al: Activation of transcription factor AP2 mediates ultraviolet-A radiation-and singlet oxygen-induced expression of the human ICAM-1 gene. *Proc Natl Acad Sci USA* 93:14586–14591, 1996.
26. Traber M, Sies H: Vitamin E in humans: demand and delivery. *Ann Rev Nutr* 16:321–347, 1996.
27. Sies H, Stahl W: Antioxidant functions of vitamins E,C, β-carotene and other carotenoids. *Amer J Clin Nutr* 62:1315S–1321S, 1995.
28. Sies H (ed): *Oxidative Stress.* London: Academic Press; 1985.
29. Sies H (ed): *Oxidative Stress: Oxidants and Antioxidants.* London: Academic Press; 1991.
30. Sies H: Strategies of antioxidant defense. *Eur J Biochem* 215: 213–219, 1993.
31. Dafré AL, Sies H, Akerboom T: Protein-S-thiolation and regulation of microsomal glutathione transferase activity by the glutathione redox couple. *Arch Biochem Biophys* 332:288–294, 1996.
32. Sies (ed): *Antioxidants in Disease Mechanisms and Therapy.* London: Academic Press; 1985.
33. Sies H: Peroxisomal enzymes and oxygen metabolism in liver. In: Reivich M, Coburn R, Lahiri S, Chance B (eds). *Tissue Hypoxia and Ischemia.* New York: Plenum Press; 51–66, 1977.

Chapter 2

Reactive Oxygen Intermediates as Mediators for Regulating Ion Channel Activity and Gene Expression in the Process of Cellular Oxygen Sensing

Helmut Acker

Introduction

Cellular oxygen sensing is a highly conserved process in evolution, most likely developed by bacteria and yeast with the first appearance of oxygen in the atmosphere, to combat the toxic effect of reactive oxygen intermediates (ROI). Signal pathways are now very well described in these systems involving ROI as second messengers to regulate ion channel open probability, as well as gene expression. The same processes seem to take place in mammalian cells using several ROI for the same purpose. The main pathway seems to be the modification of transcription factors, as well as the increase or decrease of membrane potassium and calcium currents by influencing the gating mechanism of the corresponding ion channel. The aim of our study is the identification of the oxygen sensor protein monitoring changes in oxygen partial pressure (Po_2) and the particular ROI which incites the oxygen-sensing signal pathway. We use carotid body, as well as the hepatoma cell line (HepG2), for this purpose.

From: López-Barneo, J and Weir, EK: *Oxygen Regulation of Ion Channels and Gene Expression.* Armonk, NY: Futura Publishing Company, Inc., ©1998.

These two cell systems are well known to regulate ion channel activity and gene expression in dependence on P_{O_2}. We could identify a low output cytochrome b as a putative oxygen sensor protein by means of light absorption photometry, immunohistochemistry, and Western blot analysis. This cytochrome has components similar to the one described for the high output neutrophil nicotinamide adenine dinucleotide phosphate (NADPH) oxidase. Of the different ROI, hydrogen peroxide (H_2O_2), singlet oxygen ($^1O_2$), superoxide anion ($\cdot O_2^-$), and hydroxyl radicals ($\cdot OH$) each have their distinct influence on gene expression and ion channel activity. A local Fenton reaction, observed in perinuclear structures of HepG2 cells degrading H_2O_2 to OH, seems to be involved in the regulation of the erythropoietin (EPO) and vascular endothelial growth factor (VEGF) gene. As described in the literature, potassium channels Kv 1.4, 3.3, 3.4, most likely expressed also in carotid body cells, increase the potassium current under H_2O_2 application, whereas $^1O_2$ inhibits this current. We believe, based on these facts, in a unifying concept of oxygen sensing, valid for bacteria, yeast, and mammalian cells, for regulation of ion channel activity and gene expression with a distinct action of various ROI generated by hemeproteins as a function of P_{O_2}.

Relationship Between Oxygen Partial Pressure and Gene Expression or Ion Channel Activity

To provide a constant oxygen supply to different organs, and consequently a constant energy supply maintaining highly specialized organ functions, cells that are able to sense oxygen levels in the tissue are situated at different locations in the body to stimulate various reflex pathways. This oxygen-sensing process comprises a sensor protein which undergoes conformational changes in dependence on oxygen and a signal cascade, which transfers the message stimulated by the sensor to ion channels, metabolic pathways, or specific gene regions.[1-3] For the last pathway, numerous examples are given in the literature, like the cobalt chloride ($CoCl_2$) impedible induction of phosphoenolpyruvate carboxykinase (PCK) by glucagon in hepatocytes,[4] the regulation of the glutathione peroxidase content by oxygen tension in cardiomyocytes,[5] the gene expression for tyrosin hydroxylase in carotid body type I and PC12 cells,[6] endothelin-1 gene regulation in endothelial,[7] or the production of EPO, vascular endothelial growth factor, platelet-derived growth factor A and B chains, placental growth factor, and transforming growth factor in various cell lines (see Chapters 7–10).[8,9] Metabolic pathways comprise the lactate dehydrogenase activity,[10] mainly based on an upregulation of the lactate dehydrogenase A gene[11] or pregnenolone and aldosterone synthesis.[12] Well known examples for the participation of ion channels in the oxygen-sensing process are oxygen-sensitive potassium and calcium channels of type I cells of the carotid body and PC12 cells[13-15] of cells of neuroepithelial bodies in the lung,[16] of smooth muscle cells of the lung vasculature,[17] or of central neurons.[18] Oxygen-sensitive calcium channels are also described for peripheral vascular smooth muscle (see Chapters 12–22).[19]

The oxygen level in the tissue of different organs is determined by the Po_2 and the oxygen transport capacity of the blood, as well as by the vascular structure, blood flow, oxygen consumption, and diffusion conditions of each particular organ. Characteristically, the different organs have a frequency distribution of Po_2 values ranging from about 0 to 100 mm Hg, with mean values between 20 and 50 mm Hg.[1] While in former times the meaning of this Po_2 distribution was mainly discussed in its importance for energy supply under normoxic and hypoxic conditions, it is obvious now that the Po_2 distribution expresses the different oxygen sensitivities of ion channels, metabolic pathway activities, and gene regions mentioned above. Low as well as high Po_2 values have distinct influences. Low Po_2 is accompanied by an enhanced production of EPO, endothelin-1, vascular endothelial growth factor, platelet-derived growth factor A and B chains, placental growth factor, transforming growth factor,[7-9] and tyrosine hydroxylase (TH) below a Po_2 of 20 mm Hg,[6] whereas high Po_2 incites a higher production of glutathione peroxidase[5] or PCK peaking above Po_2 values of about 70 mm Hg.[4] Lactate dehydrogenase activity is increased at low oxygen levels,[10] whereas pregnenolone and aldosterone synthesis is enhanced under high oxygen levels.[12] The potassium channels linearly decrease their open probability with decreasing Po_2 values from 150 Torr to 0 Torr, leading to membrane potential depolarization and opening of voltage-sensitive calcium channels with a subsequent increase of the intracellular calcium level inducing neurotransmitter release[14,16] or smooth muscle contraction.[17] Central neurons activate under hypoxia by this mechanism.[18] The calcium channels decrease their open probability under low oxygen levels, too, leading to peripheral vasodilatation under hypoxia.[19] The described ion channels, metabolic pathways and gene expressions, with their different Po_2 affinities, reveal the Po_2 frequency distribution as a trigger field for various cellular activities, either to optimize living conditions or to protect against hypoxic and hyperoxic damages.

Oxygen Sensing in Procaryots and Eucaryots

Whereas the oxygen-responsive elements of the genes encoding the different proteins have been partly identified,[5,8,9] the nature of the oxygen-sensing protein influencing ion channel activity, metabolic pathway activities, and gene expression is still unclear in mammalian cells. However, studies on bacteria could describe signal cascades influencing gene expression under hypoxic as well as hyperoxic conditions. Activation of the nitrogen fixation gene in *Rhizobium meliloti* under hypoxia is mediated by a cell membrane-located heme-based sensor which phosphorylates a transcription factor for facilitating its deoxyribonucleic acid (DNA) binding.[20] The OxyR transcription factor in *E. coli* and *S. typhimurium* is activated specifically by H_2O_2 to encode enzymes such as catalase and alkyl hydroperoxide reductase.[21] Furthermore, *E.coli* contains the SoxR protein, which, activated by oxygen through a variable redox state of its FeS cluster, induces transcription of the SoxS gene, which in turn increases expression of defensive genes such as Mn- containing superoxide dismutase.[22] The stability of the FeS cluster is enhanced under hypoxia, facilitating the dimerization of the transcription factor FNR in *E.coli* for regulating metabolic reponses to hypoxic stress.[23] Potassium ion channels with an increased activity under oxidizing conditions are also described in *E.coli.*[24] In *E.coli,* the soluble flavohemoglobin (HMP) was proposed as oxygen sensor protein,[2,15] where, in the presence of oxygen, NAD(P)H transfers electrons intramolecularly via flavin adenin dinucleotide (FAD) to heme iron to maintain it as Fe^{2+}. In the absence of oxygen, electrons are diverted via intermolecular transfer to reduce other electron receptors such as FeS clusters in fumerte nitrate reductase (FNR).[2] For *S.cerevisiae,* it was proposed that: 1) a heme as oxygen sensor serves as a ligand for a transcription factor, and heme concentration regulates transcription; 2) a heme is a prosthetic group of a transcription factor responding to changes in its redox state; or 3) a heme is a prosthetic group in a kinase, phosphorylating a transcription factor in dependence on the redox state or spin state of heme iron.[25,26] By adapting to the accumulation of oxygen in the earth's atmosphere about 2 billion years ago, procaryots and eucaryots seem to have invented mechanisms to sense oxygen for regulating gene expression and ion channel activity which might in part also exist in mammalian cells.

Oxygen Sensing in Mammalian Cells

The involvement of a heme-type oxygen sensor protein has been suggested to explain the molecular mechanism of the inhibitory effect of low

PO_2 on potassium conductance of carotid body, neuroepithelial bodies, and smooth musculature of lung vasculature.[1,16,17] Cross et al[27] carried out a detailed photometric analysis of the rat carotid body to gain more information about hemeprotein characteristics in this tissue. They detected, besides typical absorbtion peaks of the different cytochromes of the respiratory chain, a measurable heme signal with absorbance maxima at 558 nm, 518 nm, and 425 nm which suggests the presence of a b-type cytochrome. This was confirmed by pyridine hemochrome and carbon monoxide (CO) spectra. This heme protein is capable of H_2O_2 formation and seems to possess, therefore, similarities with cytochrome b_{558} of the NAD(P)H oxidase in neutrophils.[28] The typical components of the NADPH oxidase, $p22_{phox}$, $gp91_{phox}$, $p47_{phox}$, and $p67_{phox}$ could be identified immunohistochemically in type I cells of the human, rat, and guinea pig carotid body by Kummer and Acker,[29] as well as by Youngson et al[16] in neuroepithelial bodies of the lung, highlighting the probability of the involvement of an NAD(P)H oxidase, or a related isoform in the cellular oxygen sensing in these cell types. Of special interest in this context are findings as published by Lopez-Lopez and González,[30] showing that the hypoxia-induced decrease of the activity of potassium channels of type I cells can be inhibited by CO. This might be interpreted as CO is inducing an oxidation of a hemeprotein which interacts with potassium channels in the cell membrane of type I cells. An H_2O_2 generating hemeprotein seems to be also involved in the control of the open probability of potassium channels in the smooth musculature of lung vessels.[17] A variety of potassium channels are now described as being influenced in their inactivation current by cystein oxidation or H_2O_2, like Kv1.4, Kv3.3, Kv3.4, and HukII (see Chapter 3).[31-34] Kv1.4 and Kv3.4, however, increase the fast inactivation current under the influence of $^1O_2$.[31] Since cystein is oxidized by H_2O_2 and $^1O_2$ is scavenged by histidin, these two amino acids might mediate the different responses of the channel protein to these ROI. Figure 1 tries to give a model of the redox-dependent inactivation of the potassium channel. The α subunit of the potassium channel protein is shown in the open and inactivated state due to the position of the ball of the β subunit.[35] The β subunit as an NAD(P)H oxidoreductase[36] might produce under normoxia high, and under hypoxia low, levels of ROI, controlling cystein oxidation and position of the ball. Besides cystein oxidation, the redox state of the channel protein might be also determined by a local Fenton reaction, i.e., degradation of H_2O_2 to $\cdot OH$ mediated by iron. This mechanism might be responsible for oxygen sensing in central neurons, which seems to be mediated by a nonheme iron-containing protein.[18]

It has been shown that hypoxia-induced EPO production of HepG2 cells is mediated by a nonrespiratory heme protein as an oxygen sensor,

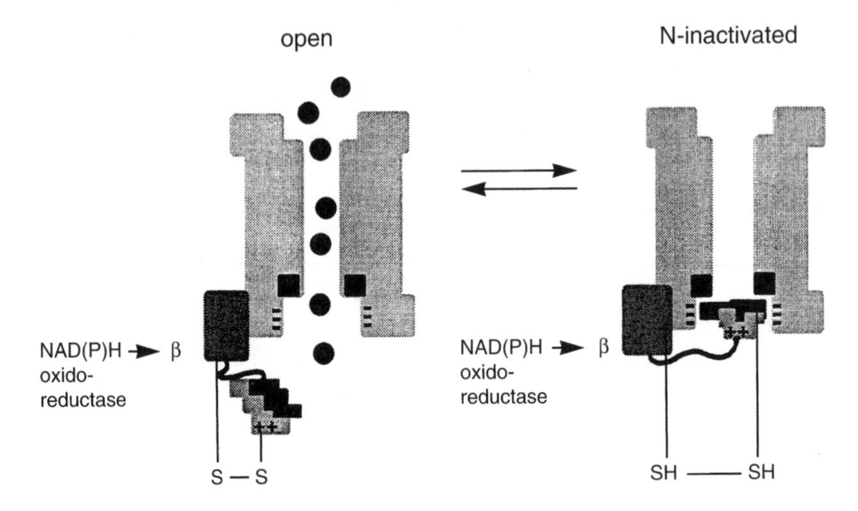

Figure 1. Model of a potassium ion channel composed of an α and β subunit for describing redox-dependent inactivation by means of a redox-dependent position of the b subunit ball.

which was proposed to be similar to the NADPH oxidase as described above.[37] This oxidase has a declining H_2O_2 formation in HepG2 cells under hypoxia which might promote the binding of the transcription factors HIF α and β as a dimer to the oxygen responsive element of the EPO gene.[38] H_2O_2 amplifies in hepatocytes the glucagon-dependent increase in PCK messenger ribonucleic acid (mRNA) stimulated above Po_2 values of 70 Torr, whereas it attenuates the hypoxic stimulated aldolase A gene expression.[39] Gleadle et al[8] underlined the importance of a flavoprotein oxidoreductase as an oxygen sensor by inhibiting the hypoxia-induced gene expression of five genes by means of diphenylene iodonium, an inhibitor of the neutrophil NADPH oxidase. This oxidase might be termed, according to Bastian and Hibbs,[40] as a low output form with respect to the rate of H_2O_2 production. This is in contrast to the stimulus-dependent respiratory burst-like activity of the high output oxidase in leucocyte defense mechanisms, which has about a 95% higher production rate than the low output form.[41] It has been shown by Ehleben et al[42] that

H_2O_2 is degraded by a local Fenton reaction close to the cell nucleus in HepG2 cells, which suggests that ·OH might control the dimerization of HIF α and β as hypothesized for FNR in *E. coli*. Figure 2 shows that the stability of the FeS cluster, which determines the dimerization of FNR, depends on the redox state of the cell. This model might also partly explain the activation of HIF under hypoxia accompanied by lower levels of ROI or depletion of iron stores by desferrioxamine (see Chapters 7 and 9).[43]

In the case of the hyperoxia-induced aldosterone production, the oxygen sensitive side is likely to be located in the mitochondrial aldosterone synthase enzyme complex.[12] A heme-protein seems not to be involved in this oxygen-sensing process.

Therefore, it might be concluded that hypoxia and hyperoxia could be sensed by different mechanisms in mammalian cells employing various ROI, as is likely to be the case in bacteria and yeast. This oxygen-sensing process might be a highly conserved evolutionary principle by which organisms adapting from anaerobic to aerobic enviromental conditions learned to measure the availibility of oxygen, as well as to cope with reactive oxygen intermediates.[21] Lack of energy or impairment of mitochondrial respiration, however, seem to be not involved in all the described cases of oxygen sensing, underlining the significance of the critical mitochondrial Po_2 value below 1 Torr for securing a constant energy supply in all cells located at different spots in the Po_2 field.

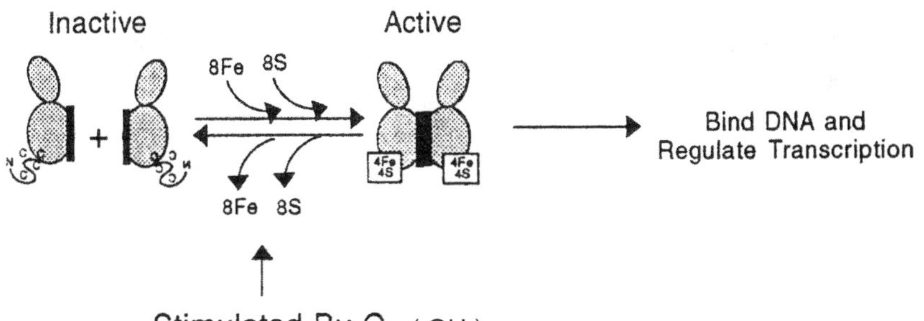

Model for the association of Fe - S cluster with FNR and regulation of FNR activity by oxygen as described for *Escherichia coli* (B.A. Lazazzera et al. 1996) might be applicable to dimerisation of HIF1α and β under hypoxia

Figure 2. Model of redox dependent dimerization of transcription factors by means of redox-dependent stability of FeS clusters.

References

1. Acker H: Mechanisms and meaning of cellular oxygen sensing in the organism. *Resp Physiol* 95:1-10, 1994.
2. Bunn HF, Poyton RO: Oxygen sensing and molecular adaptation to hypoxia. *Physiol Rev* 76:839-885, 1996.
3. Wang GL, Semenza L: Oxygen sensing and response to hypoxia by mammalian-cells. *Redox Report* 2:89-96, 1996.
4. Kietzmann T, Schmidt H, Probst I, et al: Modulation of the glucagon-dependent activation of the phosphoenolpyruvate carboxykinase gene by oxygen in rat hepatocyte cultures. *FEBS Lett* 311:251-255, 1992.
5. Cowan DB, Weisel RD, Williams WG, et al: Identification of oxygen responsive elements in the 5'flanking region of the human gluthatione peroxidase gene. *J Biol Chem* 268:26904-26910, 1993.
6. Czykzyk-Krzeska M, Furnari BA, Lawson EE, et al: Hypoxia increases rate of transcription and stability of tyrosine hydroxylase mRNA in pheochromocytoma (PC12) cells. *J Biol Chem* 7:760-764, 1994.
7. Bodi I, Bishopric NH, Discher DJ, et al: Cell-specificity and signaling pathway of endothelin-1 gene regulation by hypoxia. *Cardiovasc Res* 30:975-984, 1995.
8. Gleadle JM, Ebert BL, Firth JD, et al: Regulation of angiogenic growth factor expression by hypoxia, transition metals and chelating agents. *Am J Physiol* 268: C1362-C1368, 1995.
9. Goldberg MA, Schneider TJ: Similarities between the oxygen sensing mechanisms regulating the expression of vascular endothelial growth factor and erythropoietin. *J Biol Chem* 269:4355-4359, 1994.
10. Marti HH, Jung HH, Pfeilschifter J, et al: Hypoxia and cobalt stimulate lactate dehydrogenase (LDH) activity in vascular smooth muscle cells. *Pflügers Arch* 429:216-222, 1994.
11. Firth JD, Eberrt BL, Ratcliffe PJ: Hypoxic regulation of lactate dehydrogenase A, interaction between hypoxia-inducible factor 1 and cAMP response elements. *J Biol Chem* 270:21021-21027, 1995.
12. Raff H, Jankowski B: O_2 dependence of pregnenolone and aldosterone synthesis in mitochondria from bovine zona glomerulosa cells. *J Appl Physiol* 78:1625-1628, 1995.
13. Montoro RJ, Ureña J, Fernández-Chacón R, et al: Oxygen sensing by ion channels and chemotransduction in single glomus cells. *J Gen Physiol* 107:133-143, 1996.
14. Ureña J, Fernández-Chacón R, Benot AR, et al: Hypoxia induces voltage-dependent Ca^{2+} entry and quantal dopamine secretion in carotid body glomus cells. *Proc Natl Acad Sci USA* 91:10208-10211, 1994.
15. Zhu WH, Conforti L, Czyzyk-Krzeska MF, et al: Membrane depolarization in PC12 cells during hypoxia is regulated by an O_2-sensitive K^+ current. *Amer J Physiol Cell Physiol* 40:C658-665, 1996.
16. Youngson C, Nurse C, Yeger H, et al: Oxygen sensing in airway chemoreceptors. *Nature* 365:153-155, 1993.
17. Weir EK, Archer SL: The mechanism of acute hypoxic pulmonary vasoconstriction: the tale of two channels. *FASEB J* 9:183-189, 1995.
18. Jiang C, Haddad GG: A direct mechanism for sensing low oxygen levels by central neurons. *Proc Natl Acad Sci USA* 91:7198-7201, 1994.
19. Franco-Obregón A, Ureña J, López-Barneo J: Oxygen-sensitive calcium channels

in vascular smooth muscle and their possible role in hypoxic arterial relaxation. *Proc Natl Acad Sci USA* 92:4715-4719, 1995.

20. Gilles-Gonzalez MA, Gonzalez G: Regulation of the kinase activity of heme protein FixL from the two-component system FixL/FixJ of *Rhizobium meliloti. J Biol Chem* 268:16293-16297, 1993.
21. Pahl HL, Baeuerle PA: Oxygen and the control of gene expression. *Bio Essays* 16:497-502, 1994.
22. Hidalgo E, Demple B: An iron-sulfur center essential for transcriptional activation by the redox-sensing SoxR protein. *EMBO J* 13:138-146, 1994.
23. Lazazzera BA, Beinert H, Khoroshilova N, et al: DNA binding and dimerization of the Fe-S-containing FNR protein from *Escherichia coli* are regulated by oxygen. *J Biol Chem* 271:2762-2768, 1996.
24. Meury J, Robin A: Glutathione-gated K^+ channels of *Escherichia coli* carry out K^+ efflux controlled by the redox state of the cell. *Arch Microbiol* 154:475-482, 1990.
25. Poole PK, Ioannidis N, Orii Y: Reactions of the *Escherichia coli* flavohaemoglobin (HMP) with oxygen and reduced nicotinamide adenine dinucleotide: evidence for oxygen switching of flavin oxidoreduction and a mechanism for oxygen sensing. *Proc R Soc Lond* 225:251-258, 1994.
26. Poyton RO, Burke PV: Oxygen regulated transcription of cytochrome c and cytochrome oxidase genes in yeast. *Biochem Biophys Acta* 110:252-256, 1992.
27. Cross AR, Henderson L, Jones OTG, et al: Involvement of an NAD(P)H oxidase as a Po_2 sensor protein in the rat carotid body. *Biochem J* 272:743-747, 1990.
28. Bokoch GM: Biology of the Rap proteins, members of the ras superfamily of GTP-binding proteins. *Biochem J* 289:17-24, 1993.
29. Kummer W, Acker H: Immunohistochemical demonstration of 4 subunits of neutrophil NAD(P)H oxidase in type I cells of carotid body. *J Appl Physiol* 78: 1904-1909, 1995.
30. López-López JR, González C: Time course of $K+$ current inhibition by low oxygen in chemoreceptor cells of adult rabbit carotid body. Effects of carbon monoxide. *FEBS Lett* 299:251-254, 1992.
31. Duprat F, Guillemare E, Romey G, et al: Susceptibility of cloned $K+$ channels to reactive oxygen species. *Proc Natl Acad Sci USA* 92:11796-11800, 1995.
32. Heinemann SH, Rettig J, Wunder F, et al: Molecular and functional characterization of a rat brain Kv beta 3 potassium channel subunit. *FEBS Lett* 377:383-389, 1995.
33. Stephens GJ, Owen DG, Robertson B: Cysteine-modifying reagents alter the gating of the rat cloned potassium channel Kv1.4. *Pflügers Arch* 431:435-442, 1996.
34. Vega-Saenz de Miera E, Rudy B: Modulation of K^+ channels by hydrogen peroxide. *Biochem Biophys Res Comm* 186:1681-1687, 1992.
35. Kukuljan M, Labarca P, Latorre R: Molecular determinants of ion conduction and inactivation in $K+$ channels. *Amer J Physiol Cell Physiol* 268:C535-C556, 1995.
36. McCormack T, McCormack K: *Shaker* K^+ channel β subunits belong to an NAD(P)H-dependent oxidoreductase superfamily. *Cell* 79:1133-1135, 1994.
37. Görlach A, Holtermann G, Jellkmann W, et al: Photometric characteristics of heme proteins in erythropoietin producing hepatoma cells (HepG2). *Biochem J* 290:771-776, 1993.

38. Fandrey J, Frede S, Jelkmann W: Role of hydrogen-peroxide in hypoxia-induced erythropoietin production. *Biochem J* 303:507-510, 1994.
39. Kietzmann T, Freimann S, Bratke J, et al: Regulation of the gluconeogenic phosphoenolpyruvate carboxykinase and the glycolytic aldolase A gene expression by O_2 in rat hepatocyte cultures. Involvement of the hydrogen peroxide as mediator in the response to O_2. *FEBS Lett* 388:228-232, 1996.
40. Bastian NR, Hibbs JB Jr: Assembly and regulation of NADPH oxidase and nitric oxide synthase. *Cur Opi Immunol* 6:131-139, 1994.
41. Jones OTG, Jones SA, Wood JD: Expression of components of the superoxide generating NAD(P)H oxidase by human leucocytes and other cells. *Protoplasma* 184:79-85, 1995.
42. Ehleben W, Porwol T, Fandrey J, et al: Cobalt and desferrioxamine reveal crucial members of the oxygen sensing pathway in HepG2 cells. *Kidney Int* 51:483–491, 1997. (In press.)
43. Ho VT, Bunn HF: Effects of transition metals on the expression of the erythropoietin gene: further evidence that the oxygen sensor is a heme protein. *Biochem Biophys Res Comm* 223:175-180, 1996.

Chapter 3

Critical Cysteine Residues in the Inactivation Domains of Voltage-Activated Potassium Channels

Olaf Pongs

Introduction

Voltage-activated potassium (Kv) channels are key players in many aspects of electrical responses in the nervous system. For example, Kv channel activities are involved in the regulation of wave forms and frequencies of action potentials, of thresholds of excitation, of synaptic strength, and of the resting potential of membranes.[1] Two main types of Kv channels may be discerned: slowly or noninactivating Kv channels and rapidly inactivating (A-type) Kv channels.[2,3] A-type Kv channels may operate in the subthreshold range of action potentials and, thereby, fulfill important regulatory functions for encoding pre- and postsynaptic neural signalling. Several A-type Kv channel mediated currents have been described which differ in their voltage sensitivity of activation and inactivation, and/or in the time constants of activation, inactivation, and recovery from inactivation.[4] Thus, diverse A-type Kv channels are expressed in the nervous system suggesting that A-type Kv channels may have specialized and distinct functions related to nervous excitability.[1-4]

From: López-Barneo, J and Weir, EK: *Oxygen Regulation of Ion Channels and Gene Expression.* Armonk, NY: Futura Publishing Company, Inc., ©1998.

Structure of Voltage-Activated Potassium Channels

The characterization of cloned A-type Kv channels has indicated that they are most likely heteromultimers which are assembled from α and β subunits.[5-7] The primary sequences of Kvα subunit isoforms, which have been derived from many different cDNAs from bacteria and plants to man, are quite similar, always exhibiting a characteristic type of secondary structure.[3] Accordingly, all Kvα subunit isoforms may have comparable structures consisting of hydrophobic, membrane- spanning core domains flanked by hydrophilic amino and carboxy termini of varying lengths. It appears that the core domain is inserted into the membrane such that the amino and carboxy termini face the cytoplasm. The core domain of Kvα subunits invariably contains six hydrophobic segments (S1 to S6) which transverse the membrane and one hydrophobic segment, H5, interspersed between S5 and S6. Segment H5 is tucked into the membrane and enters and exits the plasma membrane from the extracellular side. The core domain of Kvα subunits contains the structures that are necessary to form the pore and the voltage sensor which determines the voltage sensitivity of Kv channel opening.[2] The cytoplasmic amino terminus contains the domains which are required for assembly and tetramerization (T-domains).[8] Some carboxy-termini may contain a carboxyterminal signature sequence for interaction with the members of the postsynaptic density (PSD) protein family.[9]

The β subunits appear to be peripheral proteins tightly associated with the cytoplasmic side of the α subunits.[8,10] Several β subunits have been cloned and characterized that interact with members of the Kvα subunit subfamily.[6,11-19] It is suggested that each Kv channel α subunit associates with a β subunit. We showed the Kvβ1 interaction site to be localized to a cytoplasmic amino-terminal region within the tetramerization domain T1B.[10] Possibly, four Kvβ1 subunits bind to Kv1α tetramers to form $\alpha 4\beta 4$ heteromultimers.[5] Apparently, Kvβ subunits are auxiliary subunits which may aid assembly of Kvα subunits and/or transport of the newly formed Kv channels to the plasma membrane. Another important function of Kvβ subunits can be that they confer rapid inactivation onto Kvα channels which otherwise cannot rapidly inactivate, but behave like delayed rectifiers.[7] This property is due to the presence of an amino-terminal inactivating domain in some β subunits like Kvβ1 and Kvβ3.[6,14]

Inactivation Domains in Voltage-Activated Potassium Channels

Shaker as well as some *Shaker* related K (K_V) channels, e.g., Kv1.4 and Kv3.4, contain an amino-terminal domain, approximately 25 to 35 amino acids in length, which behaves like an inactivating gate.[20,21] This domain binds to a receptor near or at the inner mouth of the Kv channel pore. Binding of the inactivating domain to this receptor site during depolarization of the membrane rapidly closes the open Kv channel pore within minutes. It has been proposed that inactivating domain binding resembles a ball-and-chain type mechanism, in which the inactivating domain would be the ball and other parts of the amino terminus the chain.[20] Therefore, this type of Kv channel inactivation is also referred to as N-type inactivation. According to the ball-and-chain model of N-type inactivation, the "ball" domain inactivates the channel in the open state by binding at or near the inner mouth of the open Kv channel pore, a process which is largely independent of membrane voltage at voltages above -40 mV.[21] Amino-terminal peptides which contain the ball domain act as pore-blocking "ball peptides."[6,20,21] When added to the bath solutions of inside-out patches expressing noninactivating Kv channels, "ball peptides" restore rapid inactivation as schematically shown in Figure 1. Thus, the ball domain does not require a covalent bond to the rest of the α-subunit protein sequence for inactivating Kv channels.

Kvβ subunits like Kvβ1 and Kvβ3 also contain an amino-terminal inactivating domain.[7] An alignment of the α and β inactivating domains showed that they are comparable in structure (and in function) (Figure 2). The domains may be divided into two subdomains: 1) which contains a cysteine residue flanked by hydrophobic residues, as well as hydrophilic serines, and 2) which contains a relatively high density of positively charged amino acids. Both subdomains are important for inactivating activity. Similarly to α subunits, removal of the Kvβ1.1 amino terminus, which contains the inactivating ball domain, eliminates rapid inactivation that is conferred on otherwise noninactivating Kv channels upon coexpression of Kv1α with Kvβ1.1 subunits.[6] Also, the addition of the amino-terminal Kvβ1.1 ball peptide to the bath solution of inside-out patches expressing nonactivating Kv channels restores rapid inactivation. These results suggested that α and β subunit inactivating domains function similarly and bind to the same receptor site that closes the Kv channel pore from the inside. Most likely, one inactivating domain is sufficient to close the inner mouth of the open Kv channel pore. Thus, coexpression of Kvα and Kvβ1.1 subunits, both of which have ball domains, should give A-type Kv channels having ball domains in excess. Then, the α and β balls might compete for the one receptor binding site. This proposition was tested by comparing the inactivation properties of A-type Kv channel possessing various ball domain combinations. When Kv1.4α subunits were expressed in 293 cells, the corresponding A-type Kv channels were inactivated with a time constant $\tau_i = 25 \pm 1.8$ ms (n = 5). Coexpression of Kv1.4α with Kvβ1.1 β subunits yielded A-type Kv channels that were

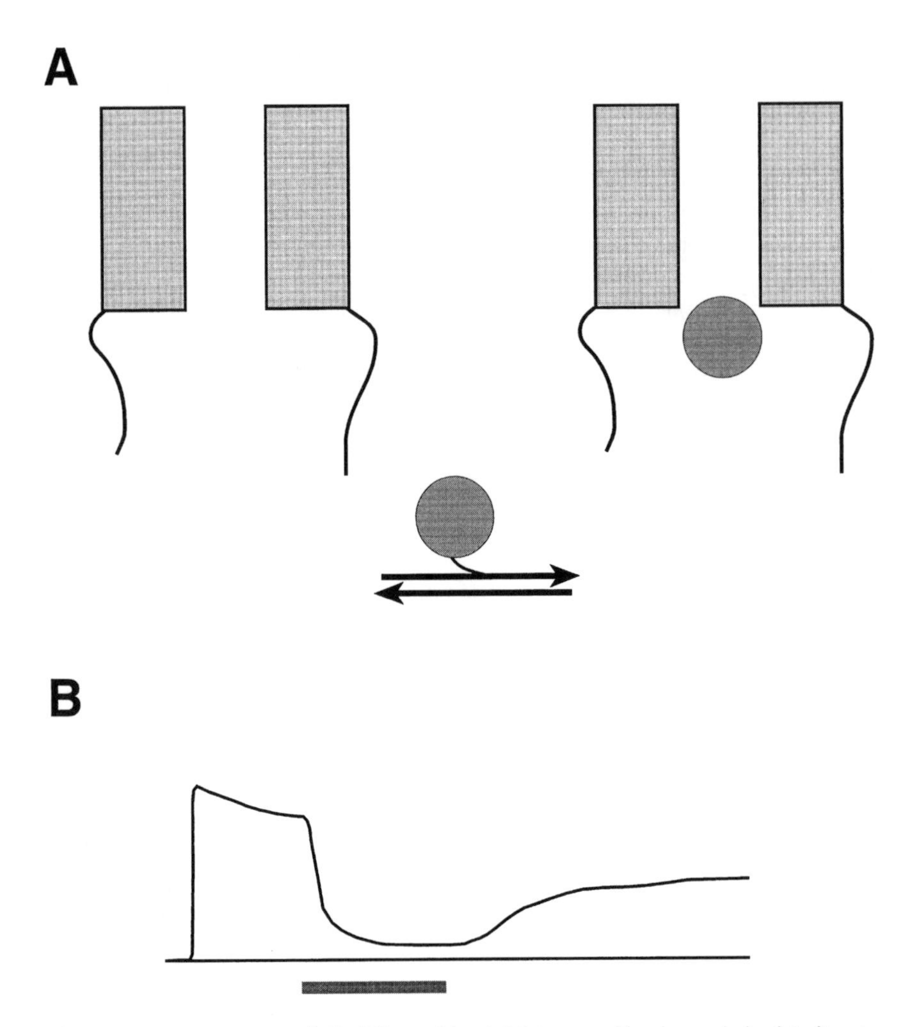

Figure 1. Amino-terminal "ball" peptides inhibit open Kv channels by binding to the cytoplasmic side of Kv subunits. In **A**, schematically binding and unbinding of ball peptide to the receptor binding site at or near the inner mouth of the pore is illustrated. Peptides, which resemble amino acid sequences 1 to 20 in *Shaker*, 1 to 37 in Kv1.4, 1 to 28 in Kv3.4, and 1 to 24 in Kvβ1.1, induced rapid Kv channel closure when added at 100 to 200 μM concentration to the bath solution of inside-out patches expressing noninactivating Kv1 type channels.[6,20,21] **B** shows representative current trace measured in inside-out patches with test pulses from -80 to +40 mV. **Thick bar** indicates application of ball peptide to the bath. After removal of the ball peptide, Kv channels reopen. (Data adapted with permission from Reference 21.)

inactivated more rapidly than Kv1.4 channels alone (τ_i = 4.6 ± 0.4 ms; n = 4). Then, we removed the α ball domain in Kv1.4 (Kv1.4 Δ 110) and coexpressed Kv1.4 Δ 110α and Kvβ1.1 subunits. This created A-type Kv channels which inactivated still faster than the previous ones (τ_i = 3.1 ± 0.1 ms; n = 4). The results suggested that β balls in Kv1.4 Δ 110/Kvβ1.1 channels represent a more efficient inactivating gate than α balls in Kv1.4 channels.[19] The presence of α and β balls in Kv1.4/Kvβ1.1 channels creates apparently an intermediate situation. This may indicate that both types

A

```
KVβ1              MQVSIACTEHNL-------KSRNGEDRLLSKQS
KVβ3              MQVSIACTEQNL-------RSRSSEDRLCGPRP
KV1.4  MEVAMVSAESSGCNSHMPYGYAAQARARERERLAHSRAA
KV3.4              MISSVCVSSY--------RGKKSGNKPPSKTC

Shaker              MAAVAGLYGL-----------GEDRQHRKKQ
```

B

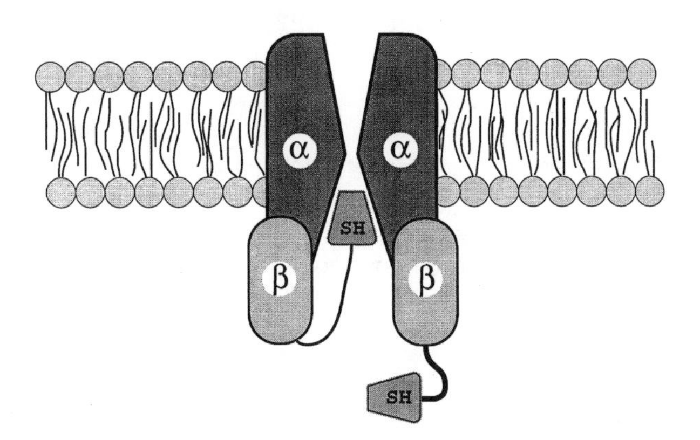

Figure 2. **A.** Alignment of the primary sequences of amino-terminal inactivating domains of Kvα and Kvβ subunits. Sequences have been divided into two domains and were aligned accordingly. The first domain has been **shaded**. This domain is enriched in alanine/serine, valine/isoleucine and, in the case of mammalian "ball" domains, contains a conserved cysteine residue. This cysteine residue is critical for inactivating activity of the ball domains. **B.** Schematic proposed ball-and-chain type mechanism to illustrate N-type inactivation of Kv channels. SH symbolizes the critical cysteine residue which is responsible for the redox sensitivity of the inactivating gate. This gate may be covalently bonded to Kvα or to Kvβ subunits.

of ball domains compete with each other for binding to the same binding site for closing the Kv channel pore. Finally, we swapped the β ball domain in Kvβ1.1 with the Kv1.4 α ball domain (KvαNβ1.1). Expression of Kv1.4 Δ 110/KvαNβ1.1 channels generated A-type Kv channels that inactivated more slowly than the Kv1.4 Δ 110/Kvβ1.1 channels. This result corroborates our notion that the Kvβ1.1 inactivating gate is more efficient than the Kv1.4 one.

Redox Modulation of Inactivation

It is well known that cysteine-containing proteins are prone to oxidation. After formation of inside-out patches and exposure to oxygen or oxidizing conditions such as hydrogen peroxide (H_2O_2), the mammalian A-type K channels like Kv1.4 or Kv1.1/Kvβ1.1 rapidly lose the fast component of inactivation (Figure 3).[6,22] The loss of inactivation was similar over the whole voltage range and for currents in inward and outward directions measured in symmetrical K^+ solution. Inactivation could not be restored in the inside-out patches by varying the pH, ionic concentration, or by adding adenosine triphosphate (ATP) or cyclic adenosine monophosphate (cAMP) to the bath solution facing the cytoplasmic side of the patch.[22] However, after addition of 5 mM glutathione or 5 mM dithiotreitol to the bath solution, rapid inactivation behavior of the A-type K channels was fully restored within 10 seconds. In contrast, *Drosophila Shaker* channels, of which the inactivating domains do not contain a cysteine residue, did not lose their rapid inactivation behavior upon patch excision. This observation is consistent with the idea that in mammalian inactivating domains, the cysteine residue is critical for their activity and must be present in a reduced form. Apparently, this cysteine was rapidly oxidized after excision of the patches, since rapid inactivation disappeared immediately after excision in less than 500 milliseconds. On

→

Figure 3. Redox sensitivity of N-type inactivation of Kv channels. **A.** Under reducing conditions (**red**) Kv1.4 channels rapidly inactivate at +50 mV with a time constant (τ_i = 26 ± 10 ms; n = 5). Rapid (N-type) inactivation is lost upon oxidation (**ox**) of Kv1.4 channels. **B.** Similarly, rapid inactivation of Kv1.4 Δ 110/Kvβ1.1 channels (τ_i = 4.2 ± 0.8 ms; n = 8) was eliminated by oxidation. **C.** When the critical cysteine in the inactivation domains was replaced with serine in Kv1.4 Δ 110/Kvβ1.1C7S channels, the corresponding A-type K channels were no longer redox-sensitive as described in Reference 6.

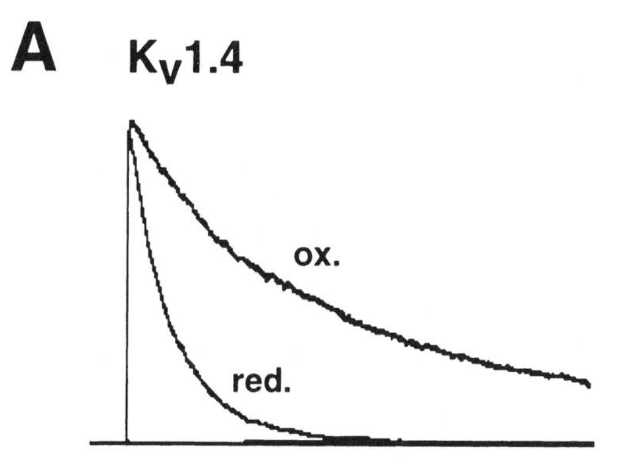

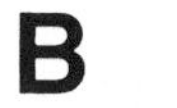

$K_V1.4\Delta110 + K_V\beta1.1$

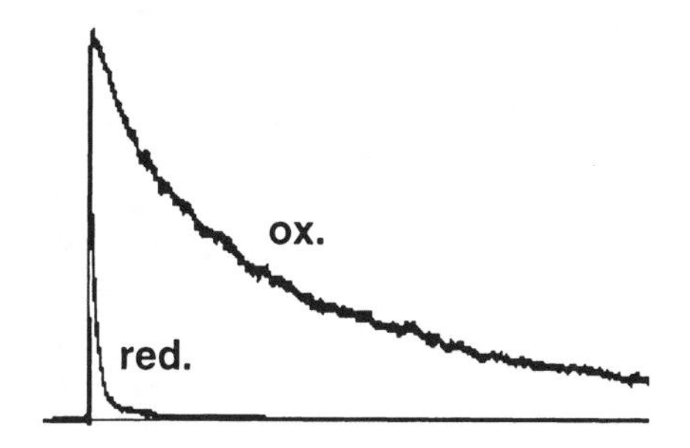

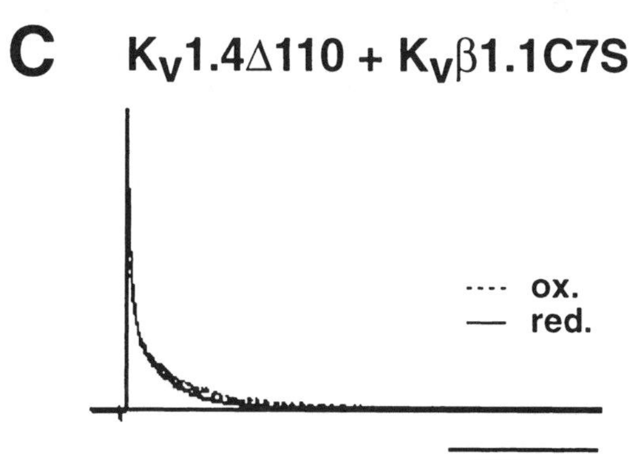

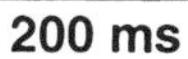

the other hand, recovery from inactivation of inactivated Kv channels was not affected and had its normal time course. This observation indicates that inactivating domains that are engaged in channel closure are resistant to oxidation.[22] The cysteines in inactivating domains may only be accessible to modification when the inactivating gate is not bound at or near the inner mouth of the Kv channel. The time course of interconversion between the oxidized and reduced states of the inactivating domains appears to occur with a time constant of the same order of magnitude as rapid inactivation. When 5 mM glutathione was applied to the bath solution facing the cytoplasmic side of the oxidized A-type K channel, the observed time course of current decay, i.e., restoration of rapid inactivation, was similar to the ones of rapid inactivation itself.[6,22]

When the critical cysteine in the inactivation domains was replaced with serine by in vitro mutagenesis, e.g., Kv1.4 - C13S and Kvβ1.1 - C7S, the redox-sensitivity of the corresponding A-type K channel was no longer observed.[6,22] N-type inactivation was not affected in inside-out patches under exactly those conditions that produced a rapid loss of ball activity. This corroborates the observation that the amino-terminal inactivating domains of mammalian A-type K channels, when they contain a cysteine residue, require this cysteine, e.g., C13 in Kv1.4 and C7 in Kvβ1.1, in a reduced form for their function. In conclusion, N-type inactivation of mammalian A-type Kv channels is regulated by cysteine oxidation. This type of regulation may have a role in vivo to link the cellular redox status or free radical-induced oxidant stress to the excitability of membrane areas containing A-type Kv channels. The oxygen-radical sensitivity may be particularly important in physiologic and pathophysiologic states related to ischemia, neurodegeneration, and some heart disease states, for example.

Recently, it has been shown that Kv channels may respond differently to different reactive oxygen species. Consistent with our H_2O_2 experiments, application of *tert*-butyl hydroperoxide removed the N-type inactivation process from Kv1.4 and Kv3.4. By contrast, the activity (current amplitude) of several Kv channels (Kv1.3 and Kv1.5) in addition to Kv1.4 and Kv3.4 was significantly inhibited (80%) by photoactivation of rose bengal as well as the inward rectifier channel IRK3.[23] The inhibitory effects, however, were not reversible. The effects of *tert*-butyl hydroperoxide and of rose bengal on Kv1.4 and Kv3.4 channels were additive. This suggests that the different reactive oxygen species, generated by *tert*-butyl hydroperoxide or rose bengal, modified the K channels differently.

Acknowledgments

O. Pongs thanks the Deutsche Forschungsgemeinschaft and the Fonds der Chemischen Industrie for generous support.

References

1. Hille B: *Ionic Channels of Excitable Membranes.* Sunderland, MA: Sinauer Associates, Inc.; 1992.
2. Jan LY, Jan YN: Structural elements involved in specific K^+ channel functions. *Annu Rev Physiol* 54:537-555, 1992.
3. Stühmer W, Ruppersberg JP, Schröter KH, et al: Molecular basis of functional diversity of voltage-gated potassium channels in mammalian brain. *EMBO J* 8: 3235-3244, 1989.
4. Chandy G, Gutman GA: Voltage-gated K^+ channels. In: North RA (ed): *Handbook of Receptors and Channels.* Boca Raton, FL: CRC Press, Inc.; 1-71, 1994.
5. Parcej DN, Scott VES, Dolly JO: Oligomeric properties of α-dendrotoxin-sensitive potassium ion channels purified from bovine brain. *Biochemistry* 31:11084-11088, 1992.
6. Rettig J, Heinemann SH, Wunder F, et al: Inactivation properties of voltage-gated K^+ channels altered by presence of β subunit. *Nature* 369:289-294, 1994.
7. Pongs O: Regulation of the activity of voltage-gated potassium channels by β subunits. *Neuroscience* 7:137-146, 1995.
8. Yu W, Xu J, Li M: NAB domain is essential for the subunit assembly of both α-α and α-β complexes of *Shaker*-like potassium channels. *Neuron* 16:441-453, 1996.
9. Kim E, Niedhammer M, Rothschild A, et al: Clustering of Shaker-type K^+ channels by interaction with a family of membrane-associated guanylate kinases. *Nature* 378:85-88, 1995.
10. Sewing S, Roeper J, Pongs O: Kvβ1 subunit binding specific for *Shaker*-related potassium channel subunits. *Neuron* 16:455-463, 1996.
11. Scott VES, Rettig J, Parcej DN, et al: Primary structure of a β subunit of α-dendrotoxin-sensitive K^+ channels from bovine brain. *Proc Natl Acad Sci USA* 91:1637-1641, 1994.
12. Chouinard SW, Wilson G, Schlimgen AK, et al: A potassium channel β subunit related to the aldo-keto reductase superfamily is encoded by the *Drosophila* hyperkinetic locus. *Proc Natl Acad Sci USA* 92:6763-6767, 1995.
13. England SK, Uebele VN, Shear H, et al: Characterization of a voltage-gated K^+ channel β subunit expressed in human heart. *Proc Natl Acad Sci USA* 92:6309-6313, 1995.
14. Heinemann SH, Rettig J, Wunder F, et al: Molecular and functional characterization of a rat brain Kvβ3 potassium channel subunit. *FEBS Lett* 377:383-389, 1995.
15. Majumder K, De Biasi M, Wand Z, et al: Molecular cloning and functional expression of a novel potassium channel β subunit from human atrium. *FEBS Lett* 361:13-16, 1995.
16. McCormack K, McCormack T, Tanouye M, et al: Alternative splicing of the human *Shaker* K^+ channel β1 gene and functional expression of the β2 gene product. *FEBS Lett* 370:32-36, 1995.
17. Morales MJ, Castellino RC, Crews AL, et al: A novel β subunit increases rate of inactivation of specific voltage-gated potassium channel subunits. *J Biol Chem* 270:6270-6277, 1995.
18. Heinemann SH, Rettig J, Graack HR, et al: Functional characterization of Kv channel β subunits from rat brain. *J Physiol* 493:625-633, 1996.
19. Leicher T, Roeper J, Weber K, et al: Structural and functional characterization

of human potassium channel subunit $\beta 1$ (KCNA1B). *Neuropharmacology* 35: 787-795, 1996.

20. Hoshi T, Zagotta WN, Aldrich R: Biophysical and molecular mechanisms of *Shaker* potassium channel inactivation. *Science* 250:533-538, 1990.
21. Ruppersberg JP, Frank R, Pongs O, et al: Cloned neuronal $I_k(A)$ channels reopen during recovery from inactivation. *Nature* 353:657-660, 1991.
22. Ruppersberg JP, Stocker M, Pongs O, et al: Regulation of fast inactivation of cloned mammalian $I_k(A)$ channels by cysteine oxidation. *Nature* 352:711-714, 1991.
23. Duprat F, Guillemare E, Romey G, et al: Susceptibility of cloned K^+ channels to reactive oxygen species. *Proc Natl Acad Sci USA* 92:11796-11800, 1995.

Section 2

OXYGEN SENSORS IN BACTERIA AND PLANTS

Chapter 4

Nitrogen Fixation and Oxygen Sensing

Eric Soupène
Pierre Boistard

Introduction

Biological reduction of atmospheric nitrogen into ammonia, together with industrial synthesis of chemical fertilizers, provides the living world with nearly all the nitrogen compounds required for biosynthetic reactions. Each molecule of ammonia produced by biological nitrogen fixation necessitates the consumption of 16 adenosine triphosphate (ATP) molecules needed for passing eight electrons, one by one, from the electron-accepting component II of the nitrogenase complex to the catalytic component I at each round of reduction. Because of this sophisticated reaction, nitrogenase shows a high degree of structural conservation in all the prokaryotic organisms which perform nitrogen fixation.[1] Component I, where substrate reduction takes place, is an iron molybdenum enzyme. Component II is an electron acceptor from low potential donors such as ferredoxins or flavodoxins and an electron donor to component I. Reduction of component II occurs at solvent-exposed iron sulphur clusters, which may be responsible for the high sensitivity of this molecule to oxygen.[2]

Because of the high sensitivity of nitrogenase to oxygen inactivation, the various prokaryotic nitrogen fixers have evolved very elaborate oxy-

From: López-Barneo, J and Weir, EK: *Oxygen Regulation of Ion Channels and Gene Expression.* Armonk, NY: Futura Publishing Company, Inc., ©1998.

gen responsive regulatory pathways which utilize a large variety of oxygen-sensing modules, for the control of nitrogenase expression. In addition, because nitrogenase synthesis can divert a large proportion of the cell metabolic resources, nitrogen-fixing microorganisms very strictly control nitrogenase synthesis according to their own needs, or to the creation of a favorable environment in the case of symbiotic nitrogen fixers. The achievement of these favorable conditions is due to the development of a specialized plant organ, the nodule. The pattern of nitrogen fixation gene expression inside the nodule is controlled by oxygen distribution, which accordingly plays a similar role to morphogen gradients in developmental processes.

Control by Oxygen of the Activity of the NifA Transcriptional Activator

In most nitrogen fixing organisms in which gene expression has been studied, *nif* genes which encode the structural components of nitrogenase, as well as products necessary for nitrogenase maturation and functioning, are transcribed by sigma 54 holoenzyme ribonucleic acid (RNA) polymerase which recognizes promoters with characteristic -12 -24 motifs.[3,4] Sigma 54 RNA polymerase holoenzyme is able to bind to these promoters and, therefore, promote the formation of closed transcription complexes. However, melting of deoxyribonucleic acid (DNA), leading to the formation of heparin-stable open complexes, needs the operation of a transcriptional activator which generally binds to upstream sequences around −100 and interacts with the transcription complex as a result of an integration host factor (IHF)-promoted loop formation.[5,6] This functional duality of sigma 54 polymerase activators is reflected at the structural level, which renders them similar to eukaryotic activators.[7,8] The C-terminal domain is a DNA binding domain, whereas the central domain is responsible for the activation of the closed transcription complexes. This activation needs the hydrolysis of a nucleoside triphosphate for which a highly conserved binding site has been identified in the N-terminal part of the central domain.[9]

In microorganisms such as *Klebsiella pneumoniae* or *Azotobacter vinelandii*, oxygen control of NifA-dependent gene expression is mediated through the NifL protein. NifL from *A. vinelandii* has been purified recently and turned out to be a flavoprotein.[10] It has been shown that NifL protein extracted from aerobically grown *A. Vinelandii* cells inhibits in vitro NifA-promoted formation of open complexes, even in anoxic conditions. The inhibitory action of NifL is relieved only in the presence of a reductant such as dithionite, which indicates that NifL senses redox state rather than oxygen itself. Contrary to other flavoproteins, the change in the redox status of the flavin moiety of NifL is not coupled to a catalytic reaction.

In a majority of nitrogen-fixing organisms in which *nif* gene expression has been studied, oxygen control of NifA activity is achieved by a completely different, although still poorly understood, mechanism. In these organisms, the NifA protein itself is responsible for oxygen sensitivity of the expression of regulated genes. This has been shown by comparing the oxygen dependence of either *K. pneumoniae* or Rhizobium NifA-driven gene expression in *Escherichia coli*, where both NifA proteins were expressed constitutively. Sensitivity of Rhizobium NifA to oxygen has been correlated with the presence of cysteine residues which could be part of a metal (Fe) binding motif located between the central and the C-terminal domains, in the so-called interdomain linker, which is absent in *K. pneumoniae* NifA.[11] A role for a bound metal in the activity of NifA is indicated by the effects of a chelating agent on the induction of NifA-dependent gene expression.[11] The isolation of NifA mutants able to activate *nifH* expression in *E.coli* in the presence of oxygen, provides an approach to understanding the mechanism of the oxygen-mediated inhibition of NifA activity.[12] All the resistant mutants isolated so far have a methionine to isoleucine change in the immediate vicinity of the ATP binding site. Therefore, it has been proposed that a change in the redox state of the metal linked to the cysteine cluster in the interdomain linker may alter the conformation of the NifA protein around the ATP binding site. The M to I mutation would maintain this site in its active configuration for either ATP binding or hydrolysis, irrespective of the redox state of the NifA-bound metal.[12]

Oxygen Control in Symbiotic Nitrogen Fixation

The FixL Paradigm

Symbiotic interaction between rhizobia and legumes results in the formation of nodules, specialized plant organs generally located on roots. Inside the nodule, bacteria encounter a microoxic environment which meets the needs of nitrogenase for its chemical stability. The high energy requirement for nitrogen reduction is provided by an ATP-generating respiratory chain whose terminal copper-containing oxidase has a high affinity for oxygen.[13]

Expression of this electron transport chain encoded by the *fixNOQP* operon is regulated by oxygen concentration, through an oxygen responsive two-component regulatory system highly conserved in three rhizobia, whose regulatory pathways have been extensively studied, namely *Rhizobium meliloti, Azorhizobium caulinodans*, and *Bradyrhizobium japonicum*. In addition, in *R. meliloti* and *A. caulinodans*, this two-component regulatory system allows the coordinate expression between nitrogenase and the respiratory chain which provides it with energy.[14,15]

The FixL/FixJ two-component regulatory system was discovered and its regulatory mechanism deciphered in *R. meliloti*.[16] The FixJ transcriptional activator is composed of two domains: a C-terminal output domain which is responsible for the activating properties, and an N-terminal domain which has a regulatory function. This latter domain is highly conserved in all regulator members of the two-component family; it is also called the receiver domain because it carries an aspartate residue which phosphorylates using a phosphoryl group carried by a histine residue in the C-terminal transmitter domain of the histidine kinase sensor partner. In the FixL/J system, phosphorylation of FixJ is required for binding to the promoter regulatory sequences of the genes it activates. FixL, in addition to the transmitter domain conserved in the sensor proteins, has an N-terminal hydrophobic region which anchors the protein to the cytoplasmic membrane and a central cytoplasmic domain. Deletion of the hydrophobic N-terminal region of FixL allowed the purification of a soluble derivative which retained the ability to phosphorylate and which was shown to carry a heme moiety.[17] Furthermore, deletion of the hydrophobic domain did not suppress the oxygen response of FixL in vivo.[18] Availability of soluble cytoplasmic FixL derivatives allowed the first in vitro reconstitution of the complete regulatory pathway from stimulus sensing to signal transduction and transcriptional activation by a two-component regulatory system.[19,20] FixJ, incubated in the presence of FixL and ATP in anoxic conditions, was able to activate target gene expression at a much lower concentration than nonincubated protein and this enhanced activity was due to phosphorylation. FixL phosphorylation, very likely at a conserved histidine residue of the transmitter domain, is regulated by oxygen.[21] When a critical histidine 194 residue in the central domain is mutated, the mutated protein no longer shows heme attached and phosphorylation is no longer dependent on the aeration status. A reasonable conclusion of these experiments is that oxygen binding to the heme moiety regulates the kinase activity of FixL.

The FixLJ two-component regulatory system described above is conserved in *A. caulinodans* and *B. japonicum*. However, in the latter species, the N-terminal domain of FixL does not show the hydrophobic region which anchors *R. meliloti* FixL to the membrane. Whether this difference reflects a different response to oxygen concentration and/or distribution or, alternatively, means that *R. meliloti* FixL responds to an additional stimulus, remains to be determined.[14,15]

Interestingly, elements of the FixLJ regulatory system have been found in other rhizobia where they seem to participate in quite different regulatory combinations. In *Rhizobium leguminosarum* biovar *phaseoli,* there is a FixL homolog showing conservation of the cytoplasmic N-terminal domain, but the histidine residue which is likely to bind the heme group has been deleted together with the surrounding residues.[22] It is not yet known whether this FixL variant responds to another stimulus than oxygen concentration and whether it is activating the FixJ homologue encoded by an adjacent open reading frame (ORF). Yet another variation on the FixL theme is provided by *Rhizobium leguminosarum* biovar *viciae* where the FixL homologue contains an additional C-terminal domain which is constituted by a regulator receiver domain.[23] This additional domain could play a regulatory role on the transmitter domain. Alternatively, it is possible that the aspartate residue of this receiver domain could donate its phosphoryl group to the histidine of the sensor component of another two-component regulatory system, which remains to be identified. Examples of such phosphorelays have been found in regulatory cascades which are able to integrate several environmental stimuli.[24]

A search in sequence data banks revealed that a homologue to the heme domain of FixL is present in an *A. caulinodans* ORF which does not encode a histidine kinase.[25] Very interestingly, this ORF is located between genes encoding two homologous two- component regulatory systems, NtrB/NtrC and NtrY/NtrX, whose mutation affects the ability to grow on nitrate as sole nitrogen source. However, the impaired phenotype of ntrY or ntrX mutants is observed only in well-aerated cultures.[26] Therefore, it is tempting to speculate that the predicted heme-binding domain of the ORF could be involved in the oxygen response of the *ntrB/ntrC, ntrY/ntrX* controlled phenotype.

Fnr Homologues

In *R. meliloti, A. caulinodans,* and *B. japonicum,* the genes encoding the high affinity oxidase and electron transport chain are not under the direct control of the FixLJ regulatory system. FixLJ activates the expression of FixK, an Fnr homologue which, in turn, activates the *fixNOQP* operon.[14,15] Fnr was originally identified as the activator of anaerobic respiratory chains in *E. coli.*[27] The 30 kDa protein Fnr binds to *cis*-regulatory sequences with dyad symmetry centered at −41.5 bp from the transcription initiation site and activates gene expression by interacting with RNA polymerase. Recently, the mechanism by which Fnr senses oxygen has started being elucidated. Three cysteine residues at positions 20, 23, and 29 in the N-terminal region and one critical central cysteine at position 122 coordinate an iron sulphur cluster, which is essential for the regulation of the DNA binding properties of Fnr in response to oxygen. Several lines of evidence indicate that the iron sulphur cluster is oxygen labile and that its presence greatly increases the affinity of the protein for DNA.[28,29] Either the presence of the active iron sulphur cluster would facilitate the dimerization of the protein, which would bind to DNA as a dimer, or it would increase the affinity of the monomer to DNA, resulting in its assembly as a dimer on the binding sites.

Rhizobia possess two categories of Fnr homologues. The first category is represented by *R. meliloti* FixK, *A. caulinodans* FixK, *R. leguminosarum* biovar *Viciae* FixK, and *B. japonicum* FixK2. These molecules are characterized by the absence of the N- terminal and central cysteine residues which coordinate the iron sulphur cluster of *E. coli* Fnr. Expression of *R. meliloti* FixK under the control of an oxygen-independent FixLJ regulatory system resulted in an oxygen-independent expression of the target genes, a strong indication that the cysteine residues are indeed needed for the oxygen response.[30] The second category is represented by *B. japonicum* FixK1 and *R. leguminosarum* biovar *viciae* FnrN. These Fnr homologues contain the cysteine residues whose presence is correlated with oxygen sensing in *E. coli* Fnr. Both proteins, when constitutively expressed in an *fnr* mutant of *E. coli*, were able to activate *fnr*-dependent genes in response to anoxic conditions, providing evidence that these proteins are oxygen-sensitive.[31,32] Interestingly, both oxygen independent FixK and oxygen-sensitive FnrN seem to cooperate in the regulation of nitrogen fixation genes in *R. leguminosarum* biovar *viciae*, since double *fnrN/fixK* mutants are deficient for nitrogen fixation, whereas single mutants have only a partially negative phenotype.[33]

Combinatorial Organization of the Oxygen-Responsive Regulatory Pathway of Nitrogen Fixation Gene Expression

Figure 1 represents the regulatory pathway which controls nitrogen fixation gene expression in *R. meliloti* and the Table summarizes the properties of the different homologous regulatory proteins in several rhi-

Table
Regulatory Molecules of Rhizobium Nitrogen Fixation Genes

Regulatory Molecule Family	O_2-Sensing Module of the Prototype	*R. meliloti*		*B. japonicum*		*A. caulinodans*		*R.l.* bv *phaseoli*		*R.l.* bv *viciae*	
		O_2 s	*target*	*O_2 s*	*target*	*O_2 s*	*target*	*O_2 s*	*target*	*O_2 s*	*target*
FixL	Heme	yes	*fixK;nifA*	yes	*fixK2*	yes	*fixK*	no	?	yes°	?
NifA	Metal?	yes	*nifHDKE* *fixABCX*	yes	*nifHDKE* *fixABCX*	yes	*nifHDKE* *fixABCX*	yes	*nifHDK* *fixABCX*	yes#	
Fnr/FixK	Iron-Sulphur cluster	no	*fixNOQP*	no* yes*	*fixNOQP;K1* ?	no	*fixNOQP;nifA*			yes* no*	*fixNOQP?* *fixNOQP?*

° FixL sensitivity to oxygen was deduced from the presence of the heme binding motif.[23]

NifA sensitivity to oxygen was deduced from the presence of the cysteine motif.[23]

* In both *B. japonicum* and *R. leguminosarum* bv *viciae,* there are at least two representatives of the FnrN/FixK family.[14,23]

O_2 s = sensitivity to oxygen

(All other data are from References 14 and 15, except those concerning *R.l.* bv *phaseoli.*[33])

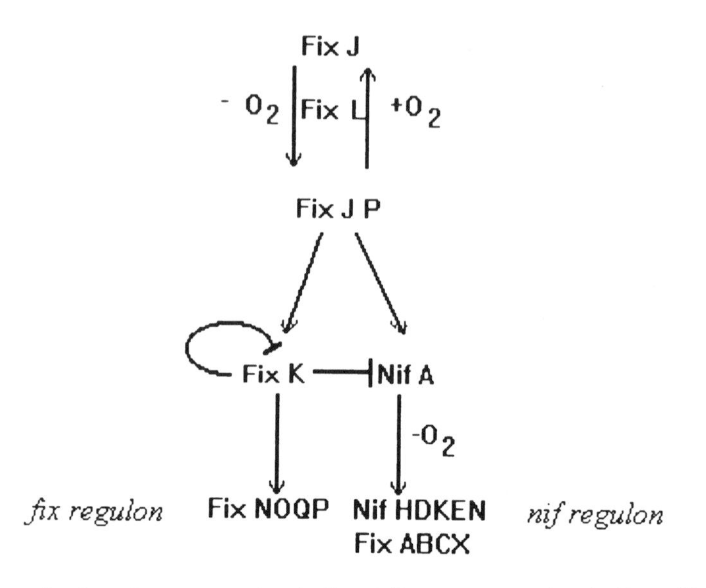

Figure 1. Regulatory cascade of *nif* and *fix* gene expression in *R. meliloti.*

zobia. In *R. meliloti,* the regulatory cascade of nitrogen fixation gene expression shows two levels of oxygen control carried out by FixLJ and NifA, respectively. Oxygen sensitivity of NifA activity allows oxygen control of *nif* gene expression in every rhizobium strain in which regulation of *nif* genes has been characterized. FixL/J allows an additional level of oxygen control in *R. meliloti* and in *A. caulinodans* through *nifA* expression, directly in *R. meliloti* and via *fixK* expression in *A. caulinodans*. In *R. meliloti,* control of *fixNOQP* expression is mediated by FixK whose activity is independent of oxygen. However, FixLJ mediated oxygen control of *fixK* expression ensures an indirect control of *fixNOQP* expression by the aeration status. The same is true for *A. caulinodans* and *B. japonicum*. On the other hand, it is likely that in *R. leguminosarum* bv *viciae, fixNOQP* expression is under the control of oxygen via the oxygen-sensitive FnrN.

In conclusion, comparison of the various oxygen-responsive regulatory molecules and regulatory pathways first shows that the same regulatory molecules can be assembled in different combinations to constitute various regulatory pathways. Second, it is likely that in a given regulatory pathway, oxygen response at a high hierarchical level of the cascade can result in a loss of oxygen response by molecules located at a lower level. Oxygen control of FixK expression would have led to the loss of oxygen sensitivity of FixK activity, initially inherent to the Fnr family.

Oxygen Concentration Determines Patterns of Nitrogen Fixation Gene Expression in the Nodule

Morphogenesis of the nodule is the result of the expression of a developmental program triggered by an exchange of signals between the Rhizobium microsymbiont and its legume host.[34,35] Successful symbiotic interaction ultimately leads to a nitrogen fixing nodule whose differentiation and activity necessitate the contribution of both partners.

In recent years, the use of molecular cytology techniques has led to the view that the expression of nitrogen fixation genes is subject to a developmental control which couples the onset of nitrogen fixation to the establishment of environmental conditions suitable for the reduction of atmospheric dinitrogen into ammonia.

Indeterminate nodules such as those induced by *R. meliloti* on alfalfa are characterized by the presence of a persistent apical meristem which generates a succession of tissues, progressively differentiating from the apex to the proximal part of the nodule (Figure 2). Immediately proximal to the meristem, also called zone I, the infection zone or zone II consists of plant cells in which the bacteria are released from the infection threads. Inside the invaded cells, bacteria differentiate into nitrogen fixing bacteroids. Nitrogen fixation takes place in zone III, the fixation zone, which is separated from zone II by a few layers of cells filled with amyloplasts.[36] In situ hybridization experiments, as well as observation of gene fusion expression, revealed that several genes essential for nitrogen fixation start being expressed in this border zone also called interzone II-III. This is true for bacterial genes, such as genes of the *nif* regulon (Figure 1), which control the synthesis and processing of nitrogenase or genes of the *fix* regulon necessary for the expression of the *fixNOQP*-encoded bacteroid respiratory chain. The plant gene encoding the high affinity oxygen transporter leghemoglobin is also expressed at the interzone II-III.[37] By combining genetic and physiologic approaches, it has been possible to show that oxygen concentration couples nitrogen fixation gene expression to nodule development.

Mutagenesis of the presumed site of phosphorylation of FixJ resulted in a FixJD54N protein whose FixL-dependent phosphorylation was no longer subject to oxygen regulation (see above and Figure 1). Accordingly, FixJD54N-mediated *nifA* and *fixK* activation was no longer dependent on oxygen concentration.[38] In nodules elicited by this FixJD54N mutant, it was found that *nifA* and *fixK* were expressed in zone II as well as in interzone II-III and in the fixation zone III. The same pattern of gene expression was observed when nodules elicited by the wild-type strain were placed in a microoxic environment.[30]

These results are strong evidence that oxygen distribution inside the nodule determines the patterns of the expression of bacterial nitrogen fixation genes *nifA* and *fixK*. As a consequence, one has to postulate the existence of a gradient of oxygen concentration along the longitudinal axis of the nodule. In order to examine the existence of this gradient, oxygen- sensitive microelectrodes were introduced at the apex of the nodule (Figure 2). There was a monotonous gradient of oxygen concentration, ranging from 250 μM at the apex to 1 μM at the distal edge of the interzone II-III, which corresponded to the threshold of sensitivity of the electrode.

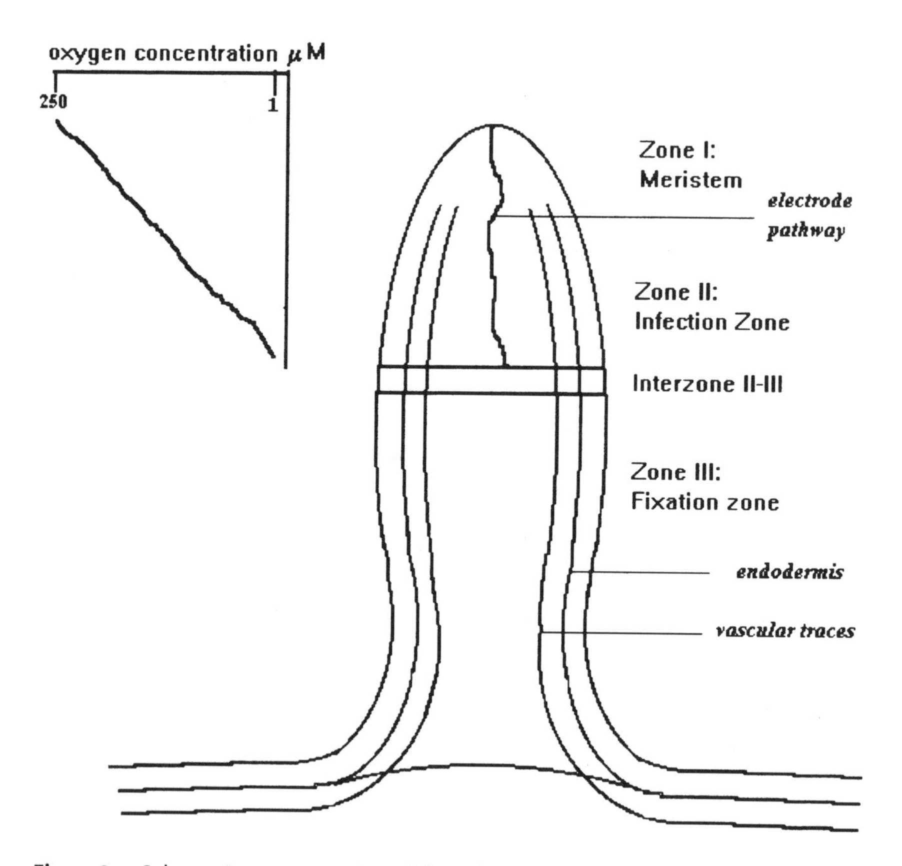

Figure 2. Schematic representation of the indeterminate nodule of alfalfa. The insert in the **upper left corner** represents the concentration gradient of oxygen measured by oxygen-sensitive electrodes.

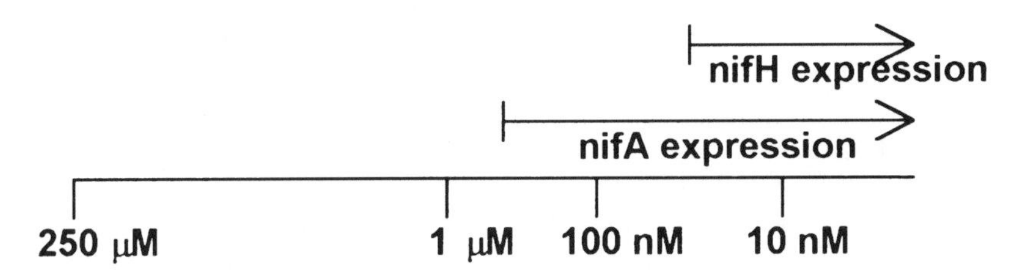

Figure 3. Hypothetical response of *R. meliloti nifH* and *nifA* expression to oxygen concentration.

Contrary to *nifA* and *fixK*, *nifH* was not expressed in zone II of nodules elicited by the FixJD54N mutant. This was not unexpected since the transcriptional activator NifA has been shown to be sensitive to oxygen. More unexpectedly, neither did wild type nor FixJD54N elicited nodules show ectopic expression of *nifH* in zone II when placed in microoxic conditions by immersion in soft agar. This result could be explained either by an exquisite sensitivity of NifA protein to oxygen or by the existence of a signal other than oxygen operating to repress *nifH* in zone II. Spectrometric measurements on leg hemoglobin have established that oxygen concentration in the fixation zone is around 10 nM, that is one hundredfold lower than the 1 μM concentration detected by the microelectrode at the apical edge of interzone II-III.[39,40] It means that there can be a dramatic decrease of oxygen concentration in a very limited area of interzone II-III. Therefore, although *nifA* and *nifH* start being expressed in the same area, their requirements for microoxic conditions could differ significantly (Figure 3). The decrease in oxygen concentration in zone II obtained by immersing the nodule in soft agar would be sufficient to induce *nifA* expression, but would not be sufficient for *nifH* expression. Although tentative, this model for the differential control of expression of *nifA* and *nifH* would be reminiscent of the differential response of developmentally regulated genes to morphogen gradients.

Conclusion

Oxygen/redox sensing in relation with genetic control of nitrogen fixation gene expression involves a variety of oygen/redox-sensing modules. The use of heme and of a flavin as sensors has been identified for the first time in nitrogen fixation regulatory pathways. This may be due to the fact that some nitrogen fixing microorganisms are among the most intensively studied prokaryotes. Another reason for this could be the drastic effect of oxygen on nitrogenase, which would have selected very efficient mechanisms of oxygen control. Because the sensing mechanisms make use of chemical motifs involved in such basic processes as electron transfer or oxygen transport, it is likely that they have been conserved in the course of evolution and will be found in eukaryotic organisms. The use for a sensing process of chemical groups involved in transfer reactions is one additional illustration of the conservative nature of evolution. It will be illuminating to decipher the allosteric transitions or chemical modifications which process oxygen concentration or redox potential into a regulatory signal.

Oxygen-sensing regulatory pathways have provided good examples of the modular nature of regulatory molecules and regulatory pathways. Furthermore, the possibility exists that recruitment of several oxygen-sensing regulatory molecules in a given regulatory pathway can lead to a loss of sensing motifs in some of the molecules as a consequence of redundancy. In this manner, one could explain that *R. meliloti* FixK activity is not modulated by the level of oxygen. Therefore, as a practical consequence, one should interpret with caution homology data between regulatory proteins until their sensory modules have been identified.

Finally, it is of interest to note the possible similarities between the oxygen gradient which determines the expression of nitrogen fixation genes along the longitudinal axis of the nodule and the morphogen gradients which organize the patterns during the developmental processes.[41] Nodule interzone II-III can be considered as the equivalent of the compartment boundary from which morphogens diffuse, generating a concentration gradient responsible for pattern formation. Another similarity, still speculative but worth considering, would reside in the differential response of *nifH* and *fixK* to the oxygen concentration gradient, similarly to the differential response of developmentally expressed genes to a given morphogen gradient.

Acknowledgments

We thank J. Batut for useful comments on the manuscript and E. Boistard for help with figures. Because of space limitation, we did not quote all the original references when reviews were available. We apologize to our colleagues whose work was not cited.

References

1. Smith BE, Roe SM, Yousafzai FK: The structures of the nitrogenase proteins: an overview. In: Tikhonovich I, Provorov N, Romanov V, et al (eds): *Nitrogen Fixa-*

tion: Fundamentals and Applications. Dordrecht, Boston, London: Kluwer Academic Publishers; 19-27, 1995.

2. Georgiadis MM, Komiya H, Chakrabarti P, et al: Crystallographic structure of the nitrogenase iron protein from Azotobacter vinelandii. *Science* 257:1653-1659, 1992.
3. Thöny B, Hennecke H: The -24/-12 promoter comes of age. *FEMS Microbiol Rev* 63:341-358, 1989.
4. Kustu S, Santero E, Keener J, et al: Expression of s^{54}(*NtrA*)-dependent genes is probably united by a common mechanism. *Microbiol Rev* 53:367-376, 1989.
5. Buck M, Cannon W, Woodcock J: Transcriptional activation of the *Klebsiella pneumoniae* nitrogenase promoter may involve DNA loop formation. *Mol Microbiol* 1:243-249, 1987.
6. Morett E, Buck M: NifA-dependent in vivo protection demonstrates that the upstream activator sequence of *nif* promoters is a protein binding site. *Proc Natl Acad Sci USA* 85:9401-9405, 1988.
7. North AK, Klose KE, Stedman KM, et al: Prokaryotic enhancer- binding proteins reflect eukaryotic-like modularity: the puzzle of nitrogen regulatory protein C. *J Bacteriol* 175:4267-4273, 1993.
8. Morett E, Segovia L: The ^{54} bacterial enhancer-binding protein family: mechanism of action and phylogenetic relationship of their functional domains. *J Bacteriol* 175:6067-6074, 1993.
9. Berger DK, Narberhaus F, Kustu S: The isolated catalytic domain of NifA, a bacterial enhancer-binding protein, activates transcription in vitro: activation is inhibited by nifL. *Proc Natl Acad Sci USA* 91:103-107, 1994.
10. Hill S, Austin S, Eydmann T, et al: *Azotobacter vinelandii* NifL is a flavoprotein that modulates transcriptional activation of nitrogen-fixation genes via a redox-sensitive switch. *Proc Natl Acad Sci USA* 93:2143-2148, 1996.
11. Fischer HM, Bruderer T, Hennecke H: Essential and nonessential domains in the *Bradyrhizobium japonicum* NifA protein: identification of indispensable cysteine residues potentially involved in redox activity and/or metal binding. *Nucleic Acids Res* 16:2207-2224, 1988.
12. Krey R, Pühler A, Klipp W: A defined aminoacid exchange close to the putative nucleotide binding site is responsible for an oxygen-tolerant variant of the *Rhizobium meliloti* NifA protein. *Mol Gen Genet* 234:433-441, 1992.
13. Preisig O, Anthamatten D, Hennecke H: Genes for a microaerobically induced oxidase complex in *Bradyrhizobium japonicum* are essential for a nitrogen fixing endosymbiosis. *Proc Natl Acad Sci USA* 90:3309-3313, 1993.
14. Fischer HM: Genetic regulation of nitrogen fixation in Rhizobia. *Microbiol Rev* 58:352-386, 1994.
15. Batut J, Boistard P: Oxygen control in Rhizobium. *Antonie van Leeuwenhoek* 66:129-150, 1994.
16. David M, Daveran ML, Batut J, et al: Cascade regulation of *nif* gene expression in *Rhizobium meliloti. Cell* 54:671-683, 1988.
17. Gilles-Gonzalez MA, Ditta GS, Helinski DR: A haemoprotein with kinase activity encoded by the oxygen sensor of *Rhizobium meliloti. Nature* 350:170-172, 1991.
18. de Philip P, Soupène E, Batut J, et al: Modular structure of the FixL protein of *Rhizobium meliloti. Mol Gen Genet* 235:49-54, 1992.
19. Agron PG, Ditta GS, Helinski DR: Oxygen regulation of *nifA* transcription in vitro. *Proc Natl Acad Sci USA* 90:3506-3510, 1993.

20. Reyrat JM, David M, Blonski C, et al: Oxygen-regulated in vitro transcription of *Rhizobium meliloti nifA* and *fixK* genes. *J Bacteriol* 175:6867-6872, 1993.
21. Monson EK, Ditta GS, Helinski DR: The oxygen sensor protein, FixL of *Rhizobium meliloti*. Role of histidine residues in heme binding, phosphorylation, and signal transduction. *J Biol Chem* 270:5243-5250, 1995.
22. D'hooghe I, Michiels J, Vlassak K, et al: Structural and functional analysis of the *Rhizobium leguminosarum* biovar *phaseoli* CNPAF512 *fixLJ* genes. *Mol Gen Genet* 249:117-126, 1995.
23. Patschkowski T, Schlüter A, Priefer U: *Rhizobium leguminosarum* bv. *viciae* contains a second *fnr/fixK*-like gene and an unusual *fixL* homologue. *Mol Microbiol* 21:267-280, 1996.
24. Appleby JL, Parkinson JS, Bourret RB: Signal transduction via the multi-step phosphorelay: not necessarily a road less traveled. *Cell* 86:845-848, 1996.
25. Kahn D: Shuffling of an oxygen sensor haem domain. *Mol Microbiol* 8:786-787, 1993.
26. Pawslowski K, Klosse U, de Bruijn FJ: Characterization of a novel *Azorhizobium caulinodans* ORS571 two-component regulatory system, NtrY/NtrX, involved in nitrogen fixation and metabolism. *Mol Gen Genet* 231:124-138, 1991.
27. Spiro S, Guest JR: FNR and its role in oxygen-regulated gene expression in *Escherichia coli*. *FEMS Microbiol Rev* 75:399-428, 1990.
28. Green J, Bennett B, Jordan P, et al: Reconstitution of the <4Fe-4S> cluster in FNR and demonstration of the aerobic- anaerobic transcription switch in vitro. *Biochem J* 316:887-892, 1996.
29. Khoroshilova N, Beinert H, Kiley PJ: Association of a polynuclear iron-sulfur center with a mutant FNR protein enhances DNA binding. *Proc Natl Acad Sci USA* 92:2499-2503, 1995.
30. Soupène E, Foussard M, Boistard, P, et al: Oxygen as a key developmental regulator of *Rhizobium meliloti* N_2-fixation gene expression within the alfalfa root nodule. *Proc Natl Acad Sci USA* 92:3759-3763, 1995.
31. Anthamatten D, Scherb B, Hennecke H: Characterization of a *fixLJ* regulated *Bradyrhizobium japonicum* gene sharing similarity with the *Escherichia coli fnr* and *Rhizobium meliloti fixK* genes. J Bacteriol 174:2111-2120, 1992.
32. Schlüter A, Patschkowski, Unden G, et al: The *Rhizobium leguminosarum* FnrN protein is functionally similar to *Escherichia coli* Fnr and promotes heterologous oxygen-dependent activation of transcription. *Mol Microbiol* 6:3395-3404, 1992.
33. Michiels J, D'Hooghe I, Verreth C, et al: Characterization of the *Rhizobium leguminosarum* biovar *phaseoli nifA* gene, a positive regulator of *nif* gene expression. *Arch Microbiol* 161:404-408, 1994.
34. Schultze M, Kondorosi E, Ratet P, et al: Cell and molecular biology of *Rhizobium*-plant interactions. *Int Rev Cytol* 156:1-75, 1994.
35. Mylona P, Pawlowski K, Bisseling T: Symbiotic nitrogen fixation. *Plant Cell* 7: 869-885, 1995.
36. Vasse J, de Billy F, Camut S, et al: Correlation between ultrastructural differentiation of bacteroids and nitrogen fixation in alfalfa nodules. J Bacteriol 172:4295-4306, 1990.
37. de Billy F, Barker DG, Gallusci P, et al: Leghaemoglobin gene transcription is triggered in a single cell layer in the indeterminate nitrogen-fixing root nodule of alfalfa. *The Plant Journal* 1:27-35, 1991.
38. Reyrat JM, David M, Batut J, et al: FixL of *Rhizobium meliloti* enhances the

transcriptional activity of a mutant FixJD54N protein by phosphorylation of an alternate residue. *J Bacteriol* 176:1969-1976, 1994.
39. Layzell DB, Hunt S, Palmer GR: Mechanism of nitrogenase inhibition in soybean nodules. *Plant Physiol* 92:1101-1107, 1990.
40. Monroe JD, Owens TG, LaRue TA: Measurement of the fractional oxygenation of leghemoglobin in intact detached pea nodules by reflectance spectroscopy. *Plant Physiol* 91:598-602, 1989.
41. Lawrence PA, Struhl G: Morphogens, compartments and patterns: lessons from drosophila? *Cell* 85:951-961, 1996.

Chapter 5

Oxygen Transducers that Regulate Behavior in Bacteria

Barry L. Taylor

Introduction

Oxygen Taxis as an Alarm Response

Bacterial aerotaxis is a rapid behavioral response to oxygen that enables bacteria to swim away from microenvironments that have too much or too little oxygen, and accumulate at oxygen concentrations that are preferable for the metabolic lifestyle of the species.[1] After a cell suspension is loaded into a glass capillary, an oxygen gradient forms with the oxygen concentration highest at the air/liquid interface. The bacteria migrate in the capillary to form sharply defined bands that may be so dense that they are visible to the unaided eye. Recent measurements determined that the facultative *Escherichia coli* accumulate at 50 μM oxygen, the microaerophilic *Azospirillum brasilense* at 4 μM oxygen, and the aerotolerant anaerobe *Desulfovibrio vulgaris* at 0.4 μM oxygen (Zhulin, Johnson, Bespalov, Taylor; unpublished observation).[2] The aerotaxis response does not require protein synthesis and probably commences within 200 ms of excitation.[3]

The observed stratification of bacterial species in a capillary is reproduced on a larger scale in aquatic environments where microorganisms

From: López-Barneo, J and Weir, EK: *Oxygen Regulation of Ion Channels and Gene Expression.* Armonk, NY: Futura Publishing Company, Inc., ©1998.

are stratified into biotopes. Ecological studies of water columns have documented many well-organized layers of bacterial species in oxic/anoxic transition zones. Each species occupies the biotope that has the preferred conditions for growth of the species. The oxygen gradient appears to be a major determinant for this stratification.[4,5]

Indirect Sensing of Oxygen for Behavior

Bacteria have multiple oxygen (redox)-sensing systems that regulate metabolism and maximize the growth rate in a given redox environment. The ArcB/ArcA system in *E. coli* is a major regulator of aerobic metabolism that controls expression of dehydrogenases, enzymes of the tricarboxylic acid cycle and terminal oxidases, in response to changes in oxygen concentration. The ArcB sensor is thought to detect redox changes rather than oxygen per se.[6] The NifL/NifA system in *Azobacter vinelandii* regulates expression of oxygen-sensitive nitrogenase, and its sensing component, NifL, is a redox-sensing flavoprotein.[7] FNR, a global transcriptional activator of anaerobic electron transport-related genes in *E. coli,* presumably senses oxygen (redox) changes via its iron sulfur center.[8] In the FixLJ system of *Rhizobium meliloti* (discussed in Chapter 4),[9] FixLJ controls expression of genes involved in nitrogen fixation under conditions of low oxygen concentration. In contrast to the ArcB/ArcA, NifL/NifA, and FNR systems, oxygen is sensed directly by binding to a heme prosthetic group of FixL.[10]

The aerotaxis sensor in *E. coli* appears to sense oxygen indirectly and is usually termed an *oxygen transducer* since it does not bind oxygen directly. The *E. coli* electron transport system has two cytochrome oxidase complexes: cytochrome *bo* and cytochrome *bd*.[11] Aerotaxis is abolished by the use of KCN to inhibit the cytochrome oxidases and in a *cyo cyd* double mutant that is deficient in both cytochrome *o* and cytochrome *d*.[12,13] Aerotaxis is observed in bacteria that have a single mutation in either cytochrome *o* or *d*. Inhibition of aerotaxis by respiratory inhibitors that act at cytochrome *b* demonstrate that a functional electron transport system is required for aerotaxis, in addition to a cytochrome oxidase.[14]

There are two respiration-associated changes that could be monitored by an aerotaxis transducer: the change in redox state of an intermediate of the electron transport system, or the proton motive force produced by electron transport-associated pumping of H^+ across the cytoplasmic membrane. Each is a good indicator of the internal energy of the cell. It is difficult to experimentally distinguish between these possible modulators of aerotaxis because they are tightly coupled and an adequate proton motive force must be maintained to provide energy for the flagellar motors.[15] Some evidence favors proton motive force as the signal,[16] other evidence favors redox potential.[17]

The selective advantage to the bacterium of a behavior that monitors the internal environment can be seen in the following scenario. *E. coli* are strongly attracted to serine and aspartate. A particle of cell debris from which serine, aspartate, and other amino acids are diffusing would create a gradient of chemoattractants. Bacteria from the surrounding microenvironment would move up the gradient to a rich supply of nutrients. The rapid multiplication of the bacteria in this rich environment could achieve a density of 10^9 cells mL^{-1} and exhaust the oxygen supply, trapping the bacteria in an anaerobic zone around the cell debris. However, as soon as the oxygen concentration becomes too low to maintain optimal energy in the cells, the aerotactic response will move the bacteria outward from the cell debris following the positive oxygen gradient that is in the opposite orientation to the serine gradient.[1]

Bacterial Energy Maximal at Preferred Oxygen Concentration

The focussed aerotaxis bands observed in the capillary oxygen gradient are the result of an aerophobic repulsion by high concentrations of oxygen and an aerophilic attraction to the preferred concentration of oxygen. Using high magnification ($\times 600$) and dark field illumination, it is possible to observe the movement of individual bacteria in the aerotaxis band. The bacteria swim vigorously in the band but if they leave the band on either side, they rapidly change direction and return to the band.[18] Clearly, an oxygen concentration that is higher or lower than the preferred concentration is a repellent for *E. coli.*

The aerophobic response of *E. coli* to oxygen has a $K_{0.5} = 1$ mM.[18] Oxygen-binding proteins have a higher affinity for oxygen. Consequently, it was suggested that the aerophobic response might be mediated by reactive products of oxygen, and not by oxygen per se.[1,18] Benov and Fridovich [19] have recently reported negative taxis of *E. coli* to hydrogen peroxide (H_2O_2). However, there is, at this time, no definitive proof that there is a tactic response of *E. coli* to any reactive oxygen derivative. We used a temporal gradient assay to evaluate this possibility. The superoxide anion does not trigger a repellent response. *E. coli sod A* and *sod B* mutants, that are deficient in superoxide dismutase, exhibited a similar repellent response to 100% oxygen in wild-type cells and in *sod* mutants, whereas the mutants were expected to have a stronger response (Johnson and

Taylor; unpublished observation). Methyl viologen (paraquat), a powerful redox-cycling (superoxide producing) agent, was not a repellent for *E. coli*, and there was no correlation between the ability of different quinones to cause negative taxis and to produce reactive oxygen species.[17] H_2O_2 elicited a smooth swimming (attractant) response in the temporal assay, perhaps due to oxygen evolution through the action of catalase. When we perfused an *E. coli* culture with 300 ppm ozone, the cells swam randomly until they lost motility and died after several minutes (Johnson and Taylor; unpublished observations). Even at high concentrations, reactive oxygen species did not seem to trigger a repellent response.

An alternative hypothesis for the mechanism of the aerophobic response originated with the unexpected observation that *A. brasilense* bacteria within the aerotactic band swam faster than the bacteria on either side of the band.[2] This suggested that the proton motive force, the energy source for the flagellar motors, was highest at the preferred oxygen concentration. The prior expectation was that as the oxygen concentration increased the proton motive force would increase with increasing respiration until it reached a plateau, where proton motive force was maximal for the cell.

In an oxygen gradient, the microaerophilic nitrogen-fixing bacterium *A. brasilense* forms a sharply defined band at a preferred oxygen concentration of 3 to 5 μM oxygen.[2] By measuring the proton motive force in *A. brasilense* as a function of the oxygen concentration, it was determined that the cellular energy level was maximal at 3 to 5 μM oxygen. The proton motive force was lower at oxygen concentrations that were higher or lower than the preferrred oxygen concentration. Bacteria swimming toward the aerotactic band would experience an increase in the proton motive force, and bacteria swimming away from the band would experience a decrease in the proton motive force. These results are consistent with a common-signal hypothesis for the mechanism of aerophobic and aerophilic aerotaxis: the bacterial aerotaxis transducers sense internal energy levels (proton motive force or redox state) and guide the bacteria to microenvironments that support the maximal energy level of the cell.

The common-signal hypothesis for aerotaxis has only been tested in one other species of bacteria, *E. coli*. The preferred oxygen concentration for *E. coli* is 50 μM, which is an order of magnitude higher than the preferred concentration for *A. brasilense*, 3 to 5 μM.[2] The motility of *E. coli* was fastest in the aerotaxis band. When the ambient oxygen concentration was varied, the membrane potential reached a maximum at oxygen concentrations that were similar to the preferred oxygen concentration and declined at higher oxygen concentrations. Preliminary studies with *D. vulgaris*, which migrates to 0.4 μM oxygen, confirm that swimming speed in that species is highest also within the aerotaxis band. Thus, an aerotolerant anaerobe, a microaerophile, and a facultative aerobe, that prefer oxygen concentrations that differ by two orders of magnitude, have aerotaxis responses that are consistent with the common signal.

Signal Transducers for Aerotaxis

The Aer protein in *E. coli* has recently been identified as a signal transducer that senses oxygen in the aerotaxis signal transduction pathway.[20] In an *aer* mutant, aerotaxis responses in a temporal aerotaxis assay are about half the duration of the aerotaxis responses in the isogenic parent. The responses to an oxygen increase or decrease are similarly affected. The aerotaxis wild-type phenotype was restored by expression of the aer^+ gene from a tightly regulated plasmid that was introduced into the *aer* mutant. When aer^+ expression was induced by increasing amounts of IPTG, the responses to oxygen were progressively lengthened. Overproduction of Aer did not increase the chemotaxis responses to serine or other chemoattractants.

The *aer* gene is located at 69.1 minutes on the *E. coli* chromosome. The predicted amino acid sequence of Aer has three recognizable domains. The N-terminal domain is similar to the N- terminal domain of NifL, the oxygen-sensing protein that regulates transcription of the nitrogen fixation genes in *A. vinelandii*.[7] There is a single 38-residue hydrophobic domain near the center of the protein sequence. The C-terminal domain has the highly conserved signaling domain motif that is present in *E. coli* chemotaxis receptors. The Aer protein was also identified as the transducer for aerotaxis by Bibikov and Parkinson (personal communication) who found evidence that the Aer transducer, like NifL, is a flavoprotein. A search of the combined protein data base revealed an extensive class of sensor proteins with homology to the N-terminal domain of Aer (Zhulin, Rebbapragada, Dixon, Taylor; unpublished data). The conserved motif is the putative binding-site for flavin-adeninedinucleotide (FAD). Our current working hypothesis is that Aer belongs to a class of signaling proteins that sense the internal environment of the cell, whereas other transmembrane signaling proteins sense the external environment. The above results are consistent with a role of Aer as a transducer for aerotaxis, and also suggest that there is an additional aerotaxis transducer in *E. coli*. Aerotaxis was absent in a *tsr aer* double mutant. No responses to oxygen are observed in a capillary or in a temporal assay, but the *tsr aer* strain responds chemotactically to aspartate and sugars.[20] These results indicate that

Tsr, the serine chemoreceptor, is also a transducer for aerotaxis. The two transducers function independently since Tsr is not essential for *aer*-mediated aerotaxis.

Redox Taxis and Energy Taxis

It was recently demonstrated that *E. coli* bacteria sense the redox potential in their surroundings and swim to a niche that has a preferred reduction potential.[7] Redox molecules, such as substituted quinones, that elicit redox taxis, interact with the bacterial electron transport system, thereby altering electron transport and the proton motive force in the bacteria. The results that were obtained were consistent with the hypothesis that the bacteria migrate in a redox gradient to the potential that supports a maximum internal energy level in the cells. This suggested that the signal transduction pathway for redox taxis monitors the change in redox state of the electron transport system, or the proton motive force.[17]

E. coli cells are attracted to glycerol in the absence of an alternative energy source.[21] The attraction is coincident with an increase in membrane potential, suggesting that this is an energy taxis in which the cells respond to the increase in internal energy and not to glycerol per se. Compelling evidence of a common signal transduction mechanism in aerotaxis, redox taxis, and energy taxis was obtained in the *aer tsr* double mutant that is deficient in both aerotaxis transducers. The *aer tsr* double mutant was completely deficient in redox taxis and glycerol taxis, indicating that the signal transducers for aerotaxis were also the signal transducers for redox and energy taxis.[20]

Convergence of the Aerotaxis and Chemotaxis Pathways

Bacteria navigate by regulating the rotation direction of the flagellar motors. Counterclockwise (CCW) rotation propels the swimming bacteria forward, whereas brief clockwise (CW) rotation of the motors causes the bacteria to change direction.[22] In chemotaxis and aerotaxis, bacteria migrate to a preferred microenvironment by suppressing direction changes (CW rotation) whenever they are swimming in a favorable direction; that is, when they are swimming toward an attractant or away from a repellent. Since chemotaxis and aerotaxis both control the flagellar motors, it is evident that these pathways must converge at, or before, the flagellar motors.

The signal transduction pathway for bacterial chemotaxis has been

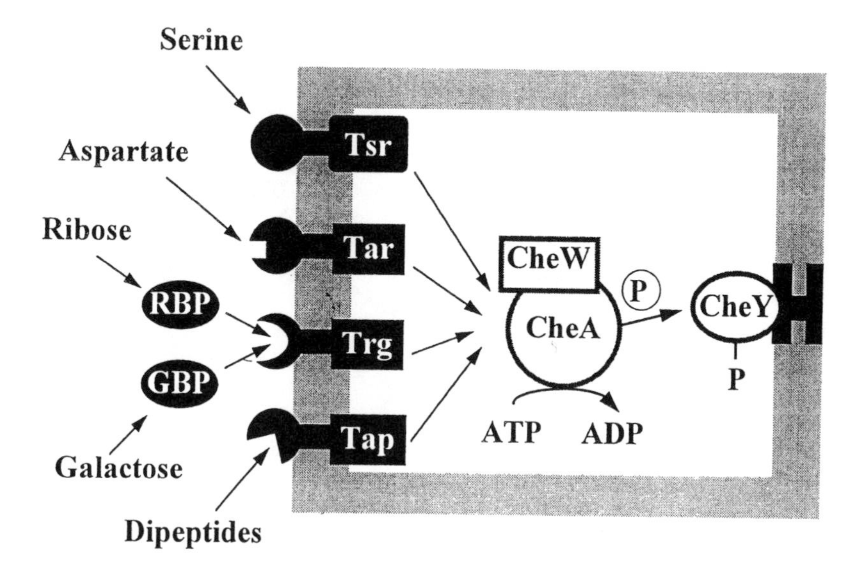

Figure 1. Scheme of signal transduction pathway for chemotaxis in *Escherichia coli*. The receptors (Tsr, Tar, Trg, Tap) form a complex with the CheA (A) and CheW (W) proteins. An attractant binding to a receptor changes the conformation of the signaling domain of the receptor to a counterclockwise (CCW)- signaling state. The CCW-signaling conformation inhibits autophosphorylation of CheA, resulting in decreased phosphorylation of CheY (Y) and CCW rotation of the flagellar motors. The motors rotate CCW, except when phospho-CheY is bound to the motor switch. The bacteria continue swimming toward the attractant without changing direction. The CheZ protein that dephosphorylates CheY, and the mechanism for adaptation to an attractant by methylating the receptor, are not shown. Repellents can increase phosphorylation of CheA and CheY, causing clockwise rotation of the motors and a change in the direction of swimming.

extensively characterized (for reviews, see References 23-25). In *E. coli*, four transmembrane receptors transduce the information from chemoattractants and repellents in the environment and transmit the information to the interior of the cell (Figure 1). Signaling between the chemoreceptor and the bacterial flagellar motor is a phospho-relay involving three soluble chemotaxis proteins: CheA, CheW, and CheY. The CheA protein is a histidine kinase that is autophosphorylated by adenosine triphosphate (ATP), and the CheY protein is phosphorylated from phospho-CheA. Binding of phospho-CheY to the switch on the flagelllar motor is the signal for CW rotation of the flagellum. A CheZ phosphatase dephosphorylates phospho-CheY and returns the motors to CCW rotation. Attractant binding to a chemotaxis receptor induces a conformational change in the receptor

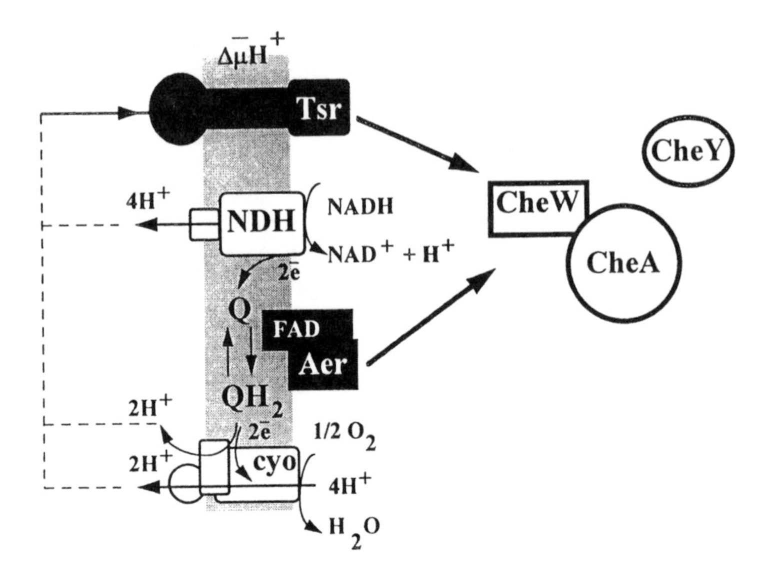

Figure 2. Model for oxygen sensing in *Escherichia coli.* Aer senses changes in the electron transport between dehydrogenases and terminal oxidases via the FAD moiety. Tsr detects changes in the proton motive force or electron transport system. Both transducers, Aer and Tsr, interact with the CheA:CheW complex to modulate activity of the CheY protein which controls the direction of flagellar rotation. Abbreviations: NDH = a coupled NADH dehydrogenase; cyo = cytochrome *o*; FAD = flavin adenine dinucleotide.

that is transmitted through the membrane, changing the cytoplasmic signaling domain to the CCW-signaling conformation. Within a CheA-CheW-receptor complex, the CCW-signaling conformation inhibits autophosphorylation of CheA. The level of phospho-CheY decreases and the cells swim smoothly (CCW flagellar rotation) without changing direction. Repellent binding to a chemoreceptor activates phosphorylation of CheA and CheY causing CW rotation and a change in the direction of swimming. Bacteria adapt to an attractant signal by methylating the cytoplasmic domain of the receptor.

Aerotaxis in *E. coli* is present in mutants that are lacking the four chemotaxis receptors.[26] Only three chemotaxis proteins, CheA, CheW, and CheY, are required for aerotaxis.[27] The C-terminal domain of the Aer aerotaxis transducer is homologous to the cytoplasmic domain of chemotaxis receptors. It is likely that CheA and CheW complex with Aer as they do with chemotaxis receptors, such as Tsr (Figure 2). Our current hypothesis for signal transduction in aerotaxis, redox taxis, and energy taxis is that FAD in the N-terminal domain of the Aer transducer is oxidized or reduced in response to redox changes in the electron transport system in *E. coli*. A resulting conformational change alters the conserved signaling domain in Aer, modulating the rate of autophosphorylation of the CheA and the phosphorylation level of the CheY. The Tsr transducer for aerotaxis also detects changes in the energy state of the cell.

Methodology for Maintaining Anoxia and Controlled Oxygen Concentrations

A critical factor in investigations of bacterial chemotaxis has been the development of methods for maintaining anoxia without the use of dithionite or a similar chemical reductant. It may be possible to adapt some of these methods for investigations of oxygen sensing in mammalian cells, and to avoid various artifacts that can be introduced by the use of dithionite to establish anoxia. In studies of *D. vulgaris*, the oxygen concentration was reproducibly alternated between anoxia and 0.04% (0.48 μM) oxygen. Prepurified grade nitrogen (99.998% minimum) is passed through two oxy-Trap (Alltech Applied Science Labs, Deerfield, Il, USA) scrubbers in series to remove traces of oxygen.[28] Stainless steel gas lines are used where possible because oxygen diffuses across the walls of flexible tubing, including butyl rubber. Only gas-tight valves are used and the valves and joints may be coated with Lubriseal (Arthur H. Thomas Co., Philadelphia, PA, USA) or nail polish to further reduce oxygen contamination.[29] In vessels that are not fully sealed, careful attention should be paid to baffling the gas flow so that the flow does not develop Bernoulli currents that can draw ambient air into the vessels. Replacement of nitrogen by heavier-than-air argon is preferable for many experiments. Biological markers provide the best surveillance for traces of oxygen. For preliminary testing of an anoxic setup, we may monitor bacteria that are nonmotile when anoxic, but motile if even traces of oxygen are present. Absorption of leghemoglobin can also be used to quantitate low concentrations of oxygen.

If sparging is not practical, the safest way to deplete oxygen from solution is via cellular respiration. The rate of diffusion of oxygen from the solution can be estimated from Fick's Law. Experiments can also be performed in an anaerobic chamber (Coy Laboratory Products, Ann Arbor, MI, USA) where the presence of 3% hydrogen and a palladium catalyst continually removes oxygen from the environment.

Conclusion

The signal transduction pathway for aerotaxis has now been elucidated, with the exception that the specific signal that is detected by the aerotaxis transducers remains to be determined. The Aer and Tsr transducers respond to the redox state of the electron transport system, the proton motive force, or another measure of the internal energy level of the cell. This information is used to regulate the CheA-CheW-CheY phosphorelay system which controls the direction of rotation of the flagellar motors.

The prototypical sensory receptor is a transmembrane protein that detects changes in the external environment and transmits a signal to the interior of the cell. The identification of Aer and Tsr as transducers that monitor the internal energy level of the cell is an important observation. The existence of a proton motive force sensor (protometer) or other sensor of internal energy has long been proposed,[1,30] including earlier models for oxygen sensing in the carotid body and a current model for oxygen sensing in pulmonary vasculature.[31,32]

Aer has a sensory input motif that has been identified in 12 proteins, six of which are known to be oxygen- or light-sensitive proteins involved in sensory transduction (Zhulin, Dixon, and Taylor; unpublished data). These sensors are found in representatives of archaea, eubacteria, fungi, and viridiplantae.

The conserved motif may include a binding domain for FAD, but this has not been conclusively demonstrated. These findings raise the possibility that sensors of internal energy are widespread in nature. Past experience has revealed in biological systems an extensive variety of mechanisms that utilize a common principle. It is likely then that cells use many different ways to sense oxygen. Two of these strategies are represented by Aer and Tsr. FixL detects oxygen directly.[10] Other strategies for detection of internal energy levels might be linked to NAD(P)H dehydrogenases, cytochromes, ubiquinone, or proton motive force-dependent orientation of histidine residues with respect to the cytoplasmic membrane. It is also to be expected that such diverse input modules will be linked to a similar diversity of output modules, including histidine kinases, serine-threonine kinases, phosphoprotein phosphatases, guanylyl cyclases, and other sensory transduction proteins.[33, 34]

Acknowledgments

Anuradha Rebbapragada, Igor Zhulin, and Mark Johnson provided unpublished observations and insightful comments that are included in this manuscript. Research in the author's laboratory is supported by a grant (GM29481) from the National Institute of General Medical Sciences, USA.

References

1. Taylor BL: How do bacteria find the optimal concentration of oxygen? *Trends Biochem Sci* 8:438-441, 1983.
2. Zhulin IB, Bespalov VA, Johnson MS, et al: Oxygen taxis and proton motive force in *Azospirillum brasilense. J Bacteriol* 178:5199-5204, 1996.
3. Segall JE, Manson MD, Berg HC: Signal processing times in bacterial chemotaxis. *Nature (London)* 296:855-857, 1982.
4. Ramsing NB, Kühl M, Jxrgensen BB: Distribution of sulfate- reducing bacteria, O_2, and H_2S in photosynthetic biofilms determined by oligonucleotide probes and microelectrodes. *Appl Environ Microbiol* 59:3840-3849, 1993.
5. Risatti JB, Capman WC, Stahl DA: Community structure of a microbial mat: the phylogenetic dimension. *Proc Natl Acad Sci USA* 91:10173-10177, 1994.
6. Iuchi S, Lin ECC: Adaptation of *Escherichia coli* to redox environments by regulation of gene expression. *Cell* 66:5-7, 1993.
7. Hill S, Austin S, Eydmann T, et al: *Azotobacter vinelandii* NIFL is a flavoprotein that modulates transcriptional activation of nitrogen-fixation genes via a redox-sensitive switch. *Proc Natl Acad Sci USA* 93:2143-2148, 1996.
8. Gunsalus RK: Control of electron flow in *Escherichia coli*: coordinated transcription of respiratory pathway genes. *J Bacteriol* 174:7069-7074, 1992.
9. Soupene E, Boistard P: Nitrogen fixation and oxygen sensing. In: Lopez-Barneo J, Weir EK (eds). *Oxygen Regulation of Ion Channels and Gene Expression.* Armonk, NY: Futura Publishing Company, Inc.; 29–43, 1998.
10. Gilles-Gonzalez MA, Gonzalez G: Regulation of the kinase activity of heme protein FixL from the two-component system FixL/FixJ of *Rhizobium meliloti. J Biol Chem* 268:16293-16297, 1993.
11. Gennis RB, Stewart V: Respiration. In: Neidhart FC, et al (eds). *Escherichia coli* and *Salmonella typhimurium. Cellular and Molecular Biology.* Washington, DC: American Society for Microbiology; 217-261, 1996.
12. Laszlo DJ, Taylor BL: Aerotaxis in *Salmonella typhimurium*: role of electron transport. *J Bacteriol* 145:990-1001, 1981.
13. Shioi J, Tribhuwan RC, Berg ST, et al: Signal transduction in chemotaxis to oxygen in *Escherichia coli* and *Salmonella typhimurium. J Bacteriol* 170:5507-5511, 1988.
14. Laszlo DJ, Niwano M, Goral WW, et al: *Bacillus subtilis* electron transport and proton motive force during aerotaxis. *J Bacteriol* 159:820-824, 1984.
15. Khan S, Macnab RM: Proton chemical potential, proton electrical potential and bacterial motility. *J Mol Biol* 138:599-614, 1980.
16. Shioi J, Taylor BL: Oxygen taxis and proton motive force in *Salmonella typhimurium. J Biol Chem* 259:10983-10988, 1984.
17. Bespalov VA, Zhulin IB, Taylor BL: Behavioral responses of *Escherichia coli* to changes in redox potential. *Proc Natl Acad Sci USA* 93:10084-10089, 1996.
18. Shioi J, Dang CV, Taylor BL: Oxygen as attractant and repellent in bacterial chemotaxis. *J Bacteriol* 169:3118-3123, 1987.
19. Benov L, Fridovich I: *Escherichia coli* exhibits negative chemotaxis in gradients of hydrogen peroxide, hypochlorite, and N-chlorotaurine: products of the respiratory burst of phagocytic cells. *Proc Natl Acad Sci USA* 93:4999-5002, 1996.
20. Rebbapragada A, Johnson MS, Zhulin IB, et al: Aer and Tsr transduce oxygen, redox, energy signals for *Escherichia coli* behavior. *Proc Natl Acad Sci USA* 94: 10541–10546, 1996.

21. Zhulin IB, Rowsell EH, Johnson MS, et al: Glycerol elicits energy taxis in *Escherichia coli* and *Salmonella typhimurium. J Bacteriol* 179:3196–3201, 1996.
22. Larsen SH, Reader RW, Kort EN, et al: Change in direction of flagellar rotation is the basis of the chemotactic response in *Escherichia coli. Nature* 249:74-77, 1974.
23. Bourret RB, Borkovich KA, Simon MI: Signal transduction pathways involving protein phosphorylation in prokaryotes. *Annu Rev Biochem* 60:401-441, 1991.
24. Manson MD: Bacterial motility and chemotaxis. *Adv Microb Physiol* 33:277-346, 1992.
25. Stock JB, Surette MG: Chemotaxis. In: Neidhart FC et al (eds). *Escherichia coli and Salmonella typhimurium. Cellular and Molecular Biology.* Washington, DC: *American Society for Microbiology*; 1103-1129, 1996.
26. Niwano M, Taylor BL: Novel sensory adaptation mechanism in bacterial chemotaxis to oxygen and phosphotransferase substrates. *Proc Natl Acad Sci USA* 79: 11-15, 1982.
27. Rowsell EH, Smith JM, Wolfe A, et al: CheA, CheW, and CheY are required for chemotaxis to oxygen and sugars of the phosphotransferase system in *Escherichia coli. J Bacteriol* 177:6011-6014, 1995.
28. Johnson MS, Zhulin IB, Gapuzan E, et al: Oxygen-dependent growth of the obligate anaerobe *Desufovibrio vulgaris* Hildenborough. *J Bacteriol* 179: 5598–5601, 1996.
29. Wong LS, Johnson MS, Zhulin IB, et al: Role of methylation in aerotaxis in *Bacillus subtilis. J Bacteriol* 177:3985-3991, 1995.
30. Baryshev VA, Glagolev AN, Skulachev VP: Sensing of μH^+ in phototaxis of *Halobacterium halobium. Nature* 292:338-340, 1981.
31. Gonzalez C, Almarez L, Obeso A, et al: Carotid body chemoreceptors: from natural stimuli to sensory discharges. *Physiol Rev* 74:829-898, 1994.
32. Archer SL, Huang J, Henry T, et al: A redox based O_2 sensor in rat pulmonary vasculature. *Circ Res* 73:1100-1112, 1993.
33. Stock JB: Signaling across membranes: a one and a two and a . . . *Science* 274: 370-371, 1996.
34. Appleby JL, Parkinson JS, Bourret RB: Signal transduction via the multi-step phosphorelay: not necessarily a road less traveled. *Cell* 86:845-848, 1996.

Chapter 6

Oxygen Sensing in Plants

Emilio Cervantes

Introduction

The evolution of vascular plants, as well as that of metazoans, in the course of the last 500 million years, has taken place in an enriched oxygen environment.[1] Plant metabolism and development are strictly adapted to atmospheric oxygen partial pressure (Po_2) values resulting in the involvement of oxygen in many plant life processes, ranging from the more general metabolic reactions (oxygen is the final electron acceptor in respiration) to very specific reactions of plant metabolism like the synthesis of phytohormones and secondary plant metabolites.[2]

Broadly, two kinds of approaches have been followed to investigate the responses of plants to varying oxygen tensions. The observation of plant species that can germinate and grow in low oxygen tensions (under water) was the basis for the first experimental approach. Several morphological and physiologic adaptations were found when investigating plants such as rice and *Echinochloa*.[3] The second approach was based on the observation of the effects that a reduced oxygen pressure has on particular biochemical, physiologic, or morphological characteristics of plants that normally grow under atmospheric Po_2.[4-6]

As a result of many experiments based on both approaches, several, either constitutive or transient, responses to low oxygen tensions have been described. These include morphological, biochemical, and metabolic

From: López-Barneo, J and Weir, EK: *Oxygen Regulation of Ion Channels and Gene Expression*. Armonk, NY: Futura Publishing Company, Inc., ©1998.

adaptations, which are accompanied by changes in gene expression. In the first part of this chapter, these different responses to altered oxygen pressures in the environment are briefly reviewed.

The existence of such a plethora of responses makes it clear that mechanisms for sensing oxygen tension must be widespread in plants. The second part of this chapter deals with these sensing mechanisms, some demonstrated, others more speculative. Among the former, an increase in particular hormones is the mechanism used by many plants to initiate the responses to low oxygen tension. Other possible mediators of the oxygen sensing may be the reactive oxygen species (ROS), (reactive oxygen species), but their role in plants has been investigated more in the context of plant defense reactions than as possible second messengers in the oxygen sensing.

Molecular oxygen binding proteins have long been recognized in plants. They were first described in root nodules of nitrogen fixing plants, where they function as oxygen transporters (see Chapter 4).[7] Recently, the occurrence of hemoglobins in diverse plant species, including cereals, as well as their reported expression in tissues other than nitrogen fixing nodules, has raised the possibility that plant hemoglobins may function as sensors of oxygen tension in the environment.[8] The possible existence of other oxygen binding proteins and oxygen receptors in plants will be discussed.

Plant Responses to Hypoxia

Constitutive Versus Transient Responses

In the course of evolution, many land plants have adapted their root systems to life under hypoxia[3-6]; they present both constitutive and inducible, morphological and physiologic, characteristics that make survival possible in these environmental conditions. Among them, rice is the plant with the highest economic importance. Its ability to grow in poorly aerated, flooded soils is due to the presence of an aerenchyma, i.e., a specialized tissue containing intercellular spaces filled with air, that allows oxygen transport from shoots to submerged roots.[9] Rice also presents root, coleoptile, and mesocotyl extension when submerged and rapid stem underwater extension in the ecotypes called deepwater rice.[4,6,10] The presence of an aerenchyma is constitutive in rice,[4,5] whereas underwater extension is induced by growth conditions due to the action of ethylene.[4] Other monocotyledons can, as rice, germinate and grow in waterlogged soils.

They present metabolic adaptations to flooding and hypoxia as discussed by Kennedy et al,[3] but the basis of tolerance to hypoxia is still not completely understood.

Effects of Hypoxia on Plant Structure

In mesophytes (plants not particularly well adapted to excess water) such as maize, wheat, barley, and oats, poor aeration promotes the formation of a cortical aerenchyma. New air spaces are formed by cell separation or cell breakdown in the cortex or in the pericycle. An aerenchyma develops constitutively in hydrophytes, even grown in well-drained soils, but it develops in mesophytes as a consequence of flooding and, at least in newly emerging adventitious roots of maize, is induced by the phytohormone ethylene. [4,11,12]

Ethylene is synthesized in plants from methionine, via SAM (S- adenosyl methionine) and ACC (amino cyclopropane carboxylic acid), by the consecutive action of ACC synthetase and ACC oxidase.[12,14] When water covers the roots, ethylene concentration increases because hydrodiffusion is much slower than aerodiffusion, thus resulting in higher ethylene concentration. Suberin and lignin layers may also be deposited in the walls of cells below the epidermis, inhibiting radial oxygen diffusion in the zone.[5,9,15]

Effects of Hypoxia on Plant Physiology and Metabolism

During the switch from aerobic to anaerobic metabolism, mitochondrial respiration is blocked and fermentation from pyruvate to lactate and ethanol is promoted.[16,17] At the onset of anaerobiosis, the lactic fermentation pathway would be predominant, with the production of lactate by the action of LDH (lactate dehydrogenase) and a subsequent decrease in cytoplasmic pH that may activate pyruvate decarboxylase (PDC), leading to ethanol production by the action of ADH (alcohol dehydrogenase). ADH, converting acetaldehyde to ethanol, is essential to keep nicotinamide adenine dinucleotide (NAD) regeneration without a notable decrease in the pH. During an extended anoxia, the final cause for cell death may be the lowering of the cytoplasmic pH.[18,19] The precise nature of the damage by low pH is not resolved, but hypoxia causes important alterations in the fine structure of meristematic cells at the mitochondria, endoplasmic reticulum, Golgi apparatus, and chromatin, as well as physiologic changes such as membrane depolarization, loss of turgor, and leakage of cell metabolites and ions.[5,20]

Effects of Hypoxia on Plant Gene Expression

When seedlings of maize were exposed to anaerobiosis, a particular group of proteins was induced in the roots. These were called the anaerobic polypeptides (ANP) or anaerobic stress polypeptides (ASP).[21] The ASPs appeared in about 90 minutes of anoxia and continued to be synthesized for many hours until death of the seedlings. Some of the ASPs were later identified as enzymes of glycolisis and fermentation: ADH, LDH, PDC, glyceraldehyde 3-P dehydrogenase, aldolase, and glucose phosphate isomerase; others included sucrose synthase and alanine aminotransferase. Three additional enzymes of this pathway show enhanced activity under oxygen deficiency.[22]

Oxygen deficiency in maize increases the amounts of mRNAs encoding ADH1 and ADH2,[23-25] aldolase,[26] PDC,[27] and sucrose synthase.[28] For ADH1, oxygen deficiency has been shown to increase the rate of transcription as well as transcript stability.[25] Other plant species showed similar ASP induction. Conserved regions in the promoters of these genes were identified that are required for anaerobically regulated gene expression.[29] These regions were called AREs (anaerobic response elements) and, in later work, proteins binding to these sequences were isolated. These DNA binding proteins belong to the family of the leucine zipper proteins, and due to their binding to the G boxes in the AREs, were termed GBFs (G box binding factors).[30] GBF1 is induced by hypoxia some time before ADH1 is induced. Further evidence for the involvement of GBF1 in the ADH gene expression comes from analysis demonstrating that GBF1 binds to the ADH1 promoter region.[30]

Mechanisms activating GBF1 expression and, in general, ASP transcription can respond either to the metabolic consequences of oxygen limitation or directly to an oxygen-binding system. Studies with transgenic tobacco plants expressing *Zymomonas nobilis* PDC support the second hypothesis.[31] In this work, the inhibition of the respiratory chain or of the entrance of pyruvate into the TCA cycle, thus artificially creating an anaerobic metabolism under normal oxygen tension, did not result in the induction of ADH transcripts.

Mechanisms Sensing Environmental Oxygen Partial Pressure in Plants

Hormonal Mediators to Low Oxygen Tension

According to Jackson,[4] the involvement of ethylene in triggering developmental changes after plant submergence and waterlogging resulted in "the clearest available evidence for mediation of a hormone in plant responses to environmental stress." The reader is referred to this review for a record of the experimental evidence that leads to this statement. Ethylene, in cooperation with gibberellic acid, is also responsible for internode growth in deepwater rice.[6,32,33]

Other Possible Mechanisms for Oxygen Sensing in Plants

In many animal systems, evidence in favor of the implication of ROS (reactive oxygen species) as second messengers in signal transduction is accumulating.[34] In animal cells, it has been suggested that Po_2 may be one of the signals that triggers the production of ROS.[35] In plants, there is evidence in favor of free radicals regulating gene expression[36] and also in the induction of plant SAR (systemic acquired resistance) by salicylic acid.[37] Indeed, the salicylic acid signal acts through the production of hydrogen peroxide (H_2O_2) which acts as a second messenger in the activation of defense-related genes. Evidence in favor of ROS as mediators of oxygen sensing in plants is lacking at the moment.

Oxygen Binding Proteins

A Hypothesis on Oxygen Signal Transduction in Plants

In many biological systems, the sensation of environmental or hormonal stimuli involves the binding to a membrane receptor protein that is modified and initiates a signal transduction chain that will end with modifications in gene expression, cell morphology, and/or physiology in response to the initial stimulus.

Many proteins reacting with oxygen do so via a heme moiety. This allows a change in protein conformation from the deoxy state (tense) to the oxy state (relaxed)[38] as reported for bacterial, yeast, plant, and animal systems.[39] This conformational change may be the trigger for an enzymatic activity that initiates the response to a change in oxygen tension, as has been demonstrated with the kinase activity of the bacterial oxygen sensor protein NifL in *Rhizobium meliloti* (see Chapter 4).[40] Oxygen sensors based on heme proteins are also described in mammalian cells.[41] Hemoglobin in plants was first discovered in the nitrogen fixing root nodules of legumes. In the nodule, its function is to facilitate the diffusion of oxygen to the respiring bacteroids.[7] Later on, hemoglobins had been discovered in many divergent plant groups, including genera that never form nitrogen fixing nodules. Also, transcripts for hemoglobin were found in stems, roots, and cotyledons.[8] For these nonsymbiotic hemoglobins, two possible functions were proposed: as carriers in oxygen transport or as sensors of oxygen concentrations. However, the nonsymbiotic hemoglobins were discovered on the basis of previously known sequences for the oxygen carrier, symbiotic hemoglobins. Thus, it is also possible that other oxygen-binding proteins may exist with amino acid sequences unrelated to the symbiotic hemoglobins.

FixL, the reported oxygen sensor of *Rhizobium meliloti*,[40] is homologous to ETR1, the putative ethylene receptor of *Arabidopsis*.[42] Five amino acid sequences homologous among them are involved in kinase activity (Figure 1). The binding site for ethylene has been proposed to contain a

FIXL: 505 aminoacids

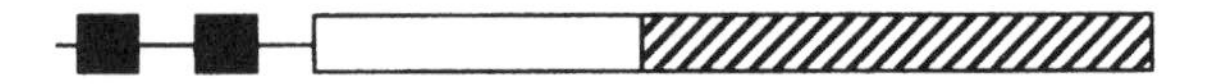

ETR1: 738 aminoacids

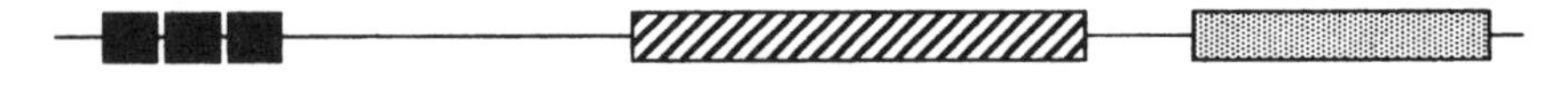

Figure 1. Schematic representations comparing ETR1, the putative ethylene receptor of *Arabidopsis* with FIXL, the reported oxygen sensor protein of *R.meliloti*. **Black boxes:** hydrophobic, probable membrane-spanning domains.[48] **Dashed:** region containing protein kinase conserved domains.[42] **White box** in FIXL: heme binding domain.[49] **Dotted** in ETR1: homologous region to bacterial response regulators.[42]

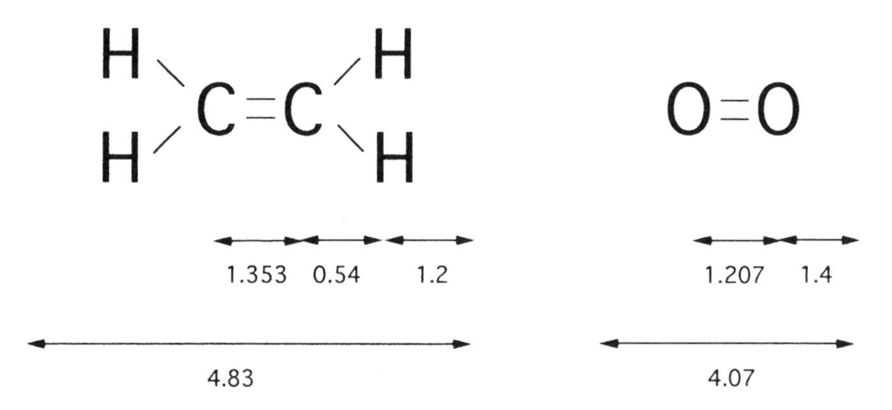

Figure 2. Schematic representation of the oxygen and ethylene molecules. (Interatomic and van der Vaals distances taken from Reference 50.)

transition metal such as zinc or copper.[43,44] The reactivities of oxygen and ethylene with metals are related, giving synthetic compounds like Zeise's salt in the case of ethylene[45] and several complexes of iridium, rodium, and cobalt in the case of oxygen.[46] According to the proposed mechanism of oxygen binding to hemoglobin, the oxygen molecule in oxyhemoglobin has a structure isoelectronic with that of ethylene.[46] As their molecular sizes are in the same range of magnitude (Figure 2), it seems likely that under some circumstances, oxygen may be able to interact with an ethylene receptor and/or vice versa. Our recent results with a cysteine proteinase gene transcript of chickpea (*Cicer arietinum*, L.), previously reported to be regulated by ethylene,[47] indicate that it may also be oxygen responsive, supporting the hypothesis that ethylene and oxygen may have common pathways in their sensing mechanisms in plants.

Acknowledgments

I thank Vicente Rives and Iñigo Zabalgogeazcoa for critically reading the manuscript.

References

1. Canfield DE, Teske A: Late proterozoic rise in atmospheric oxygen concentration inferred from phylogenetic and sulphur- isotope studies. *Nature* 382:127-132, 1996.

2. Prescott AG, John P: Dioxygenases: molecular structure and role in plant metabolism. *Ann Rev Plant Physiol Plant Mol Biol* 47:245-272, 1996.
3. Kennedy RA, Rumpho ME, Fox TC: Anaerobic metabolism in plants. *Plant Physiol* 100:1-6, 1992.
4. Jackson MB: Ethylene and responses of plants to soil waterlogging and submergence. *Ann Rev Plant Physiol* 36:145-174, 1985.
5. Drew MC: Sensing soil oxygen. *Plant, Cell and Environment* 13:681-693, 1990.
6. Perata P, Alpi A: Plant responses to anaerobiosis. *Plant Sci* 93:1-17, 1993.
7. Appleby, C: Leghemoglobin and *Rhizobium* respiration. *Ann Rev Plant Physiol* 35:443-478, 1984.
8. Andersson CR, Ostergard Jensen E, Llewellyn DJ, et al: A new hemoglobin gene from soybean: a role for hemoglobin in all plants. *Proc Natl Acad Sci USA* 93: 5682-5687, 1996.
9. Clark LH, Harris WM: Observation of the root anatomy of rice. *Am J Bot* 68: 154-161, 1981.
10. Vergara BS, Jackson B, De Datta SK: Deep water rice and its response to deep water stress. In: *Climate and Rice*. Los Baños: Int Rice Res Inst; 301-319, 1976.
11. Jackson MB, Fenning TM, Drew MC, et al: Stimulation of ethylene production and gas space (aerenchyma) formation in adventitious roots of *Zea mays* L. by small partial pressures of oxygen. *Planta* 165:486-492, 1995.
12. He C-J, Morgan PW, Drew MC: Transduction of an ethylene signal is required for cell death and lysis in the root cortex of maize during aerenchyma formation induced by hypoxia. *Plant Physiol* 112:463-472, 1996.
13. Yang SF, Hoffman EN: Ethylene biosynthesis and its regulation in higher plants. *Ann Rev Plant Physiol* 35:155-189, 1984.
14. Zarembinski TI, Theologis A: Ethylene biosynthesis and action: a case for conservation. *Plant Mol Biol* 26:1579-1597, 1994.
15. Armstrong J, Armstrong W: Phragmites australis: a preliminary study of soil-oxidizing sites and internal gas transport pathways. *New Phytol* 108:373-382, 1988.
16. Davies DD, Crego S, Kenworth P: The control of the production of lactate and ethanol in higher plants. *Planta* 118:297-310, 1974.
17. Menegus F, Cattaruza E, Mattana M, Beffagna N, Ragg E: Response to anoxia in rice and wheat seedlings. Changes in the pH of intracellular compartments, glucose 6-phosphate level, and metabolic rate. *Plant Physiol* 95:760-767, 1991.
18. Roberts JKM, Callis J, Jardeztki O, Walbot V, Freeling M: Cytoplasmic acidosis as a determinant of flooding intolerance in plants. *Proc Natl Acad Sci USA* 81: 6029-6033, 1984.
19. Roberts JKM, Andrade FH, Anderson IC: Further evidence that cytoplasmic acidosis is a determinant of flooding intolerance in plants. *Plant Physiol* 77:492-494, 1985.
20. Aldrich HC, Ferl RJ, Hils MH, et al: Ultrastructural correlates of anaerobic stress in corn roots. *Tissue Cell* 17:341, 1985.
21. Sachs MM, Freeling M, Okimoto R: The anaerobic proteins of maize. *Cell* 20: 761-767, 1980.
22. Bailey-Serres J, Kloeckener-Gruissem B, Freeling M: Genetic and molecular approaches to the study of the anaerobic response and tissue specific gene expression in maize. *Plant, Cell Environment* 11:351-357, 1988.
23. Ferl RJ, Brennan M, Schwartz D: In vitro translation of maize ADH: evidence for the anaerobic induction of mRNA. *Biochem Genet* 18:681-691, 1980.

24. Gerlach WJ, Pryor AJ, Dennis ES, et al: cDNA cloning and induction of the alcohol dehydrogenase (ADH1) gene of maize. *Proc Natl Acad Sci USA* 79: 2981-2985, 1982.
25. Rowland LJ, Strommer JN: Anaerobic treatment of maize roots affects transcription of Adh1 and transcript stability. *Mol Cel Biol* 6:3368-3372, 1986.
26. Dennis ES, Gerlach WJ, Walker JC, et al: Anaerobically regulated aldolase gene of maize: a chimaeric origin? *J Mol Biol* 202:759-767, 1988.
27. Kelley, PM: Maize pyruvate decarboxylase mRNA is induced anaerobically. *Plant Mol Biol* 13:213-222, 1989.
28. Springer B, Werr W, Starlinger P, Bennett DC, Zokolika M, Freeling M: The shrunken gene on chromosome 9 of *Zea mays L.* is expressed in various plant tissues and encodes an anaerobic protein. *Mol Gen Genet* 205:461-468, 1986.
29. Walker JC, Howard EA, Dennis ES, et al: DNA sequences required for anaerobic expression of the maize alcohol dehydrogenase 1 gene. *Proc Natl Acad Sci USA* 84:6624-6628, 1987.
30. De Vetten NC, Ferl RJ: Characterization of a maize G-box binding factor that is induced by hypoxia. *Plant J* 7(4):589-601, 1995.
31. Bucher M, Brändle R, Kuhlemeier C: Ethanolic fermentation in transgenic tobacco expressing *Zymomonas mobilis* pyruvate decarboxylase. *EMBO J* 13(12): 2755-2763, 1994.
32. Raskin Y, Kende H: Role of gibberellin in the growth response of deep water rice. *Plant Physiol* 76:947-950, 1984.
33. Sauter M, Kende H: Gibberellin induced growth and regulation of the cell division cycle in deep water rice. *Planta* 188:362-368, 1992.
34. Sen CK ,Packer L: Antioxidant and redox regulation of gene transcription. *FASEB J* 10:709-719, 1996.
35. Schreck R, Baeuerle PA: A role for oxygen radicals as second messengers. *Trends Cell Biol* 1:39-42, 1991.
36. Matters GL, Scandalios JG: Effect of the free radical- generating herbicide paraquat on the expression of the superoxide dismutase (SOD) genes in maize. *Biochem Biophys Acta* 882:29-38, 1986.
37. Chen Z, Silva H, Kleesing DF: Active oxygen species in the induction of plant systemic acquired resistance by salicylic acid. *Science* 262:1883-1886, 1993.
38. Perutz, MF: Hemoglobin structure and respiratory transport. *Sci Am* 239(6):92-125, 1978.
39. Zhu H, Riggs AF: Yeast flavohemoglobin is an ancient protein related to globins and a reductase family. *Proc Nat Acad Sci USA* 84:5015-5019, 1992.
40. Gilles Gonzalez MA, Ditta GS, Helinski DR: A hemoprotein with kinase activity encoded by the oxygen sensor of *Rhizobium meliloti*. *Nature* 350:170-172, 1991.
41. Goldberg MA, Dunning JP, Franklin Bunn H: Regulation of the erytropoietin gene: evidence that the oxygen sensor is a heme protein. *Science* 242:1412-1415, 1988.
42. Chang C, Kwok SF, Bleecker AB, et al: Arabidopsis ethylene response gene ETR1: similarity of product to two component regulators. *Science* 262:539-544, 1993.
43. Burg SP, Burg EA: Molecular requirements for the biological action of ethylene. *Plant Physiol* 42:144-148, 1967.
44. Sisler EC: Ethylene binding components in plants. In: Matoo AK, Shuttle JC (eds). *The Plant Hormone Ethylene*. Boca Raton, FL: CRC Press; 82-99, 1991.

45. Bailar JC, Emelens HJ, Nyholm R, et al: *Comprehensive Inorganic Chemistry* (5 vol). Pergamon Press; 1973.
46. Klevan L, Peone J, Madan SK: Molecular oxygen adducts of transition metal complexes: structure and mechanism. *J Chem Ed* 50(10):670-675, 1973.
47. Cervantes E, Rodriguez A, Nicolas G: Ethylene regulates the expression of a cysteine proteinase gene during germination of chickpea (*Cicer arietinum*, L.). *Plant Mol Biol* 34:207-215, 1994.
48. David M, Daveran ML, Batut J, et al: Cascade regulation of nitrogen fixation genes in *Rhizobium*. *Cell* 54:671-683, 1988.
49. Gilles Gonzalez MA, Gonzalez G, Perutz MF: Kinase activity of oxygen sensor FixL depends on the spin state of its heme iron. *Biochemistry* 34:232-236, 1995.
50. Weast RC (ed). *Handbook of Chemistry and Physics.* 61st ed. Boca Raton, FL: CRC Press; 1981.

Section 3

OXYGEN SENSING AND EUCHARYOTIC GENE EXPRESSION

Chapter 7

Oxygen-Regulated Gene Expression: A Widely Operative System Recognized Through Studies of Erythropoietin Regulation

Peter J. Ratcliffe
Jonathan M. Gleadle
Patrick H. Maxwell
John F. O'Rourke
Christopher W. Pugh
S. Morwenna Wood

Introduction

The provision of oxygen to the respiring tissues presents a fundamental physiologic challenge which is approached in different ways by different organisms.[1] For instance, many bacteria live in diverse chemical environments, and in hypoxia they regulate gene expression to provide enzymes which utilize a variety of alternate electron acceptors, such as nitrate or fumarate, instead of the more energy efficient oxygen. In higher animals, alternate electron acceptors are not used in this way. Some form of aerobic environment is obligatory, and specialized systems (lungs, heart, vessels, and blood) have evolved to provide oxygen in optimal concentrations for cellular respiration. Since oxygen in excess is potentially toxic, the matching of oxygen supply with cellular metabolism must

From: López-Barneo, J and Weir, EK: *Oxygen Regulation of Ion Channels and Gene Expression.* Armonk, NY: Futura Publishing Company, Inc., ©1998.

be precise. Comparative anatomists and physiologists have demonstrated many examples of this precision. For instance, among muscles from different species and different parts of the body, there is a striking concordance of measures of capillary and mitochondrial volume density, implying a close coordination of oxygen supply and demand.[2] Despite the detail of this type of organization, physiologic texts have tended to stress the importance of chemoreceptors with control over major functions such as ventilatory rate, cardiac output, or red cell production. Relatively little consideration has been given to the implications of the detailed organization of oxygen supply and demand at the microscopic level for cellular oxygen sensing. It now seems likely that recent advances arising from the study of one of the major systemic regulators, erythropoietin (EPO) production, may also shed light on the transcriptional processes underlying these local responses to oxygenation.

Erythropoietin Regulation

The study of any sensing mechanism is dependent on the existence of a dynamic response which is easily measured. It was the unusual, or even unique, hormonal operation of the hematopoietic growth factor EPO which enabled the classic physiologic studies on which the idea of an underlying oxygen sensor was established. These experiments showed that production of EPO was increased by reduction in blood oxygen availability (which might arise from reduced arterial oxygen partial pressure [Po_2] or increased hemoglobin affinity, as well as anaemia), but that beyond this, the stimulus response range is narrow.[3] For instance, production is not increased by metabolic inhibitors such as cyanide, or stresses such as heat shock, indicating that the system is most likely responding to hypoxia itself rather than some secondary consequence of impaired cellular respiration, or cell damage.

Cloning of the EPO gene opened the way for further studies. Increased production is based on new protein synthesis, arising at least in part from increased gene transcription.[4] Oxygen-dependent EPO gene expression could be observed in the hepatoma cell lines Hep3B and HepG2, providing a tissue culture model.[5] Induction of EPO messenger ribonucleic acid (mRNA) is blocked by cycloheximide, implying that new protein synthesis is required at some point in the activation mechanism. Gene expression is also induced by certain metal ions (cobalt, manganese, and nickel)[5] and by exposure of cells to selective iron chelators.[6] These distinctive features of the inducible response, which are clearly represented in a tissue culture system, have led many investigators to approach analysis of the regulatory mechanism from a consideration of the gene itself.

One of the first steps in this approach is to define the control sequences at the EPO locus which mediate the oxygen-regulated expression. Using transient transfection of hepatoma cells, we and others defined a control sequence lying 3′ to the gene (the EPO 3′enhancer) which could confer oxygen-regulated expression on heterologous reporter genes (see Chapter 8).[7–9] Although this sequence is only one of several elements mediating regulation of the EPO, its operation reproduced the main features of regulation of the endogenous gene rather precisely. The enhancer can also be activated by cobaltous ions and iron chelating agents, but otherwise showed the same narrow stimulus response characteristic that had been defined for the endogenous gene. These studies indicated that analysis of regulatory mechanisms underlying activation of the 3′ enhancer could be expected to shed light on physiologically relevant sensing and signal transduction pathways. An important step was, therefore, the identification of hypoxia inducible factor-1 (HIF-1) as a deoxyribonucleic acid (DNA) binding transcriptional complex which was critical for enhancer function.[10]

A Similiar System of Gene Regulation by Oxygen Operates Widely

Although the definition of a regulatory element by transfection of EPO-producing hepatoma cells was a useful step toward understanding the mechanism of regulation by oxygen, it was not unexpected. Implicit in the regulation of the EPO gene in these cells, was the existence of sequences which could convey the response. What was more surprising was that the EPO 3′ enhancer defined in these experiments was able to convey similar oxygen-regulated responses when transfected into a wide variety of other cells, which do not express the EPO gene and were not derived from tissues which make the hormone.[11] An example of such an experiment is illustrated in Figure 1. In each of the cell types, the expression of two plasmids was compared; one plasmid contained the mouse EPO 3′ enhancer linked to a human α-globin reporter gene, the other was identical except for omission of the enhancer sequence. In the EPO-producing HepG2 cells (lanes 1–4), a large increase in reporter gene expression was observed in hypoxic cells (lane 2), which was dependent on the presence of the EPO 3′ enhancer. Essentially identical responses can be seen in the non-EPO-producing Chinese hamster ovary cells. In further experiments, similar behavior was observed in each of 17 cell lines

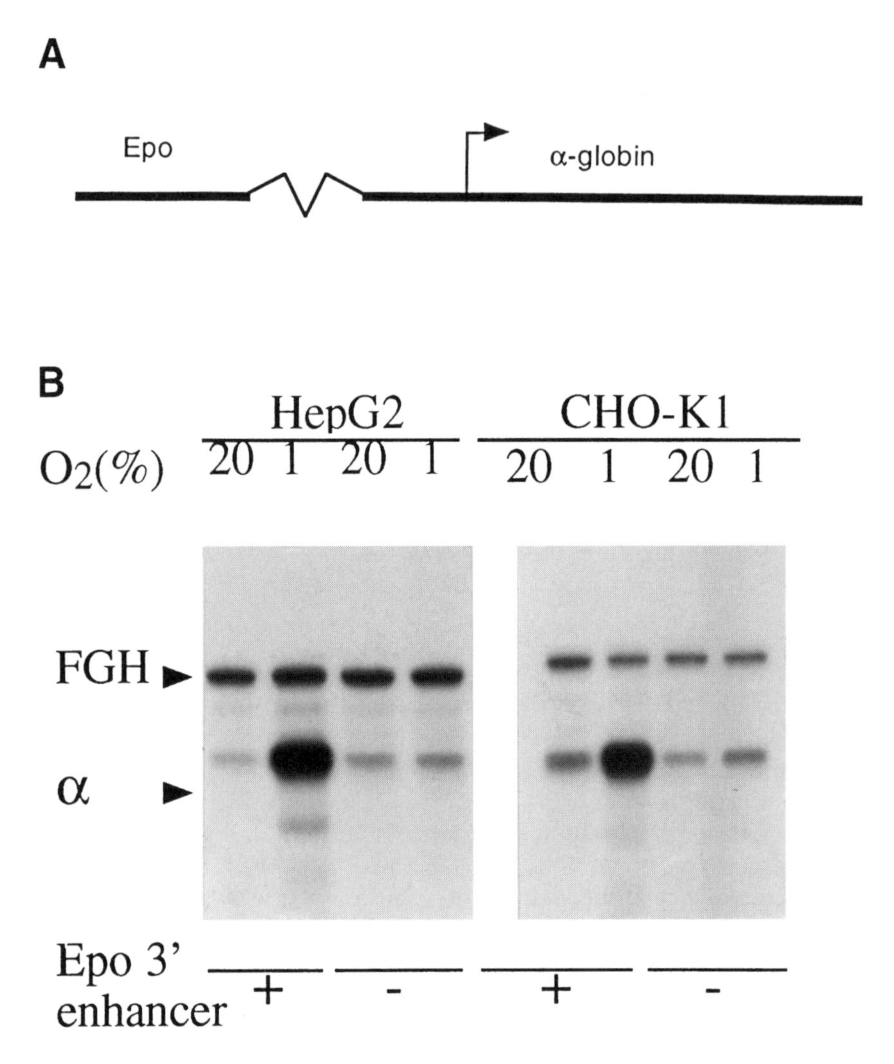

Figure 1. The erythropoietin (EPO) 3′ enhancer confers responses to hypoxia in both EPO producing cell types (HepG2, hepatoma) and non-EPO producing cell types (K1, Chinese hamster ovarian fibroblast). **A.** Schematic (not to scale) showing the EPO 3′ enhancer linked to the *α*-globin reporter gene. **B.** Expression of reporter (*α*) and control (FGH) plasmids in transfected cells. Alternate lanes are from hypoxic and normoxic cells. Alternate pairs of lanes show results for reporter plasmids containing (+) or not containing (−) the EPO 3′ enhancer. (Data from Reference 11.)

tested. As with the endogenous EPO gene, responses to hypoxia could be mimicked by cobalt. The findings indicated that an identical or closely similar sensing and signal transduction system was present in all the cells, and that it could interact with DNA sequences within the EPO 3′ enhancer. The implication was that the system was operating on other genes in non-EPO-producing cells and that such genes should possess similar DNA control sequences. Shortly after this, it was demonstrated that the inducible transcription factor HIF-1, which had been shown to be critical for the operation of the EPO 3′ enhancer in hepatoma cells, was indeed widely expressed.[12,13] Subsequently, other genes were defined which showed hypoxically inducible characteristics similar to EPO, and detailed examination of the cis-acting control elements by transient transfection and DNA binding studies did demonstrate that HIF-1 binding sites were important in conveying these responses. Perhaps, surprisingly, the first of these turned out to be genes involved in glucose metabolism, phosphoglycerate kinase-1, and lactate dehydrogenase-A (LDH-A).[14] That such genes, so functionally dissimilar from EPO, are linked to a common control system suggested that this system of gene regulation might be very widely operative in biology. In keeping with this, a large number of genes have now been identified which show functionally similar inducible responses to EPO (for instance induction by cobaltous ions and iron chelation, as well as hypoxia), or where functional characterization of the regulatory elements has demonstrated the importance of HIF-1 binding sites (see Chapter 9). These genes include several examples with important roles in cellular metabolism and vascular growth, supporting the view that this system of gene regulation has an important role in coordinating these processes (Table).

Although the relevance of oxygen supply to these processes is clear, it is not immediately obvious how the same or even a very similar mechanism of sensing and transcriptional activation could satisfy the precise requirements of regulated gene expression in each case. In general terms, the precise regulation of gene transcription is thought to be dependent on the variability which can be produced by combinatorial interactions between multiple transcription factors.[15] Some insight as to how this might be achieved in this system has been provided by detailed mutational analysis of the cis-acting elements. For the two oxygen regulated cis-acting sequences which have been analyzed in detail by scanning mutations (the EPO 3′ enhancer[10,16] and the LDH-A promoter[17]), activity is critically dependent on three sites, the HIF-1 recognition sequence, and two other sequences. For the EPO 3′ enhancer, one of these sites has been identified as binding the tissue-specific transcription factor hepatic nuclear factor-4 (HNF-4);[18] in the case of the LDH-A promoter, one of the

Table

Some Processes in Which Functional Similarities with Erythropoietin Regulation Have Been Defined or Gene Regulation by HIF-1 Has Been Demonstrated

Vasomotor control:	endothelial nitric oxide synthase[32]; endothelin[33]; platelet derived growth factor[25,34]
Angiogenesis:	vascular endothelial growth factor[25,35]; placental growth factor, platelet derived growth factor
Wound repair/inflammation:	transforming growth factor β_1[36]; inducible nitric oxide synthase[37]
Glucose metabolism:	glucose transporters[38]; glycolytic enzymes[14,39]; gluconeogenesis (phosphoenolpyruvate carboxykinase)[40]
High energy phosphate metabolism:	adenylate kinase-3[26]
Catecholamine metabolism:	tyrosine hydroxylase[41]
Iron metabolism:	transferrin[42]

other critical sites conforms to the consensus sequences for a cyclic adenosine monophosphate (cAMP) response element (CRE)[17] (Figure 2). Neither the HNF-4 binding site nor the CRE appear to convey inducible responses to hypoxia themselves. In each case, mutation at these sites abolishes or severely reduces the inducible activity of the natural enhancer, although artificial enhancers composed of multimers of the shorter sequences omitting these sites, but retaining the HIF-1 site, are active.[10,16,17] Thus, it appears likely that these cooperative factors influence the transcriptional activity of the HIF-1 complex in a way which contributes to shaping of the overall characteristics of gene expression.

Hypoxically Inducible Gene Expression in Mutant Cells

In addition to HIF-1, regulation by hypoxia or related metabolic changes has been reported for a number of widely expressed transcription factors including NF-kB,[19] some members of the Fos/Jun family,[20] p53,[21] and NF Il-6, implying that a large number of transcriptional systems may contribute to the response to hypoxia. In view of this, it has been rather surprising that the transfection studies of cis-acting regulatory elements have so commonly implicated HIF-1 in conveying responses to hypoxia on different genes. An important opportunity to determine the role of HIF-1 in transcriptional responses to hypoxia using different methodology was, therefore, provided, following the cloning of HIF-1,[22] by the availabil-

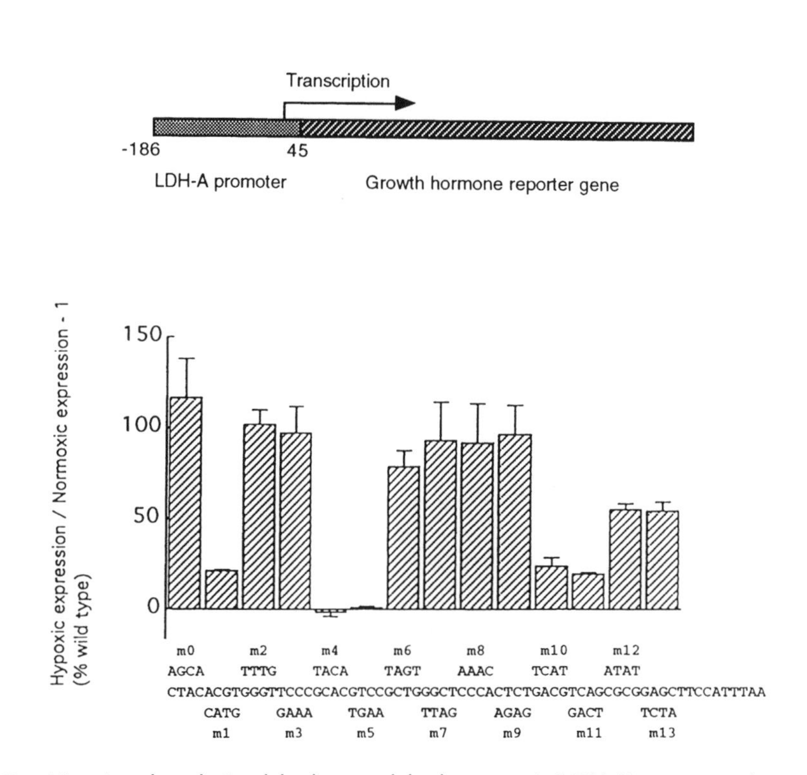

Figure 2. Mutational analysis of the lactate dehydroganse-A (LDH-A) promoter. **A.** Schematic diagram of the LDH-A promoter fused to the growth hormone reporter gene. The LDH-A promoter was found to convey hypoxia inducible expression on the growth hormone reporter. **B.** Effect of scanning mutations on hypoxia inducible promoter activity. Successive 4 base pair mutations were assayed. Three sites, corresponding to m1, m4/m5, and m10/m11 were found to be of importance. m1 and m4/m5 are HIF-1 binding sites; m10/m11 is a cyclic adenosine monophosphate response element. These sites cooperate to generate the hypoxia-inducible promoter function.

ity of mutant cells which are defective for one component of the DNA binding complex.

Affinity purification and molecular cloning of HIF-1 by Semenza and colleagues[22] demonstrated that the DNA binding complex is composed of two basic-helix-loop-helix PAS (termed PAS for Per, Arnt, and Sim) proteins termed HIF-1α and HIF-1β. HIF-1α was a newly defined member of this family, whereas HIF-1β had previously been identified as the aryl hydrocarbon nuclear receptor translocator (ARNT), a molecule previously identified by mutation and complementation studies as essential for the transcriptional response to certain environmental hydrocarbons termed the xenobiotic response.[23] In this capacity, ARNT forms a heterodimer with another basic helix-loop-helix PAS protein, the ligand binding subunit termed the aryl hydrocarbon receptor (AHR). This complex binds the xenobiotic responsive element, a control sequence for genes such as *CYP1A1*, a cytochrome P450 which can convert aryl hydrocarbons to toxic or carcinogenic metabolites.[24] This connection between two inducible responses to apparently distinct environmental stimuli raises important questions as to the functional and evolutionary links between the responses. It also provided an important resource for the analysis of hypoxic gene regulation in the form of mutant mouse hepatoma (Hepa-1) cells, originally selected for a defective xenobiotic response by survival in the presence of benzo(a)pyrene. One group of these mutants was shown to be defective in the nuclear translocation of the ligand binding complex and provided the original basis for cloning of the gene encoding ARNT by complementation.[23] Since ARNT and HIF-1β are identical, the ARNT deficient cells have now provided a powerful tool for the analysis of hypoxic gene regulation.

A comparison of HIF-1 DNA binding activity in the wild-type Hepa-1 cells and the ARNT-line, c4 is shown in Figure 3A. The absence of the inducible HIF-1 complex in c4 cells indicates that ARNT is an essential component of HIF-1. Following this, we surveyed the expression of a large number of genes in a panel of wild type, mutant, complemented, and revertant Hepa-1 cells.[25,26] An example is shown in Figure 3B. There were striking differences between wild type and ARNT cells. For some genes, such as LDH-A, the response to hypoxia was almost totally abrogated in the ARNT cells. In other cases, such as vascular endothelial growth factor (VEGF), there was a clear reduction in the regulation of mRNA levels by hypoxia, but a definite inducible response persisted. A third pattern of response was defined for HIF-1α itself, where the induction of mRNA by hypoxia appeared to be significantly greater in the ARNT cells than in the wild type.

These responses clearly define both ARNT-dependent and ARNT-independent mechanisms of gene regulation by hypoxia. When cells were exposed to the iron chelator desferrioxamine (DFO), patterns of response for the different genes were closely similar to those defined for hypoxia, supporting the view that the actions of the iron chelator are closely connected with the mechanism(s) of oxygen sensing underlying both ARNT-dependent and ARNT-independent mechanisms of gene regulation.

The profound abnormality of hypoxically inducible gene expression

Figure 3. **A.** DNA binding assay for hypoxia inducible factor-1 (HIF-1) in wild-type Hepa-1 cells and the mutant derivative c4 which lacks a functional HIF-1b/ARNT gene product. Nuclear extract was incubated with double stranded oligonucleotide containing the HIF-1 binding site from the mouse erythropoietin (EPO) 3′ enhancer. Species binding the oligonucleotide retard the mobility with respect to the free probe (FP). Both constitutive (Cons) and inducible (Ind) binding complexes are observed. The inducible complex corresponding to HIF-1 is not observed in c4 cells.

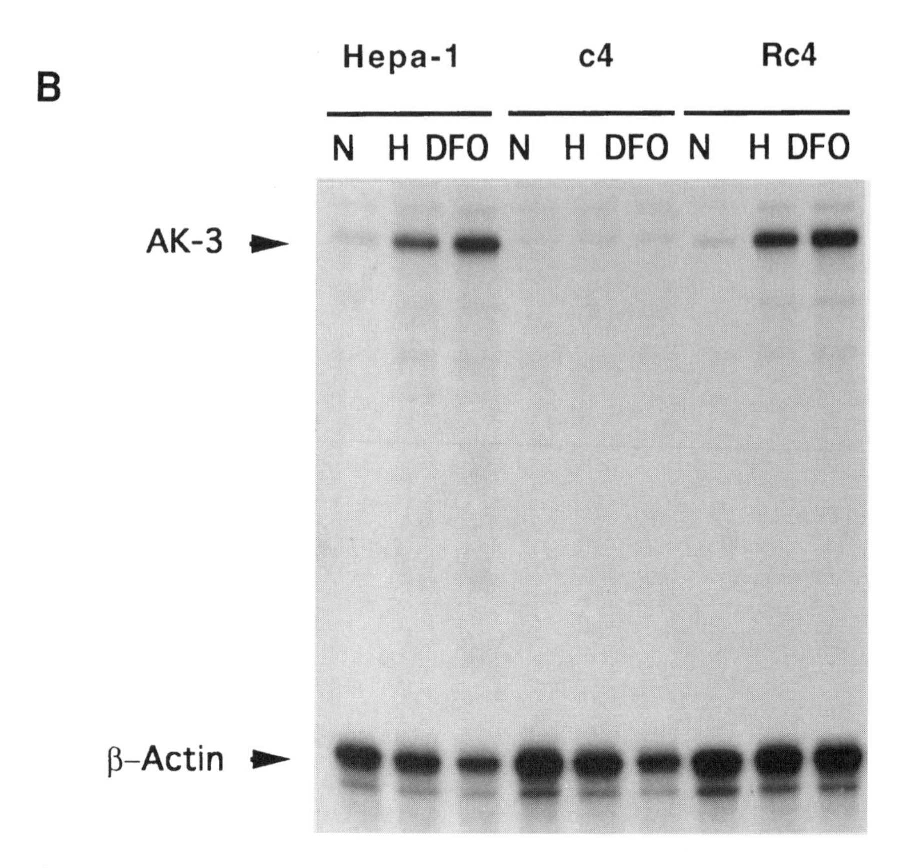

Figure 3. *(continued)* **B.** RNAse protection assay showing inducible expression of the adenylate kinase-3 (AK-3) gene in wild-type Hepa-1 cells, mutant (c4) cells, and revertant (Rc4) cells. Inducible responses to both hypoxia and desferrioxamine (DFO) are clearly dependent on HIF-1*β*/ARNT. The AK-3 gene had previously been identified as a hypoxia inducible gene by differential display polymerase chain reactions (PCR).[26] It catalyses the interconversion of Mg-GTP and AMP to Mg-GDP and ADP and provides an example of a gene with no clear functional relationship to erythropoietin, but which nevertheless shares the HIF-1 dependent control mechanism. *β*-actin mRNA signal provides an internal control.

observed in ARNT cells indicates that studies of these cells should provide important insights into the role of this system of gene regulation in cell physiology. We have not observed a clear difference in cell growth as tissue culture monolayers, between wild-type Hepa-1 and c4 cells either at 20% oxygen or at 1% oxygen. In contrast, in experiments performed in collaboration with Dr. Gabi Dachs and Dr. Ian Stratford (Medical Research

Council Radiobiology Unit, Oxon, UK), we have found that tumor growth following transplantation to nude mice was markedly different between the wild type, mutant, and revertant cells. Although initial growth rates were similar, beyond a certain size, wild-type tumors grew more rapidly, and had better developed vasculature than tumors of c4 cells. It, therefore, appears likely that, in keeping with the existence of profound hypoxia within many types of tumor, HIF-1 or a related transcriptional complex which is dependent on ARNT, has a major role in tumor biology.

Evolutionary Origins of the Transcriptional Response to Hypoxia

A Hypoxia-Inducible Factor-1 Homologue in *Drosophila*

Since functional sites of interaction between two or more molecules are often highly conserved, we sought evidence for the evolutionary conservation of HIF-1 using oligonucleotides from HIF-1 binding sites at mammalian EPO and phosphoglycerate kinase-1 loci in binding reactions with nuclear extract prepared from insect cells (the *Drosophila melanogaster* SL2 cell line).[27] Nuclear extracts were prepared from insect cells grown in normoxic (20% oxygen) or hypoxic (1% oxygen) tissue culture conditions. The extracts from insect cells were shown to form an hypoxically inducible complex (HIF-D) which has similar DNA binding specificity, and mobility, to mammalian HIF-1. Interestingly, as has been described for HIF-1,[28] HIF-D is very sensitive to redox conditions. Omission of the sulfhydryl reducing agent, dithiothreitol from the preparative buffers, or treatment with the sulfhydryl oxidising agent diamide, abolished DNA binding of HIF-D in a reversible way. The remarkable in vitro sensitivity to such reagents makes it tempting to suggest that sulfhydryl redox changes might be an important mechanism of oxygen-regulated activity of these complexes in vivo. Unfortunately, determination of the redox conditions which pertain in the intracellular microenvironment of these proteins is not straightforward and there is, as yet, insufficient data to confirm or refute this possibility.

Several other issues are raised by the demonstration of a HIF-1 homologue in *Drosophila*. The function and molecular identity of HIF-D in *Drosophila* cells are unknown. The defining members of the PAS groups of transcription factors were the *Drosophila* genes Per and Sim. Neither are likely candidates for involvement in HIF-D. Nevertheless, given the potential importance of oxygen in the organization of growth in higher animals, it is interesting that the Drosophila PAS genes for which function has so far been defined are involved in the spatial and temporal aspects of growth control.

Oxygen Sensing and Transciptional Regulation of Hypoxia-Inducible Factor-1

Since the first recognition of this system of gene regulation in the control of EPO production, understanding of the mechanism of oxygen sensing has been an important goal. In theory, any process that is affected by oxygen in a concentration-dependent manner could form the basis of sensing, although in the case of this system, many candidates might reasonably be excluded by the failure of mitochondrial inhibitors to mimic the response. In the broadest sense, molecular interactions with oxygen are of two types: redox-based systems, in which oxygen acts as an electron acceptor, and the reversible liganding of dioxygen to metal ions as occurs in oxygen carrying proteins such as hemoglobin (Figure 4). In the case of redox-based systems, a number of different types of sensing mechanisms are possible. The reaction products (either a partially reduced active oxygen species, such as superoxide, or an oxidized product such as a steroid molecule) could act as signal pathway intermediates. Alternatively, a redox enzyme could signal through redox-based conformational changes. Since a chain of redox reactions may take place with oxygen as the terminal acceptor, signals could be generated by the redox status of components quite distant from the reaction with oxygen. Quite possibly, the action of oxygen could be to divert electron flow from an alternate (signalling) electron acceptor so that, effectively, a switch of sign is achieved with high rates of electron flow potentially able to signal hypoxia. This long list of theoretical possibilities, together with the large number of known oxidases make direct analysis of the mechanism of sensing difficult. Nevertheless, several interesting insights have already been obtained. Based on the pharmacologic characteristics of gene induction (particularly sensitivity to carbon monoxide) the involvement of a hemoprotein has been postulated with the constitutive action of cobalt being explained by the formation of constitutively-deoxy cobalt protoporphyrin.[5] Although it seems difficult to accommodate all the characteristics of the system in the operation of a simple hemoglobin-like molecule reversibly binding oxygen, the involvement of hem-containing groups in more complex redox-based sensing mechanisms remains very plausible. Inhibition of gene induction by hydrogen peroxide and has led to the suggestion that this partially reduced reactive oxygen species could function as a signal

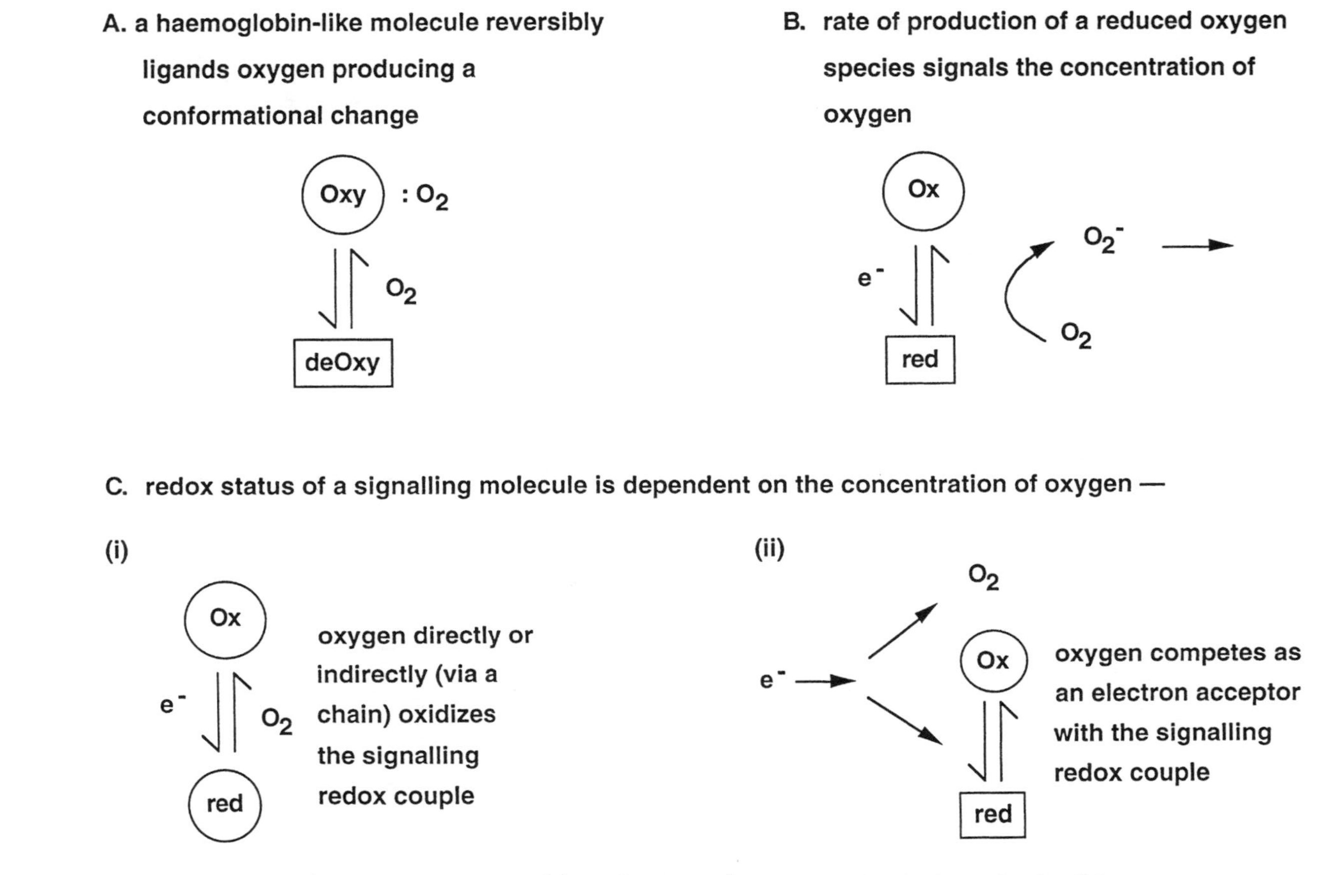

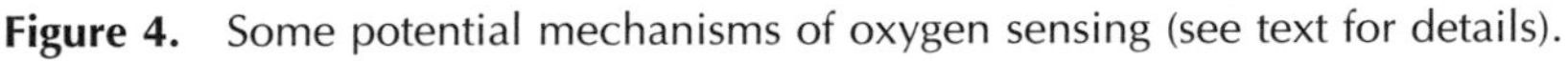

Figure 4. Some potential mechanisms of oxygen sensing (see text for details).

pathway intermediate with oxygen dependent production providing a sensing mechanism.[29] In this model, it has been proposed that the action of iron chelators might then be explicable through inhibition of iron-dependent catalysis of radical production by the Fenton reaction. We have noted that induction of the system by hypoxia, but not cobalt, is very sensitive to the flavoprotein inhibitor diphenylene iodonium.[30] This implies some difference in cobalt-induced activation, and also that the system might involve the operation of a flavoprotein oxido-reductase. Such molecules are often coupled to hem proteins in electron transport systems; for instance, the flavoprotein cytochrome P450 reductase is coupled to many different hem-containing cytochrome P450s which perform a wide variety of oxygen-dependent reactions. One or more of such reactions could be involved in the oxygen-sensing process. Since the HIF-1 related AHR is a ligand-binding transcription factor activated by the binding of certain aryl hydrocarbons,[24] and an influence of P450 induction on EPO regulation has previously been demonstrated,[31] it is tempting to speculate that oxygen-dependent generation of a P450 oxygenase reaction product might provide a regulatory ligand for HIF-1. Although the possibility of direct definition of the signalling molecules by pharmacologic probing is, therefore, attractive, the potential complexity of biological reactions with oxygen remains formidable.

Analysis of the molecular mechanism(s) underlying the activation of HIF-1 allows a potentially more secure route to understanding the proximal mechanisms involved in oxygen sensing and signal transduction. We have not observed hypoxic induction of the mRNAs encoding either HIF-1α or HIF-1β, indicating that the major regulatory mechanisms are either translational or post-translational (see Chapter 9). Many transcription factors contain distinct domains involved with DNA binding, dimerization, or transcriptional activation,[15] and regulatory mechanisms could be involved in some or all of these processes. To define regulatory interactions in transcriptional activation by HIF-1, we have created series of chimeric genes in which the whole or portions of the HIF-1 coding sequence are fused to the DNA binding domain of another transcription factor. In the first series of experiments, HIF-1α, HIF-1β/ARNT, and AHR coding sequences were fused to the N terminal DNA binding domain of the glucocorticoid receptor, and the inducible activity of the chimeric gene was tested by cotransfection of cells together with a reporter plasmid containing a glucocorticoid responsive promoter linked to the luciferase reporter gene. HIF-1α sequences, but not those encoding the dimerization partner HIF-1β/ARNT, or the related PAS protein, AHR, conveyed hypoxically inducible regulation on the glucocorticoid receptor reporter system, indicating that one or more sequences in the HIF-1α protein have a regulatory

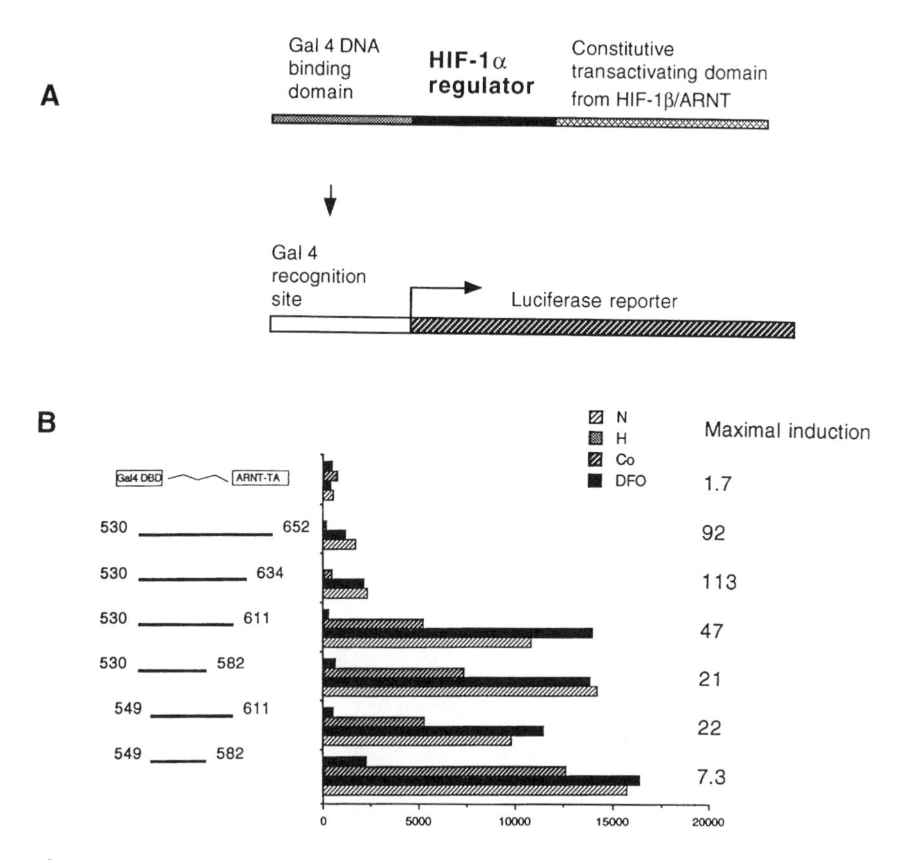

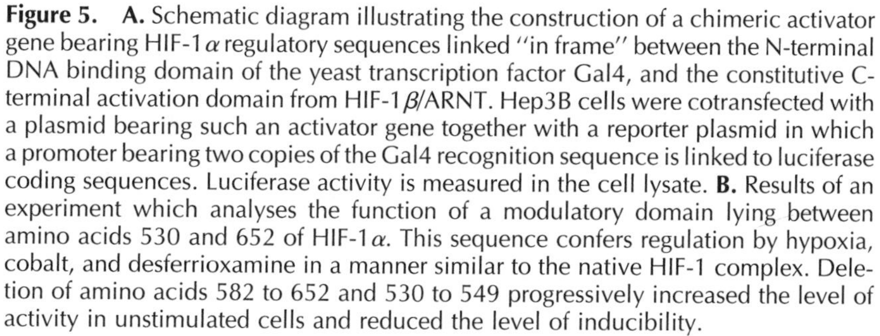

Figure 5. **A.** Schematic diagram illustrating the construction of a chimeric activator gene bearing HIF-1*α* regulatory sequences linked "in frame" between the N-terminal DNA binding domain of the yeast transcription factor Gal4, and the constitutive C-terminal activation domain from HIF-1*β*/ARNT. Hep3B cells were cotransfected with a plasmid bearing such an activator gene together with a reporter plasmid in which a promoter bearing two copies of the Gal4 recognition sequence is linked to luciferase coding sequences. Luciferase activity is measured in the cell lysate. **B.** Results of an experiment which analyses the function of a modulatory domain lying between amino acids 530 and 652 of HIF-1*α*. This sequence confers regulation by hypoxia, cobalt, and desferrioxamine in a manner similar to the native HIF-1 complex. Deletion of amino acids 582 to 652 and 530 to 549 progressively increased the level of activity in unstimulated cells and reduced the level of inducibility.

function. When other conditions were tested, this response was found to mimic the inducible characteristic of HIF-1; induction was observed with cobaltous ions and desferrioxamine, but not with the metabolic inhibitors cyanide and azide. Such a system has great advantages for the analysis of a regulatory mechanism, since the portion of the molecule responsible for the inducible property can be isolated from other functions. Deletion and mutational analysis have been performed to define more accurately the regulatory sites and mechanisms. These experiments have defined a C-terminal transactivation domain in HIF-1α which itself is regulated by oxygen, but further regulatory regions were also defined lying 5′ to this region.

An example of the analysis of one such domain, lying between amino acids 530 and 652 is shown in Figure 5. A constitutively active chimeric transcription factor was first constructed by linking the DNA binding domain lying in the N-terminal portion of the yeast transcription factor Gal4 to a noninducible transactivation domain from the C-terminus of HIF-1β (Gal/ARNT). The potential of HIF-1α sequences (which need not necessarily have intrinsic transactivating activity) to convey oxygen-dependent regulation was tested by placing the HIF-1α sequence to be tested between these domains. Figure 5(B) shows data for a number of activator plasmids bearing HIF-1α sequence from the domain and shows that this sequence contains elements which convey strongly regulated behavior on the otherwise constitutive activity of the Gal/ARNT fusion gene. Comparison of levels of the fusion protein products of these chimeric genes showed that inclusion of the HIF-1α sequence also greatly reduced the expressed protein level in normoxic cells. Whereas levels of the Gal4/ARNT fusion protein were similar in transfected cells exposed to normoxia, hypoxia, cobalt, and desferrioxamine, the inclusion of the HIF-1α sequences was associated with marked regulation of the expressed protein level. Since the chimeric gene is expressed from a heterologous promoter and translational initiation site, this strongly suggested that the modulatory sequences from HIF-1α reduce the stability of the chimeric gene in a manner which contributes to its regulated activity. Although this is an unusual mechanism of post-translational regulation, studies of HIF-1 protein levels show a very rapid reduction when hypoxic cells are reoxygenated, implying that HIF-1 is unstable in normoxia. Furthermore, the modulatory domain of HIF-1α contains sequences enriched in PEST (proline, glutamic acid, serine, and threonine) residues which have been implicated as signals for rapid proteolysis. Analysis of the precise mechanism is the subject of ongoing studies which are intended ultimately to provide a route to the mechanism of oxygen sensing itself.

Acknowledgments

This work was supported by the Wellcome Trust and the Medical Research Council, UK. The Hepa-1-derived mutant cells were kindly provided by Professor Oliver Hankinson, Department of Pathology and Laboratory Medicine and Jonsson Comprehensive Cancer Center, UCLA, California 90095. Expert technical assistance was provided by S.M. Bartlett, L.G. Nicholls, and K. Yeates.

References

1. Bunn HF, Poyton RO: Oxygen sensing and molecular adaptation to hypoxia. *Physiol Rev* 76:839–885, 1996.
2. Weibel ER, Taylor CR, Hoppeler H: Variations in function and design: Testing symmorphosis in the respiratory system. *Respir Physiol* 87:325–348, 1992.
3. Jelkmann W: Erythropoietin: Structure, control of production, and function. *Physiol Rev* 72:449–489, 1992.
4. Schuster SJ, Badiavas EV, Costa-Giomi P, et al: Stimulation of erythropoietin gene transcription during hypoxia and cobalt exposure. *Blood* 73:13–16, 1989.
5. Goldberg MA, Dunning SP, Bunn HF: Regulation of the erythropoietin gene: evidence that the oxygen sensor is a heme protein. *Science* 242:1412–1415, 1988.
6. Wang GL, Semenza GL: Desferrioxamine induces erythropoietin gene expression and hypoxia-inducible factor 1 DNA-binding activity: implications for models of hypoxia signal transduction. *Blood* 82:3610–3615, 1993.
7. Semenza GL, Nejfelt MK, Chi SM, et al: Hypoxia-inducible nuclear factors bind to an enhancer element located 3′ to the human erythropoietin gene. *Proc Natl Acad Sci USA* 88:5680–5684, 1991.
8. Beck I, Ramirez S, Weinmann R, et al: Enhancer element at the 3′-flanking region controls transcriptional response to hypoxia in the human erythropoietin gene. *J Biol Chem* 266:15563–15566, 1991.
9. Pugh CW, Tan CC, Jones RW, et al: Functional analysis of an oxygen-related transcriptional enhancer lying 3′ to the mouse erythropoietin gene. *Proc Natl Acad Sci USA* 88:10553–10557, 1991.
10. Semenza GL, Wang GL: A nuclear factor induced by hypoxia via de novo protein synthesis binds to the human erythropoietin gene enhancer at a site required for transcriptional activation. *Mol Cell Biol* 12:5447–5454, 1992.
11. Maxwell PH, Pugh CW, Ratcliffe PJ: Inducible operation of the erythropoietin 3′ enhancer in multiple cell lines: evidence for a widespread oxygen sensing mechanism. *Proc Natl Acad Sci USA* 90:2423–2427, 1993.
12. Wang GL, Semenza GL: General involvement of hypoxia-inducible factor 1 in transcriptional response to hypoxia. *Proc Natl Acad Sci USA* 90:4304–4308, 1993.
13. Beck I, Weinmann R, Caro J: Characterization of hypoxia-responsive enhancer in the human erythropoietin gene shows presence of hypoxia-inducible 120-Kd nuclear DNA-binding protein in erythropoietin-producing and nonproducing cells. *Blood* 82:704–711, 1993.

14. Firth JD, Ebert BL, Pugh CW, et al: Oxygen-regulated control elements in the phosphoglycerate kinase 1 and lactate dehydrogenase A genes: similarities with the erythropoeitin 3′ enhancer. *Proc Natl Acad Sci USA* 91:6496–6500, 1994.
15. Pabo CO, Sauer RT: Transcription factors: structural families and principles of DNA recognition. *Annu Rev Biochem* 61:1053–1095, 1992.
16. Pugh CW, Ebert BL, Ebrahim O, et al: Characterisation of functional domains within the mouse erythropoietin 3′ enhancer conveying oxygen-regulated responses in different cell lines. *Biochim Biophys Acta* 1217:297–306, 1994.
17. Firth JD, Ebert BL, Ratcliffe PJ: Hypoxic regulation of lactate dehydrogenase A: interaction between hypoxia inducible factor 1 and cAMP response elements. *J Biol Chem* 270:21021–21027, 1995.
18. Galson DL, Tsuchiya T, Tendler DS, et al: The orphan receptor hepatic nuclear factor 4 functions as a transcriptional activator for tissue-specific and hypoxia-specific erythropoietin gene expression and is antagonized by EAR3/COUP-TF1. *Mol Cell Biol* 15:2135–2144, 1995.
19. Koong AC, Chen EY, Giaccia AJ: Hypoxia causes the activation of nuclear factor kB through the phosphorylation of IkBa on tyrosine residues. *Cancer Res* 54: 1425–1430, 1994.
20. Webster KA, Discher DJ, Bishopric NH: Regulation of fos and jun immediate-early genes by redox or metabolic stress in cardiac myocytes. *Circ Res* 74: 679–86, 1994.
21. Graeber TG, Peterson JF, Tsai M, et al: Hypoxia induces accumulation of p53 protein, but activation of a G1-phase checkpoint by low-oxygen conditions is independent of p53 status. *Mol Cell Biol* 14:6264–6277, 1994.
22. Wang GL, Jiang B-H, Rue EA, et al: Hypoxia-inducible factor 1 is a basic-helix-loop-helix-PAS heterodimer regulated by cellular O_2 tension. *Proc Natl Acad Sci USA* 92:5510–5514, 1995.
23. Reyes H, Reisz-Porszasz S, Hankinson O: Identification of the Ah receptor nuclear translocator protein (Arnt) as a component of the DNA binding form of the Ah receptor. *Science* 256:1193–1195, 1992.
24. Hankinson O: The Aryl Hydrocarbon Complex. *Annu Rev Pharmacol Toxicol* 35:307–340, 1995.
25. Wood SM, Gleadle JM, Pugh CW, et al: The role of aryl hydrocarbon receptor nuclear translocator (ARNT) in hypoxic induction of gene expression: studies in ARNT deficient cells. *J Biol Chem* 271:15117–15123, 1996.
26. O'Rourke JF, Pugh CW, Bartlett SM, et al: Identification of hypoxically inducible mRNAs in Hela cells using differential display PCR. *Eur J Biochem* 241:403–410, 1996.
27. Nagao M, Ebert BL, Ratcliffe PJ, et al: *Drosophila melanogaster* SL2 cells contain a hypoxically inducible DNA binding complex which recognises mammalian HIF-1 binding sites. *FEBS Lett* 387:161–166, 1996.
28. Wang GL, Jiang B-H, Semenza GL: Effect of altered redox states on expression and DNA-binding activity of hypoxia-inducible factor 1. *Biochem Biophys Res Commun* 212:550–556, 1995.
29. Fandrey J, Frede S, Jelkmann W: Role of hydrogen peroxide in hypoxia-induced erythropoietin production. *Biochem J* 303:507–510, 1994.
30. Gleadle JM, Ebert BL, Ratcliffe PJ: Diphenylene iodonium inhibits the induction of erythropoietin and other mammalian genes by hypoxia: implications for the mechanism of oxygen sensing. *Eur J Biochem* 234:92–99, 1995.

31. Fandrey J, Seydel FP, Siegers C-P, et al: Role of cytochrome P450 in the control of the production of erythropoietin. Life Sci 47:127–134, 1990.
32. McQuillan LP, Leung GK, Marsden PA, et al: Hypoxia inhibits expression of eNOS via transcriptional and posttranscriptional mechanisms. *Am J Physiol* 267: H1921-H1927, 1994.
33. Kourembanas S, Marsden PA, McQuillan LP, et al: Hypoxia induces endothelin gene expression and secretion in cultured human endothelium. *J Clin Invest* 88: 1054–1057, 1991.
34. Kourembanas S, Hannan RL, Faller DV: Oxygen tension regulates the expression of the platelet-derived growth factor—b chain gene in human endothelial cells. *J Clin Invest* 86:670–674, 1990.
35. Levy AP, Levy NS, Wegner S, et al: Transcriptional regulation of the rat vascular endothelial growth factor gene by hypoxia. *J Biol Chem* 270:13333–13340, 1995.
36. Gleadle JM, Ebert BL, Firth JD, et al: Regulation of angiogenic growth factor expression by hypoxia, transition metals, and chelating agents. *Am J Physiol* 268:C1362-C1368, 1995.
37. Melillo G, Musso T, Sica A, et al: A hypoxia-responsive element mediates a novel pathway of activation of the inducible nitric oxide synthase promoter. *J Exp Med* 182:1683–1693, 1995.
38. Ebert BL, Firth JD, Ratcliffe PJ: Hypoxia and mitochondrial inhibitors regulate expression of glucose transporter-1 via distinct *cis*-acting sequences. *J Biol Chem* 270:29083–29089, 1995.
39. Webster KA: Regulation of glycolytic enzyme RNA transcriptional rates by oxygen availability in skeletal muscle cells. *Mol Cell Biochem* 77:19–28, 1987.
40. Kietzmann T, Schmidt H, Unthan FK, et al: A ferro-heme protein senses oxygen levels, which modulate the glucagon-dependent activation of the phosphoenolpyruvate carboxykinase gene in rat hepatocyte cultures. *Biochem Biophys Res Commun* 195:792–798, 1993.
41. Norris ML, Millhorn DE: Hypoxia-induced protein binding to O_2-responsive sequenes on the tyrosine hydroxylase gene. *J Biol* Chem 270:23774–23779, 1995.
42. Rolfs A, Kvietikova I, Gassman M, Wenger RH: Oxygen regulated transferrin expression is mediated by hypoxia-inducible factor-1. *J Biol Chem* 272: 20055–20062, 1997.

Chapter 8

Hypoxic Control of Erythropoietin Gene Expression

Jaime Caro
Susana Salceda

Introduction

As it accumulated in the atmosphere more than a billion years ago, oxygen, as a final acceptor of electrons in the respiratory chain, became an evolutionary advantage by allowing a more complete utilization of energy sources. Although less recognized, but equally as important, it also provided a new and highly versatile biochemical reagent for biosynthetic and degradative reactions. Cholesterol and unsaturated fatty acids, fundamental components of eukaryotic cell membranes, could only be synthesized under an oxygen-enriched environment. Since then, organisms developed complex cardiopulmonary systems to secure an adequate oxygen supply. Furthermore, vertebrates evolved a specialized cell type, the erythrocyte, for a more efficient delivery of oxygen. Erythrocyte production is controlled by a glycoprotein hormone, erythropoietin (EPO), which adjusts the red cell mass to the oxygen needs of the tissues and responds to changes of oxygen concentration in the environment. Tissue hypoxia is the main stimulus for EPO production. Besides stimulating EPO, hypoxia elicits a series of systemic, local, and intracellular responses which tend to ameliorate the detrimental effects of the lack of oxygen to

From: López-Barneo, J and Weir, EK: *Oxygen Regulation of Ion Channels and Gene Expression.* Armonk, NY: Futura Publishing Company, Inc., ©1998.

the organism. These adaptive responses include, among others, adjustments in cardiac and respiratory rate, vascular tones, development of collateral blood vessels, and stimulation of anaerobic glycolytic pathways. Important for these adaptive responses to hypoxia is the activation of genes whose expression is stimulated under low oxygen tension. Although our understanding of the molecular mechanisms that control gene expression under hypoxia is still incomplete, there is mounting evidence that most of these genes likely utilize common mechanisms for oxygen sensing and possibly very similar mechanisms for transcriptional activation.

Erythropoietin and Red Cell Production

Under physiologic conditions, the circulating red blood mass is maintained at a size optimal for oxygen transport by proper adjustment of the rate of red cell production. The fundamental role of EPO in controlling erythropoiesis was definitively established in the early 1950s by the pioneer work of Reissman[1] in parabiotic rats and the conclusive findings of an EPO stimulating factor in the plasma[2] or urine[3] of anemic animals. In 1957, Jacobson and coworkers[4] established the renal origin of EPO and the physiologic feedback loop that controls the red cell mass which was initially formulated (Figure 1). It took, however, more than 30 years before the cloning of the EPO gene[5,6] allowed the complete elucidation of the structure of the EPO molecule.

Analysis of the EPO gene reveals that it encodes a polypeptide of 193 amino acids with a peptide molecular weight of 18,389 Da. The protein also undergoes extensive glycosylation which brings its total molecular weight to about 30,000 Da. The three-dimensional array predicted from the amino acid sequence suggests a 4-helix bundle array, very similar to the structure of the growth hormone. EPO acts in the bone marrow by stimulating the proliferation and differentiation of early and late erythroid committed precursor cells, thus determining the rate of red cell production.

In agreement with the postulated model of regulation shown in Figure 1, plasma EPO levels have been found to be greatly elevated in patients with various anemias.[7] In contrast, inappropriately low levels are found in patients with renal diseases.[8] Elevated levels are also found in patients with chronic hypoxemia and compensatory erythrocytosis. Experimental animals exposed to acute hypobaric hypoxia present a rapid induction of EPO mRNA in the kidneys which is followed by a rapid decay after discontinuation of the hypoxic stimulus (Figure 2).[9] Similar induction of

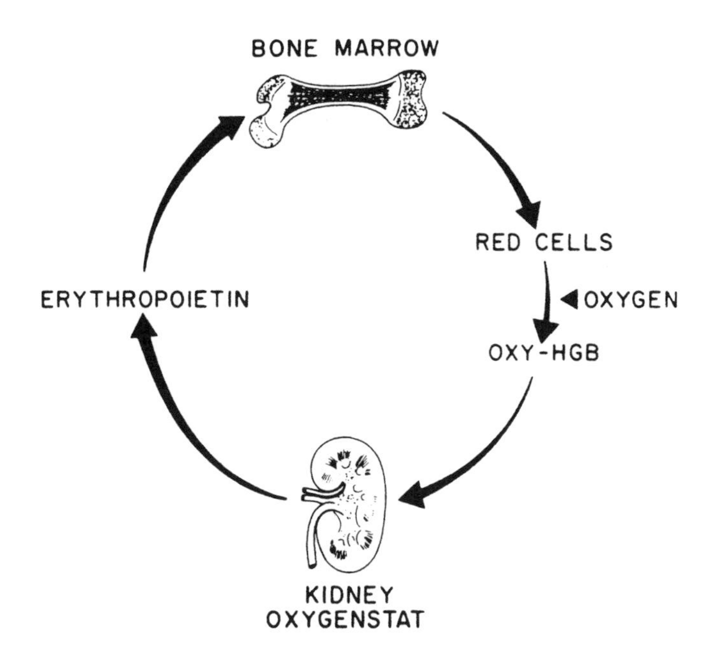

Figure 1. Schematic representation of the feedback loop that regulates erythropoiesis.

EPO mRNA is observed in the kidneys of animals subjected to bleeding anemia or exposed to carbon monoxide.[10]

The cell origin of EPO in the kidney has been a matter of continuing controversy. Initial studies using cell separation techniques indicated a nonglomerular origin. More recent work, utilizing in situ hybridization techniques, points to a peritubular interstitial cell in the renal cortex.[11,12] The exact cell identification is not yet clear, but is likely to be of fibroblastic origin. In the liver, there is evidence for both hepatocyte and interstitial cells, although the predominant cell seems to be the hepatocyte.[13]

Molecular Aspects of Hypoxic Erythropoietin Stimulation

The studies of the molecular mechanisms that regulate the EPO production in response to hypoxia have been greatly facilitated by the identification of human hepatoma cell lines (HepG2 and Hep3B) that produce EPO in a hypoxia-regulated way.[14] Unfortunately, no equivalent cell line

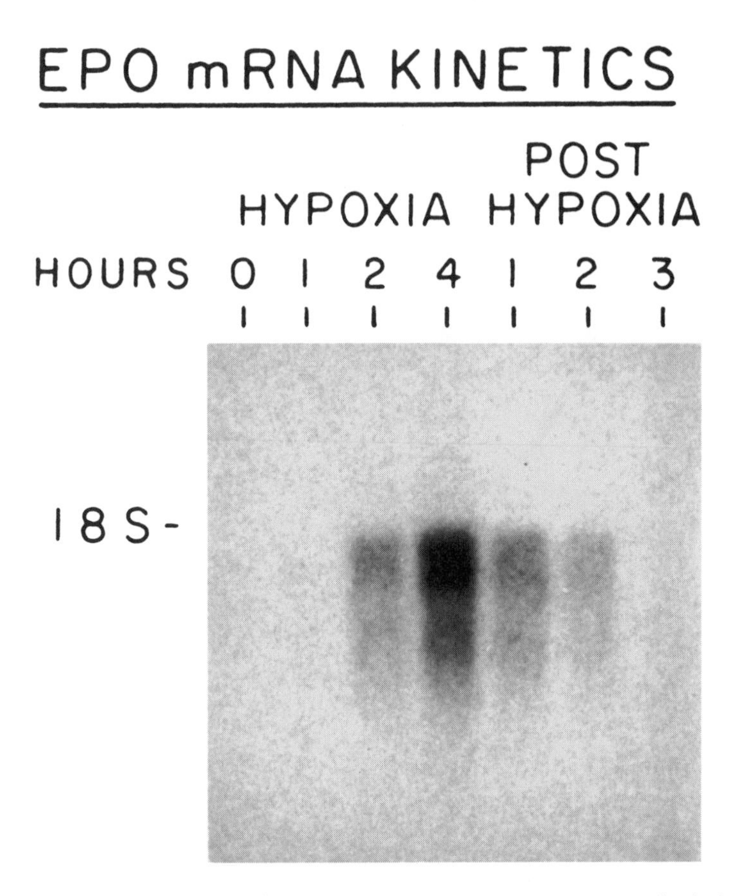

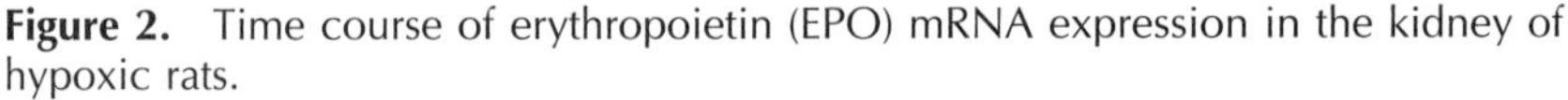

Figure 2. Time course of erythropoietin (EPO) mRNA expression in the kidney of hypoxic rats.

has yet been identified for the kidney. Hep3B cells exposed to hypoxia show an induction of EPO production that is inversely correlated to the oxygen tension utilized. At 1% oxygen, EPO production is stimulated 50 to 100 times. Moreover, the cells also respond to cobalt chloride, a known pharmacologic stimulator of EPO production. Nuclear run-on experiments have shown that hypoxia primarily stimulates the rate of transcription of the EPO gene.[15] The use of cycloheximide, an inhibitor of transcription, blocks transcriptional activation and subsequent messenger accumulation, indicating that ongoing protein synthesis is necessary for the transcriptional response. Although it has been suggested that hypoxia may also stabilize the EPO messenger,[16] there has not yet been conclusive evidence to support this effect.

The *cis*-acting elements and trans-acting factors that regulate the EPO gene response to hypoxia have recently been elucidated.[17-19] Using transient transfection assays, several groups have identified an enhancer sequence in the 3′ flanking region of the EPO gene that is responsible for hypoxia responsiveness (see Chapter 7). The initial studies using a human mini-gene construct showed that a complete deletion of 5′ flanking sequences had no significant effect on the hypoxia response, whereas deletions of the 3′ flanking region completely abolished it. Further studies delineated the enhancer to about 40 bp located 116 nucleotides downstream of the polyadenylation site of the human gene. A similar enhancer, with highly conserved sequences, has been located at an equivalent position in the mouse EPO gene. The hypoxia-responsive enhancer is able to act in a position- and orientation-independent way and confer hypoxia responsiveness to a number of heterologous promoters. Detailed mutational analysis revealed the presence of three areas which are functionally important in the response to hypoxia (Figure 3). The two most proximal areas of the enhancer, sites 1 and 2, appear to be absolutely necessary for the hypoxia response, while the most distal area, site 3, seems to be required for amplification of the response.

Site 1 is the binding site for a hypoxia-inducible transcriptional activation complex, designated as hypoxia inducible factor-1 (HIF-1).[20,21] This deoxyribonucleic acid (DNA) binding complex is present only in nuclear extracts of hypoxic cells and is not found in normal cells. HIF-1 is also induced by cobalt or by exposure to iron chelating agents. HIF-1 induction

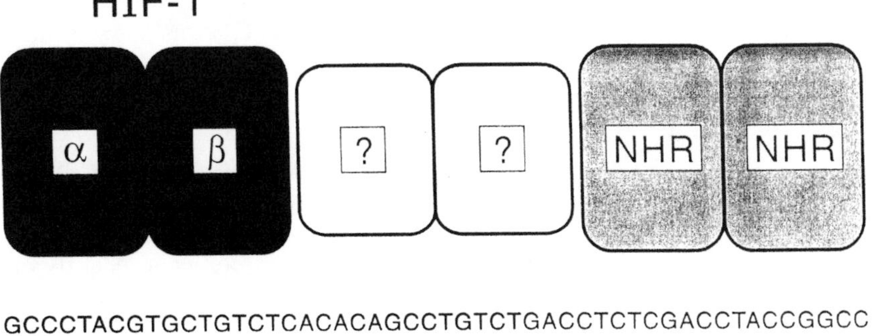

Figure 3. Schematic representation of the 3′ hypoxia responsive enhancer and its DNA binding proteins. HIF-1 = hypoxia inducible factor-1. (Modified with permission from Reference 18.)

precedes EPO mRNA accumulation. The appearance of the inducible complex is inhibited by cycloheximide, confirming that ongoing protein synthesis is necessary for the hypoxia response. Discontinuation of the hypoxic stimulus results in rapid decay of the HIF-1 complex, indicating a very short half-life of the complex and a tight regulation by oxygen tension. Most interestingly, HIF-1 induction by hypoxia and cobalt was observed also in cells that did not produce EPO, thus suggesting that it was part of a more generalized mechanism for hypoxia sensing and response.[20-23] These findings indicated that HIF-1, or closely related proteins, were probably involved in the hypoxia responsiveness of genes other than EPO. Indeed, recent studies have shown that several of the genes encoding enzymes of the glycolytic pathway, such as enolase, pyruvate kinase, and lactate dehydrogenase, are regulated by hypoxia and cobalt through enhancer sequences which are highly homologous to the ones of the EPO gene enhancer (see Chapter 7).[24,25] A core sequence 5′-(C/T/G)ACGTGC(G/T)-3′, which corresponds to the binding site of HIF-1, was found to be present in the flanking region of all the glycolytic enzyme genes which were hypoxia responsive. Moreover, those sequences were able to bind purified HIF-1 complex and to induce hypoxia transcriptional activation to reporter sequences in transient transfection assays. Besides hypoxia, all these genes, like EPO, were also induced by cobalt and desferrioxamine. Another of the well-characterized hypoxia responsive genes is the one encoding for vascular endothelial growth factor (VEGF), a potent and specific mediator of angiogenesis. Increased VEGF mRNA was found in the most ischemic areas of tumors, suggesting that local hypoxia was a stimulus for its production.[26] Further studies in vitro showed that hypoxia greatly stimulated VEGF expression in normal and malignant cells.[27] Again, it was found that VEGF was also induced by cobalt and iron chelating agents. A hypoxia- responsive enhancer with characteristics similar to the EPO enhancer was found in the 5′ flanking region of the rat VEGF gene.[28] It thus appears that most of the known hypoxia-regulated genes utilize similar mechanisms for oxygen sensing (responsive also to cobalt and iron chelators), and are likely to utilize the same or similar transcription factors.

The biochemical purification of the HIF-1 complex was recently accomplished by Wang and Semenza[28] and revealed the presence of two protein subunits: one of about 120 kDa (HIF-1α) and the other in the range of 91 to 95 kDa (HIF-1β). Cloning of both subunits revealed them to be part of the group of basic-helix-loop-helix (bHLH) transcription factor proteins containing a PAS domain (termed PAS for Per, Arnt, and Sim).[29] This PAS domain has been defined by its presence in the *Drosophila* Per and Sim and in the mammalian aryl hydrocarbon receptor (AHR) and aryl hydrocarbon nuclear translocator (ARNT) proteins. The PAS domain shares an approximately 250 amino acid-long region of similarity between these proteins, and it is believed to be necessary for the heterodimerization process. The HIF-1α cDNA predicts an 826-aa polypeptide with an estimated molecular weight of 93 kDa. This subunit is most similar to AHR, also known as the dioxin receptor. AHR is a cytoplasmic receptor protein which translocates to the nuclei after the binding of certain halogenated aromatic hydrocarbons that are widely distributed in nature. In the nuclei, it dimerizes with ARNT to form the active aryl hydrocarbon receptor complex (AHRC) which induces transcription of cytochrome p-450 (CYP1A1) genes.[30] The peptide sequence of the HIF-1β polypeptide corresponded exactly with that of ARNT. As mentioned, ARNT dimerizes with AHR to activate transcription of genes containing the so-called xenobiotic responsive element (XRE), present in several genes of the CYP family. It thus appears that the response to hypoxia involves the activation of two proteins: one subunit, which is a common partner for other DNA-binding complexes (ARNT), and a second one, which appears to be specific for hypoxia (HIF-1). Both subunits seem to be absolutely necessary for the hypoxia response, since (Figure 4) cell lines which are deficient in ARNT expression do not form HIF-1 complex in response to hypoxia, cobalt, or desferrioxamine stimulation. More importantly, these cells which lack HIF-1 complex do not upregulate known hypoxic responsive genes, like aldolase A or VEGF, thus confirming the primordial role of HIF-1 in the hypoxia response.[34] The mechanisms of activation of the HIF 1 complex are not yet well defined. Hypoxia, cobalt, or desferrioxamine do not affect the mRNA levels of either member of the complex (Figure 5), suggesting that the regulation is at the protein level (see also Chapter 9).

Mechanisms of Oxygen Sensing in Mammalian Cells

Examples of adaptive responses to changing oxygen concentrations are found in all forms of life, from bacteria to mammals. Studies in *E. coli* and *R. meliloti* have identified various mechanisms for oxygen sensing that allow the regulated expression or repression of multiple genes involved in energy generation and nitrogen fixation.[31,32] In the baker's yeast *S. cerevisiae*, there is also a group of genes which encode oxygen-dependent functions, such as alternate cytochrome subunits and oxydases, that are induced at low oxygen tension. In this organism, the molecule of heme plays a central role as an intermediate in the signaling mechanism for oxygen levels. Oxygen is an absolute requirement for heme biosynthesis and the concentration of free heme is an indirect reflection of oxygen availability. Hypoxic genes are suppressed in the presence of heme in a process that involves a class of transcriptional regulators known as HAPs (heme-activated proteins).[33]

The mechanisms for hypoxia sensing in higher organisms are much less defined than in bacteria or yeast. However, indirect evidence has suggested that a heme-containing protein may act as an oxygen sensor. Many proteins that interact with oxygen do so via a heme moiety, hemoglobin being a classic example. Desaturation of hemoglobin results in changes in conformation from the oxy, or relaxed state, to the deoxy, or tense state. Goldberg and coworkers showed that transition metals, such as cobalt, nickel, and manganese, were able to stimulate EPO production in a way similar to hypoxia.[35] On the other hand, inhibitors of the respiratory chain, such as cyanide, azide, and antimycin, did not. Moreover,

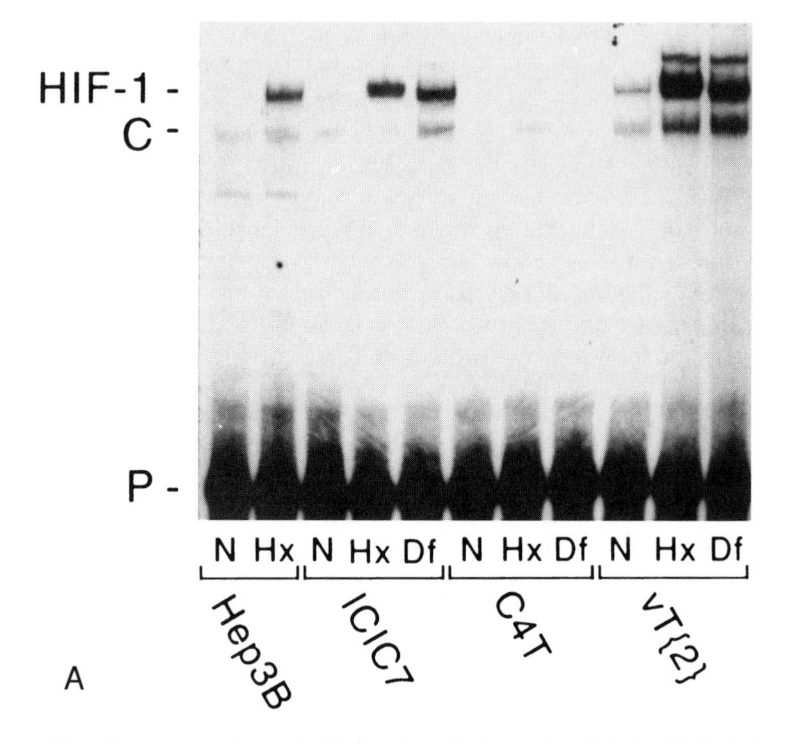

Figure 4A. Response to hypoxia (Hx) and desferrioxamine (Df) in ARNT-deficient cells. Nuclear extracts from normal (N) and Hx or Df stimulated control (ICIC7); ARNT-deficient (C4T) or ARNT-reconstituted (vT2) cells were analyzed by gel retardation using an hypoxia inducible factor-1 (HIF-1) probe.

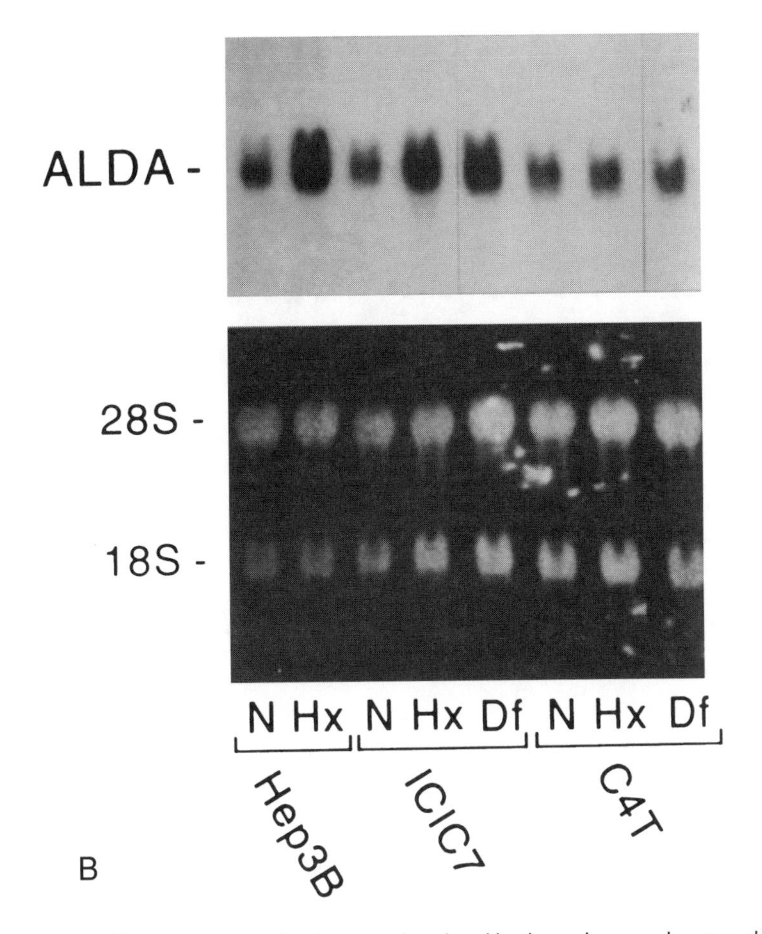

Figure 4B. Aldolase A expression in control and aryl hydrocarbon nuclear translocator (ARNT)-deficient cells.

EPO production in response to hypoxia was markedly decreased in the presence of carbon monoxide or by the use of heme synthesis inhibitors. A unifying hypothesis for these apparently unrelated observations suggested that the sensor could be a rapidly turning-over heme-containing protein with a functional capability dependent on the oxygen tension. Oxygen dissociation would result in a conformational change, as in hemoglobin, and allow the transduction of an appropriate downstream signal. The transition metals that stimulate EPO production, and other genes' activation, would replace iron in the porphyrin of heme, and since they bind oxygen with very low affinity, would lock the sensor in the deoxy

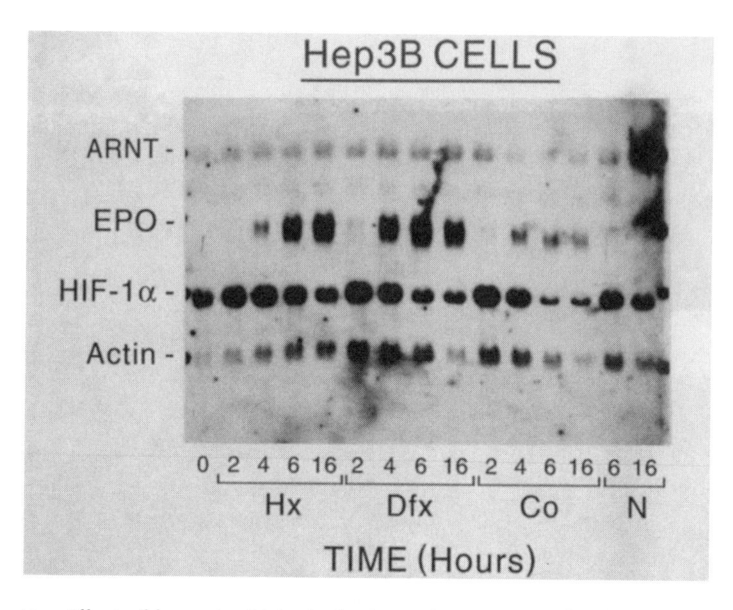

Figure 5. Effect of hypoxia (Hx), desferrioxamine (Dtx), and cobalt (Co) on gene expression in Hep3B cells. Cells were exposed to the different agents and analyzed by Northern blots using human EPO, ARNT, HIF-1α, and actin.

conformation. Carbon monoxide would be expected to block the response to hypoxia by binding with high affinity to the heme group and, lastly, inhibitors of heme synthesis would affect the synthesis of the sensor itself. Although the heme-sensor hypothesis is an attractive one, there is still no direct evidence for the existence of such a sensor. Alternative or complementary hypotheses have suggested that oxygen sensing and signal transduction may involve the detection of hydrogen peroxide (H_2O_2) and/or other reactive oxygen species. Under low oxygen conditions, there is a decrease in the generation of superoxide ions, which could act as an indirect redox-signal of oxygen availability. Fandrey and coworkers have shown that the exogenous addition of H_2O_2, or the accumulation of endogenous peroxides by the addition of catalase inhibitors, have an inhibitory effect on the EPO response to hypoxia.[36] The redox signal could possibly be generated in the respiratory chain by "leakage" of reactive oxygen species or may be the result of a nicotinamide adenine dinucleotide phosphate (NADPH)-like activity. Gorlach and coworkers have described in HepG2 cells the presence of a hypoxia and carbon monoxide-sensitive, but cyanide and antimycin- insensitive, b-type cytochrome with maximal absorption at 558 and 427 nm which could act as an oxygen sensor.[37]

This cytochrome may be part of an electron transfer chain, similar to the NADPH system present in neutrophils, and may modulate peroxide production according to oxygen concentrations. A similar type of cytochrome has been implicated in oxygen sensing by the carotid body.[38] The concentration of peroxide/oxygen radicals could act as a second messenger or directly regulate the redox state of transcription factors. As to this effect, it is interesting to note that HIF-1 activity is very sensitive to its redox state.[39] Recent findings indicate that redox changes regulate the degradation rate of the HIF-1α protein.[40] Unfortunately, there is still no direct evidence as to which and how an NADPH system may be involved in oxygen sensing.

Acknowledgments

Some of the work presented in this manuscript has been supported by grants from NIH (34642), the American Heart Association, and the Juvenile Diabetes Foundation International (195009).

References

1. Reissman KR: Studies on the mechanism of erythropoietic stimulation in parabiotic rats during hypoxia. *Blood* 5:372-380, 1950.
2. Erslev A: Humoral regulation of red cell production. *Blood* 8:349-357, 1953.
3. Hodgson G, Toha J: The erythropoietic effect on urine and plasma of repeatedly bled rabbits. *Blood* 9:299-309, 1954.
4. Jacobson LO, Goldwasser LF, Fried W, Plzak L: Role of the kidney in erythropoiesis. *Nature* 179:633-634, 1957.
5. Lin F-K, Suggs S, Lin C-H, Browne JK, Smalling R, Egrie JC, et al: Cloning and expression of the human erythropoietin gene. *Proc Natl Acad Sci USA* 82:7580-7584, 1985.
6. Jacobs K, Shoemaker C, Rudersdorf R , Neill SD, Kaufman RJ, Mufson A, et al: Isolation and characterization of genomic and cDNA clones of human erythropoietin. *Nature* 313:806-810, 1985.
7. Erslev AJ, Caro J, Miller O, Silver R: Plasma erythropoietin in health and disease. *Ann Clin Lab Sci* 10:250-257, 1980.
8. Caro J, Erslev AJ: Uremic inhibitors of erythropoiesis. *Semin Nephrol* 5:128-132, 1985.
9. Schuster SJ, Wilson JH, Erslev AJ, Caro J: Physiologic regulation and tissue localization of renal erythropoietin messenger RNA. *Blood* 70:316-318, 1987.
10. Koury ST, Koury MJ, Bondurant MC, Caro J, Graber SE: Quantitation of erythropoietin producing cells in kidneys of mice by in situ hybridization: correlation with hematocrit, renal erythropoietin RNA, and serum erythropoietin concentration. *Blood* 74:645-651, 1989.
11. Koury ST, Bondurant MC, Koury MJ: Localization of erythropoietin synthesizing cells in murine kidneys by in situ hybridization. *Blood* 71:524-527, 1988.

12. Lacombe C, Da SJL, Bruneval P, Fournier JG, Wendling F, Casadevall N, et al: Peritubular cells are the site of erythropoietin synthesis in the murine hypoxic kidney. *J Clin Invest* 81:620-623, 1988.
13. Schuster SJ, Koury ST, Bohrer M, Salceda S, Caro J: Cellular sites of extrarenal and renal erythropoietin production in anaemic rats. *Br J Haematol* 81:153-159, 1992.
14. Goldberg MA, Glass GA, Cunningham JM, Bunn HF: The regulated expression of erythropoietin by two human hepatoma cell lines. *Proc Natl Acad Sci USA* 84:7972-7976, 1987.
15. Schuster SJ, Badiavas EV, Costa-Giomi P, Weinmann R, Erslev AJ, Caro J: Stimulation of erythropoietin gene transcription during hypoxia and cobalt exposure. *Blood* 73:13-16, 1989.
16. Goldberg MA, Gaut CC, Bunn HF: Erythropoietin mRNA levels are governed by both the rate of gene transcription and post-transcriptional events. *Blood* 77: 271-277, 1991.
17. Beck I, Ramirez S, Weinmann R, Caro J: Enhancer element at the 3′ flanking region controls transcriptional response to hypoxia in the human erythropoietin gene. *J Biol Chem* 266:15563- 15566, 1991.
18. Semenza GL, Nejfelt MK, Chi SM, Antonarakis SE: Hypoxia- inducible nuclear factors bind to an enhancer element located 3′ to the human erythropoietin gene. *Proc Natl Acad Sci USA* 88:5680-5684, 1991.
19. Pugh CW, Tan CC, Jones RW, Ratcliffe PJ: Functional analysis of an oxygen-regulated transcriptional enhancer lying 3′ to the mouse erythropoietin gene. *Proc Natl Acad Sci USA* 88:10553-10557, 1991.
20. Beck I, Weinmann R, Caro J: Characterization of hypoxia responsive enhancer in the human erythropoietin gene reveals presence of hypoxia inducible 120 kDa nuclear DNA-binding protein in erythropoietin producing and nonproducing cells. *Blood* 82:704-711, 1993.
21. Semenza GL, Wang GL: A nuclear factor induced by hypoxia via de novo protein synthesis binds to the human erythropoietin gene enhancer at a site required for transcriptional activation. *Mol Cell Biol* 12:5447-5454, 1992.
22. Wang GL, Semenza GL: General involvement of hypoxia-inducible factor 1 in transcriptional response to hypoxia. *Proc Natl Acad Sci USA* 90:4304-4308, 1993.
23. Maxwell PH, Pugh CW, Ratcliffe PJ: Inducible operation of the erythropoietin 3′ enhancer in multiple cell lines: evidence for a widespread oxygen-sensing mechanism. *Proc Natl Acad Sci USA* 90:2423-2427, 1993.
24. Semenza GL, Roth PH, Fang H-M, Wang GL: Transcriptional regulation of genes encoding glycolytic enzymes by hypoxia-inducible factor 1. *J Biol Chem* 269: 23757-23763, 1994.
25. Firth JD, Ebert BL, Pugh CW, Ratcliffe PJ: Oxygen-regulated control elements in the phosphoglycerate kinase 1 and lactate dehydrogenase A genes: similarities with the erythropoietin 3′ enhancer. *Proc Natl Acad Sci USA* 91:6496-6500, 1994.
26. Shweiki D, Itin A, Soffer D, Keshet E: Vascular endothelial growth factor induced by hypoxia may mediate hypoxia-initiated angiogenesis. *Nature* 359:843-845, 1992.
27. Minchenko A, Bauer T, Salceda S, Caro J: Hypoxic stimulation of vascular endothelial growth factor (VEGF) expression in vitro and in vivo. *Lab Invest* 71:374-379, 1994.

28. Wang GL, Semenza GL: Purification and characterization of hypoxia-inducible factor 1. *J Biol Chem* 270:1230-1237, 1995.
29. Wang GL, Jiang B-H, Rue EA, Semenza GL: Hypoxia-inducible factor 1 is a basic-helix-loop-helix-PAS heterodimer regulated by cellular O_2 tension. *Proc Natl Acad Sci USA* 92:5510-5514, 1995.
30. Hankinson O: The aryl hydrocarbon receptor complex. *Annu Rev Pharmacol Toxicol* 35:307-340, 1995.
31. Spiro S: The FNR family of transcriptional regulators. *Antonie van Leeuwenhoek* 66:23-36, 1994.
32. Gilles-Gonzalez MA, Gonzalez G, Perutz MF: Kinase activity of oxygen sensor FixL depends on the spin state of its heme iron. *Biochemistry* 34:232-236, 1995.
33. Zitomer RS, Lowry CV: Regulation of gene expression by oxygen in *Saccharomyces cerevisiae. Microbiol Rev* 56:1-11, 1992.
34. Salceda S, Beck I, Caro J: Absolute requirement of ARNT for gene activation by hypoxia. *Arch Biochem Biophys* 334:389-394, 1996.
35. Goldberg MA, Dunning SP, Bunn HF: Regulation of the erythropoietin gene: evidence that the oxygen sensor is a heme protein. *Science* 242:1412-1415, 1988.
36. Fandrey J, Frede S, Jelkmann W: Role of hydrogen peroxide in hypoxia-induced erythropoietin production. *Biochem J* 303:507-510, 1994.
37. Gorlach A, Holtermann G, Jelkmann W, Hancock JT, Jones SA, Jones OTG: Photometric characteristics of heme proteins in erythropoietin-producing hepatoma cells (Hep G2). *Biochem J* 290:771-776, 1993.
38. Cross AR, Henderson L, Jones OTG, Delpiano MA, Hentschel J, Acker H: Involvement of an NAD(P)H oxidase as a pO_2 sensor protein in the rat carotid body. *Biochem* 272:743-747, 1990.
39. Wang GL, Jiang B-H, Semenza GL: Effect of altered redox states on expression and DNA-binding activity of hypoxia- inducible factor 1. *Biochem Biophys Res Commun* 212:550-556, 1995.
40. Salceda S, Caro J: Hypoxia-inducible factor 1α (HIF-1α) protein is rapidly degraded by the ubiquitin-proteasome system under normoxic conditions: its stabilization by hypoxia depends on redox-induced changes. *J Biol Chem* 272: 22642–22647, 1997.

Chapter 9

Regulation of Hypoxia Inducible Factor-1 Activity

L. Eric Huang
H. Franklin Bunn

Introduction

Adaptation to hypoxia is fundamental to the survival of all forms of life. Diverse mechanisms have evolved to activate transcription factors in response to specific environmental signals. There is growing evidence that hypoxia regulates transcription of a broad repertoire of biologically important genes through a common mechanism of oxygen sensing, signal transduction, and transactivation.[1] Among these extensively studied genes is the one which encodes human erythropoietin (EPO), a glycoprotein hormone that regulates red blood cell formation. Recently, a collective effort from several laboratories has identified a 3′ enhancer to the human EPO gene,[2-5] to which two transcription factors bind: in response to low oxygen tension, hypoxia inducible factor-1 (HIF-1) binds to the upstream portion,[2] whereas hepatic nuclear factor 4 interacts downstream in a constitutive manner (see Chapters 7 and 8).[6]

HIF-1 is composed of a 120-kD α subunit and a 91-94 kD β subunit.[7] Accordingly, HIF-1 binding can be supershifted with anti-HIF-1α antibodies and with an anti-HIF-1β antibody.[8] When activated, the HIF-1 heterodimer recognizes an 8-base pair deoxyribonucleic acid (DNA) sequence

From: López-Barneo, J and Weir, EK: *Oxygen Regulation of Ion Channels and Gene Expression*. Armonk, NY: Futura Publishing Company, Inc., ©1998.

5′-TACGTGCT-3′ in the EPO enhancer, interacting with both DNA strands in the major groove.[9] HIF-1 DNA binding can be induced by cobaltous ion and desferrioxamine with kinetics similar to that of hypoxia induction.[9,10] Recent cloning of HIF-1α and β genes showed that they are members of the basic-helix-loop-helix-PAS (termed PAS for Per, Arnt, and Sim) family of transcription factors[11]; HIF-1α is a novel protein, whereas HIF-1β is the previously cloned and characterized aryl hydrocarbon receptor nuclear translocator.[12]

Although HIF-1 was originally identified in an EPO-producing cell line (Hep3B), HIF-1 activity can also be induced by hypoxia in a wide variety of non-EPO producing cells. This was demonstrated by specific binding to oligonucleotides containing an HIF-1 response element[10] and by transactivation of reporter genes,[3] suggesting general involvement of HIF-1 in the response to hypoxia. Indeed, functional HIF-1 binding sites have also been identified in promoters/enhancers of a number of genes important in adaptation to hypoxia, such as those encoding tyrosine hydroxylase,[13] vascular endothelial growth factor,[14] glycolytic enzymes,[15-17] and glucose transporters.[18] Therefore, elucidation of the mechanism by which HIF-1 activity is regulated becomes crucial in the understanding of molecular adaptation to hypoxia.

Activation of Hypoxia Inducible Factor-1 Depends Primarily Upon Stabilization of Its α-Subunit

To investigate the mechanism underlying regulation of HIF-1 activity, we determined levels of HIF-1α and β transcripts by ribonuclease protection analysis of Helen Lake (HeLa) cells maintained at 21% oxygen (Figure 1A, lane 1) or those incubated for 4 hours under 1% oxygen (lane 2). Contrary to the initial report on the cloning of the HIF-1 subunits,[11] we found that both HIF-1α (Figure 1A) and HIF-1β transcripts (not shown) were readily detectable under normoxic conditions and were not significantly increased by exposure to hypoxia. Moreover, RNA obtained from Hep3B cells gave the same results. In agreement with our observations, Gradin et al reported recently that both HIF-1α and HIF-1β genes are constitutively expressed.[19] In contrast, hypoxia has a marked effect at the level of HIF-1α protein expression. When HeLa cells were incubated for 4 hours in 1% oxygen, the expected induction in HIF-1 DNA binding activity (Figure 1B, lane 2) was accompanied by a striking increase in HIF-1α protein from barely detectable (Figure 1C, top panel lane 1) to abundant expression (lane 2), whereas HIF-1β protein was constitutively expressed

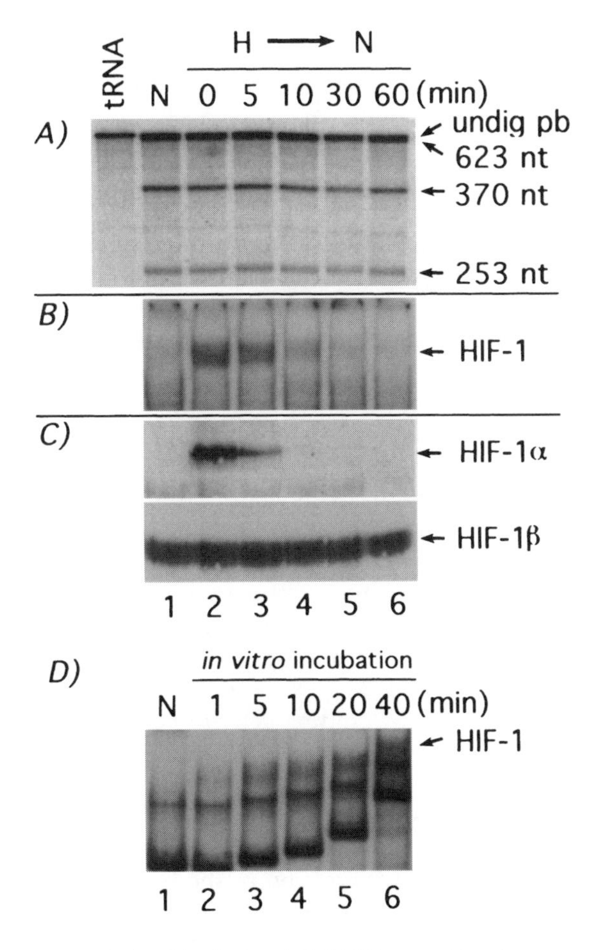

Figure 1. Hypoxia Inducible Factor-1 (HIF-1) is sensitive to oxygen in vivo but stable in vitro. After 4-hour hypoxia treatment, Helen Lake (HeLa) cells were placed in a 21% oxygen incubator for 0, 5, 10, 30, and 60 minutes, respectively (lanes 2-6). **A.** Total ribonucleic acid (RNA) was isolated to quantify HIF-1α mRNA by RNase protection analysis. Undigested riboprobes (undig pb) and protected HIF-1α fragments (623 nucleotides from incomplete digestion, 370 and 253 nucleotides from complete digestion) are marked. **Lane 0** shows yeast tRNA mixed with the riboprobe. Cell extracts were prepared and analyzed by (**B**) EMSA to examine HIF-1 binding; and **C.** Western blot to determine abundance of HIF-1α and HIF-1β. **D.** Hypoxic extracts were incubated with ^{32}P-labeled W18 oligonucleotide (containing the HIF-1 binding site) at room temperature for 1, 5, 10, 20, or 40 minutes and then loaded onto an EMSA gel.

at a high level with no significant change in abundance following exposure to hypoxia (lower panel).

One mechanism for the accumulation of HIF-1α protein is that at low oxygen tension, the subunit is stabilized but is rapidly degraded when oxygen is replete. To address this question, cells were incubated under 1% oxygen for 4 hours to produce maximal HIF-1 activation, and were then placed in a 21% oxygen chamber for 5, 10, 30, or 60 minutes. As shown in Figure 1B, we noted a precipitous drop in HIF-1 DNA-binding after exposure to normoxia (lanes 2-6), as reported previously.[9] The rapid decrease of HIF-1 DNA-binding correlated closely with the rate of decay of HIF-1α abundance ($T_{1/2}$ 5 minutes) as demonstrated by Western blot analyses of the same cell extract preparations, whereas HIF-1β abundance remained unchanged when the same blot was reprobed with anti-HIF-1β (Figure 1C, lanes 2-6). To confirm that the disappearance of HIF-1α was not due to lack of HIF-1α messenger ribonucleic acid (mRNA), total RNA was prepared from cells treated under the same conditions as above and analyzed by Rnase protection. Once again, HIF-1α mRNA levels were unaffected (Figure 1A, lanes 2-6). Therefore, these results indicate that HIF-1α protein decays very rapidly under normoxic conditions and becomes stabilized by hypoxia. To investigate whether normoxia directly destabilizes HIF-1, hypoxic extracts were incubated at room temperature, 21% oxygen, for 1, 5, 10, 20, or 40 minutes and loaded onto an electrophoretic mobility shift assay (EMSA) gel at respective time points. Results in Figure 1D showed that HIF-1 binding activity persisted throughout the course, suggesting that the instability of HIF-1α depends on cell integrity.

To confirm further that HIF-1α protein is sensitive to oxygen, a full-length HIF-1α cDNA was cloned into a eukaryotic expression vector downstream of the strong cytomegalovirus enhancer and promoter.[8] Despite the robust constitutive expression of the exogenous HIF-1α gene, no appreciable increase of HIF-1α protein was detected under normoxic conditions as analyzed by Western blotting.[8] In contrast, at low oxygen tension, significant increases in HIF-1α protein were detected in the transfected cells. Therefore, oxygen decreased the levels of both exogenous and endogenous HIF-1α protein, further supporting the notion that regulation occurs at a level distal to gene expression and protein synthesis.

To test whether oxygen-dependent regulation of HIF-1α protein is due to alterations in translation, HIF-1 was activated in HeLa cells by incubation for a total of 3 hours in 1% oxygen, and at 150 minutes cycloheximide was added anaerobically.[8] As shown in Figure 2A, the preaddition of cycloheximide completely abolished HIF-1 DNA binding (lane 3),[2] but post-addition failed to do so (lane 4). In addition, the sustained HIF-1 DNA-binding was also oxygen-dependent (compare lanes 4 and 5). These

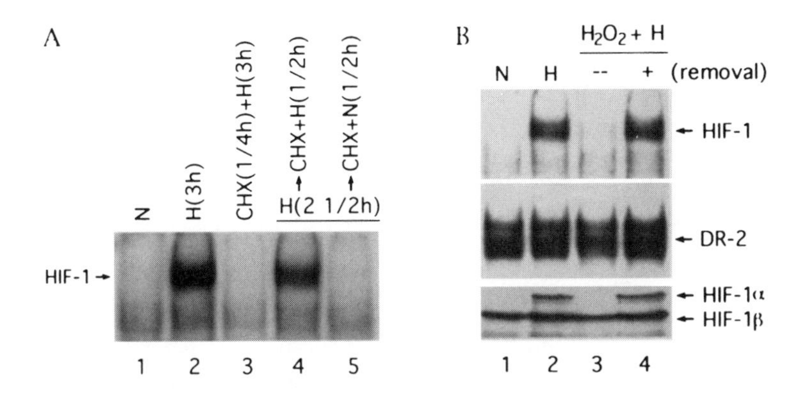

Figure 2. Cycloheximide (CHX) fails to abolish activated hypoxia inducible factor 1(HIF-1) deoxyribonucleic acid (DNA) binding, and the effect of hydrogen peroxide (H_2O_2) is reversible. **A.** Helen Lake (HeLa) cells were incubated in a hypoxic chamber for a total of 3 hours (lanes 2-4), and were either pretreated for 15 minutes (lane 3) or treated at 2.5 hours (lane 4) with 100 μg/mL of CHX. Cells in lane 5 were incubated in a hypoxic chamber for 2.5 hours, added with the same concentration of CHX, and placed in a normoxic chamber for another 30 minutes. Cell extracts were prepared and analyzed by EMSA to determine HIF-1 binding activity. **B.** Cells were pretreated 1 mM H_2O_2 for 20 minutes, and then subjected to hypoxia for 4 hours (lane 3) or prior to hypoxia treatment H_2O_2 was removed by rapidly rinsing cell twice with media (lane 4). Whole cell extracts were analyzed by EMSA to examine HIF-1 binding (**top panel**) and by Western blotting to quantify abundance of HIF-1α and β (**bottom panel**). The **middle panel** shows an EMSA analysis of proteins binding to DR-2, a tandem repeat of hormone response elements on the 3′ end of the EPO enhancer.

results indicate that alterations in translation cannot be the sole mechanism responsible for the increased level of HIF-1α during hypoxia.

Exogenous addition of hydrogen peroxide (H_2O_2) has been shown to inhibit hypoxic induction of the EPO gene through specific inhibition of HIF-1 DNA binding.[8] To elucidate the mechanism by which pretreatment with H_2O_2 inhibits HIF-1 DNA binding, levels of both HIF-1α and HIF-1β protein were quantified by Western blot analyses. The bottom panel of Figure 2B shows that expression of HIF-1α protein was hypoxia inducible (lane 2), but that this induction was inhibited by H_2O_2 treatment (lane 3). In contrast, the abundance of HIF-1β protein was not significantly affected. To further determine the effect of H_2O_2 on the expression of HIF-1α, total RNA was isolated from cells treated under the same conditions as above, and analyzed by ribonuclease protection. Despite the inhibition of HIF-1α protein accumulation, no significant changes in HIF-1α transcripts were observed.[8]

Interestingly, the inhibitory effect of H_2O_2 is fully reversible. After exposure of HeLa cells to H_2O_2 for 20 minutes, the medium was removed and the adherent cells were rinsed twice with normal (unmodified) medium. As shown in the upper panel of Figure 2B, the removal of H_2O_2 fully restored HIF-1 DNA binding (lane 4) with no significant effects on binding of nuclear receptors to the DR-2 site (middle panel), a functionally important *cis*-acting element located downstream of HIF-1 site in the EPO 3′ enhancer.[6] Moreover, the removal of H_2O_2 also fully restored HIF-1α protein accumulation (bottom panel). Taken together, these results show that, just like normoxia, pretreatment with H_2O_2 inhibits hypoxia-induced activation of HIF-1 via blocking the accumulation of HIF-1α protein, without affecting either HIF-1α mRNA expression or expression of HIF-1β protein.

Regulation of Hypoxia Inducible Factor-1 Activity Through Post-Translational Modifications

Phosphorylation

Although, as demonstrated above, the binding of HIF-1 to DNA is primarily controlled at the level of HIF-1α accumulation, there is little information on whether post-translational modifications are necessary for this activation. Previously, Wang and Semenza[9] reported that HIF-1 activation is blocked by 2-aminopurine, a protein kinase inhibitor. In addition, treatment of hypoxic cell extracts with alkaline phosphatase[9] or potato acid phosphatase[20] abolishes DNA binding. Thus, these results suggest that phosphorylation may be required for HIF-1 DNA binding.

Reduction-Oxidation

The reversible inhibitory effects of H_2O_2 on HIF-1 activity strongly suggest that redox chemistry is an important determinant of the stability of HIF-1α. Whereas *N*-ethylmaleimide (NEM) irreversibly modifies thiol groups, diamide promotes reversible disulfide bond formation.[21,22] When hypoxic extracts were incubated with NEM or diamide prior to addition of probe, HIF-1 DNA binding was significantly inhibited in a dose-dependent fashion,[8] suggesting that sulfhydryl alkylation or oxidation prevents DNA binding, in agreement with recently published results.[23] Consistent with the chemical properties of these reagents, subsequent addition of dithiothreitol (DTT) fully reversed the inhibitory effect of diamide but not that of NEM.[8] Furthermore, we investigated whether sulfhydryl reductants could stimulate HIF-1 DNA binding. Contrary to the conclusions of others,[23] we found that when oxidized thioredoxin purified from *Escherichia coli* was added in the presence of DTT, a clear stimulation in HIF-1 DNA binding was reproducibly detected in hypoxic extracts. Moreover, in the presence of DTT, thioredoxin not only reversed the inhibitory effect of diamide, but also enhanced HIF-1 DNA binding.[8] In contrast, oxidized thioredoxin had no effect in the absence of DTT.

To define the role of thiol groups involved in HIF-1 DNA binding, we determined whether HIF-1, once bound to DNA, is still sensitive to sulfhydryl alkylation and oxidation. After preincubation with HIF-1 DNA probe, cell extracts were much less sensitive to NEM and diamide than those that were not preincubated.[20] This result suggested that the binding of DNA to HIF-1 hindered alkylation and oxidation of the relevant thiol groups. We noticed, however, that despite the above difference, HIF-1 DNA binding was nevertheless diminished by NEM and diamide even when cell extracts were preincubated with the DNA probe. This is probably attributable to the fast off-rate of HIF-1 DNA binding previously reported.[9] As shown in Figure 3A, after incubation with ^{32}P/W18 oligonucleotide, cell extracts were further incubated with one hundredfold excess of unlabeled W18 oligonucleotide for 1, 5, 10, or 20 minutes, and loaded on an EMSA gel at each time point. HIF-1 ^{32}P/DNA complexes were gradually displaced by unlabeled W18 oligonucleotide (top panel, lanes 3-6), whereas further incubation for 20 minutes in the absence of unlabeled W18 oligonucleotide did not affect HIF-1 DNA binding (lane 7), suggesting that the decreased DNA binding (lanes 3-6) was not due to the instability of DNA-protein complexes during the further incubation. In like manner, NEM also gradually decreased HIF-1 DNA binding when incubated with HIF-1 ^{32}P/DNA complexes for 1 to 20 minutes (bottom panel, lanes 3-6). In fact, the rate of decay of the HIF-1 DNA complex following addition of excess unlabeled W18 oligonucleotide was in good agreement with the decay following the addition of NEM (Figure 3B).

To assay the functional effect of redox potential as a modulator of HIF-1 activity in intact cells, we transfected HeLa cells with a vector expressing human thioredoxin (pCMV-ADF) along with a luciferase reporter (pEPOE-luc) containing the human EPO HIF-1 binding site. It has been shown that exogenous expression of thioredoxin stimulates AP-1 activity, but inhibits NF-kB.[24,25] Overexpression of thioredoxin markedly potentiated the hypoxic induction of luciferase gene expression.[8] Ref-1, a nuclear protein possessing both redox and apurinic endonuclease DNA repair activities,[26,27] has also been shown to facilitate AP-1 binding activ-

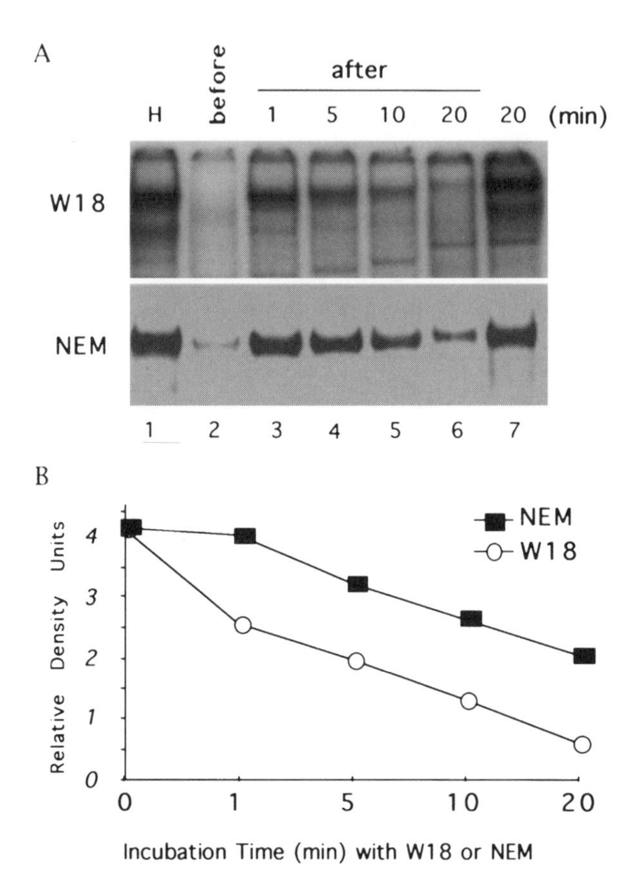

Figure 3. Correlation of dissociation of hypoxia inducible factor-1 (HIF-1) deoxyribonucleic acid (DNA) complexes with inhibitory effects of N-ethylmaleimide (NEM). **A.** Ten minutes after addition of ^{32}P-labeled W18 to hypoxic extracts, HIF-1 DNA complexes were treated with one hundredfold unlabeled W18 (**top**) or 5 mM NEM (**bottom**) for 1, 5, 10, or 20 minutes (lanes 3-6). The reaction mixtures were loaded onto an ongoing gel at each time point. Addition of one hundredfold unlabeled W18 or 5 mM NEM before DNA binding reaction is indicated in lane 2, and the further incubation of HIF-1 DNA complexes for 20 minutes in the absence of either unlabeled W18 or NEM is in lane 7. **B.** HIF-1 DNA binding activity shown above in lanes 1, and 3, 4, 5, and 6 was quantified using Phosphor Imaging. The density of these complexes was plotted in relative density units.

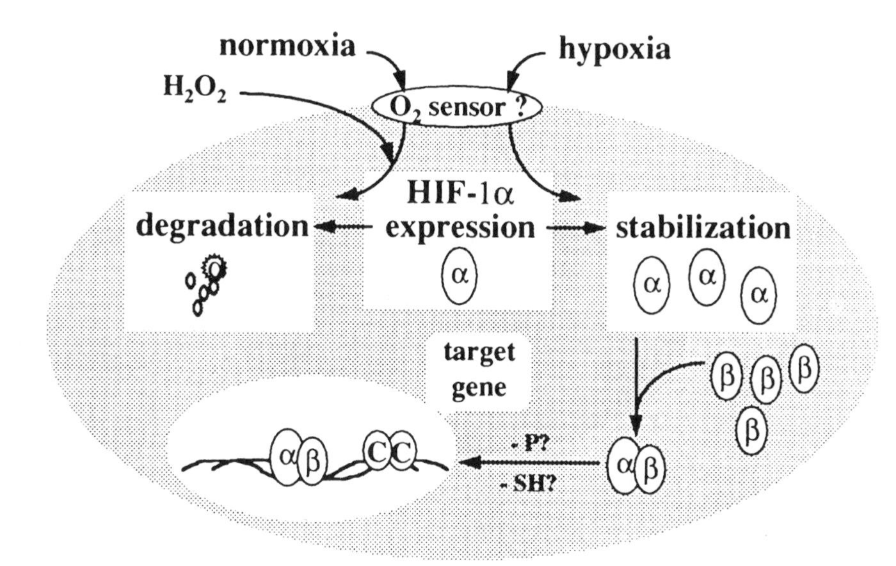

Figure 4. Oxygen-sensitive hypoxia inducible factor-1α (HIF-1α) protein determines hypoxic response. When the cell is oxygenated or treated with hydrogen peroxide, HIF-1α protein decays rapidly, preventing formation of the HIF-1 heterodimer and activation of gene expression. In contrast, hypoxia stabilizes HIF-1α, allowing formation of HIF-1 $\alpha\beta$ heterodimer and, in conjunction with other constitutively bound transcription factors (**C**) and coactivators (see text), transactivation of genes containing functional HIF-1 elements.

ity.[28] When Ref-1 expression vector (pCMV-APE) was cotransfected with the reporter, like thioredoxin, it further enhanced the hypoxic induction of the reporter.[8] Moreover, when the HIF-1 binding site was mutated, no potentiation was observed with either thioredoxin or Ref-1, indicating that the effect of these proteins was HIF-1 dependent. Because of high redox buffering capacity of cells, it is likely that both thioredoxin and Ref-1 were in the reduced form.

Conclusion

Taken together, our results indicate, as depicted in Figure 4, that the pathway leading from the sensing of hypoxia to the activation of HIF-1 is critically dependent on the relative abundance of its α subunit, and that hypoxia-induced accumulation of HIF-1α is primarily attributable to increased protein stability. The effect of oxygen in acutely lowering levels of

HIF-1α is mimicked by H_2O_2, a finding which is consistent with a large body of experimental work implicating reactive oxygen intermediates in the signaling process.[1] We present both in vitro and in vivo experiments that indicate that redox chemistry contributes importantly to HIF-1 activation.

Further investigation of the mechanism underlying oxygen- sensitive degradation of HIF-1α protein should lead to an understanding of oxygen sensing and the subsequent signaling pathway. Moreover, Arany et al[29] demonstrated that the C-terminal portion of HIF-1α binds specifically and functionally to p300/CBP, that participates in the transactivation of a fast-growing number of genes.[30-32] This transcriptional coactivator plays a critical role in regulating HIF-1 activity through protein-protein interactions.

Acknowledgments

We are grateful to Zolton Arany, David M. Livingston, Markus R. Probst, and Oliver Hankinson for antibodies, and Greg L. Semenza, Patrick Baeuerle, Lynn Harrison, and Bruce Demple for constructs. We thank members of the Bunn laboratory for helpful suggestions. This work was supported by NIH grant RO1-DK41234 (H.F.B). L.E.H. is a recipient of the National Research Service Award (DK09365-02) from the National Institutes of Health.

References

1. Bunn HF, Poyton RO: Oxygen sensing and molecular adaptation to hypoxia. *Physiol Rev* 76:839-885, 1996.
2. Semenza GL, Wang GL: A nuclear factor induced by hypoxia via de novo protein synthesis binds to the human erythropoietin gene enhancer at a site required for transcriptional activation. *Mol Cell Biol* 12:5447-5454, 1992.
3. Maxwell PH, Pugh CW, Ratcliffe PJ: Inducible operation of the erythropoietin 3′ enhancer in multiple cell lines: evidence for a widespread oxygen-sensing mechanism. *Proc Natl Acad Sci USA* 90:2423-2427, 1993.
4. Madan A, Curtin PT: A 24-base-pair sequence 3′ to the human erythropoietin gene contains a hypoxia-responsive transcriptional enhancer. *Proc Natl Acad Sci USA* 90:3928-3932, 1993.
5. Blanchard KL, Acquaviva AM, Galson DL, et al: Hypoxic induction of the human erythropoietin gene: cooperation between the promoter and enhancer, each of which contains steroid receptor response elements. *Mol Cell Biol* 12:5373-5385, 1992.
6. Galson DL, Tsuchiya T, Tendler DS, et al: The orphan receptor hepatic nuclear factor 4 functions as a transcriptional activator for tissue-specific and hypoxia-specific erythropoietin gene expression and is antagonized by EAR3/COUP-TF1. *Mol Cell Biol* 15:2135-2144, 1995.

7. Wang GL, Semenza GL: Purification and characterization of hypoxia-inducible factor-1. *J Biol Chem* 270:1230-1237, 1995.
8. Huang LE, Arany Z, Livingston DM, et al: Activation of hypoxia-inducible transcription factor depends primarily upon redox-sensitive stabilization of its α subunit. *J Biol Chem* 271:32253-32259, 1996.
9. Wang GL, Semenza GL: Characterization of hypoxia-inducible factor 1 and regulation of DNA binding activity by hypoxia. *J Biol Chem* 268:21513-21518, 1993.
10. Wang GL, Semenza GL: General involvement of hypoxia-inducible factor 1 in transcriptional response to hypoxia. *Proc Natl Acad Sci USA* 90:4304-4308, 1993.
11. Wang GL, Jiang B-H, Rue EA, et al: Hypoxia-inducible factor 1 is a basic helix-loop-helix-PAS heterodimer regulated by cellular O_2 tension. *Proc Natl Acad Sci USA* 92:5510-5514, 1995.
12. Hoffman EC, Reyes H, Chu F-F, et al: Cloning of a factor required for activity of the Ah (dioxin) receptor. *Science* 252:954-958, 1991.
13. Norris ML, Millhorn DE: Hypoxia-induced protein binding to O_2-responsive sequences on the tyrosine hydroxylase gene. *J Biol Chem* 270:23774-23779, 1995.
14. Levy A, Levy N, Wegner S, et al: Transcriptional regulation of the rat vascular endothelial growth factor gene by hypoxia. *J Biol Chem* 270:13333-13340, 1995.
15. Firth JD, Ebert BL, Pugh CW, et al: Oxygen-regulated control elements in the phosphoglycerate kinase 1 and lactate dehydrogenase A genes: similarities with the erythropoietin 3′ enhancer. *Proc Natl Acad Sci USA* 91:6496-6500, 1994.
16. Firth JD, Ebert BL, Ratcliffe PJ: Hypoxic regulation of lactate dehydrogenase A: interaction between hypoxia inducible factor 1 and cAMP response elements. *J Biol Chem* 270:21021-21027, 1995.
17. Semenza GL, Roth PH, Fang HM, et al: Transcriptional regulation of genes encoding glycolytic enzymes by hypoxia- inducible factor 1. *J Biol Chem* 269: 23757-23763, 1994.
18. Ebert BL, Firth JD, Ratcliffe PJ: Hypoxia and mitochondrial inhibitors regulate expression of glucose transporter-1 via distinct cis-acting sequences. *J Biol Chem* 270:29083-29089, 1995.
19. Gradin K, McGuire J, Wegner RH, et al.: Functional interference between hypoxia and dioxin signal transduction pathways: competition for recruitment of the Arnt transcription factor. *Mol Cell Biol* 16:5221-5231, 1996.
20. Huang LE, Bunn HF: Unpublished data.
21. Kosower NS, Kosower EM: Thiol labeling with bromobimanes. *Methods Enzymol* 143:76-84, 1987.
22. Kosower NS, Kosower EM: Formation of disulfides with diamide. *Methods Enzymol* 143:264-270, 1987.
23. Wang GL, Jiang BH, Semenza GL: Effect of altered redox states on expression and DNA-binding activity of hypoxia-inducible factor 1. *Biochem Biophys Res Commun* 212:550-556, 1995.
24. Meyer M, Schreck R, Baeuerle PA: H_2O_2 and antioxidants have opposite effects on activation of NF-kappa B and AP-1 in intact cells: AP-1 as secondary antioxidant-responsive factor. *EMBO J* 12:2005-2015, 1993.
25. Schenk H, Klein M, Erdbrugger W, et al: Distinct effects of thioredoxin and

antioxidants on the activation of transcription factors NF-kappa B and AP-1. *Proc Natl Acad Sci USA* 91:1672-1676, 1994.

26. Xanthoudakis S, Curran T: Identification and characterization of Ref-1, a nuclear protein that facilitates AP-1 DNA-binding activity. *EMBO J* 11:653-665, 1992.
27. Harrison L, Ascione G, Menninger JC, et al: Human apurinic endonuclease gene (APE): structure and genomic mapping (chromosome 14q11.2-12). *Hum Mol Genetics* 1:677-680, 1992.
28. Xanthoudakis S, Miao G, Wang F, et al: Redox activation of Fos-Jun DNA binding activity is mediated by a DNA repair enzyme. *EMBO J* 11:3323-3335, 1992.
29. Arany Z, Huang LE, Eckner R, et al: Participation by the p300/CBP family of proteins in the cellular response to hypoxia. *Proc Natl Acad Sci USA* 93:12969-12973, 1996.
30. Eckner R, Ewen ME, Newsome D, et al: Molecular cloning and functional analysis of the adenovirus E1A-associated 300-kD protein (p300) reveals a protein with properties of a transcriptional adaptor. *Genes Dev* 8:869-884, 1994.
31. Lundblad JR, Kwok RPS, Laurance ME, et al: Adenoviral E1A- associated protein p300 as a functional homologue of the transcriptional co-activator CBP. *Nature* 374:85-88, 1995.
32. Janknecht R, Hunter T: A growing coactivator network. *Science* 383:22-23, 1996.

Chapter 10

Evidence for Hydrogen Peroxide as a Signal Transduction Molecule in Oxygen-Dependent Regulation of Gene Expression

Maria F. Czyzyk-Krzeska
Sandra L. Kroll
Waltke R. Paulding

Introduction

Mammalian organisms hyperventilate when exposed to reduced oxygen tension (hypoxia). This is a basic, adaptive mechanism that compensates for decreased oxygen availability in the environment by increasing oxygen partial pressure (P_{O_2}) in the blood. Hyperventilation results from the activity of specialized oxygen-sensitive type I cells in the carotid body which sense reduced P_{O_2} in the arterial blood and communicate this information to the central nervous system respiratory networks. One of the major neurotransmitters released from carotid body cells during hypoxia is the catecholamine dopamine (DA). Dopamine metabolism is tightly regulated by P_{O_2}. Hypoxia stimulates DA release[1,2] and DA synthesis[3] in type I cells. The increase in DA synthesis results from augmented activity of tyrosine hydroxylase (TH),[4,5] the rate-limiting enzyme in catecholamine

From: López-Barneo, J and Weir, EK: *Oxygen Regulation of Ion Channels and Gene Expression.* Armonk, NY: Futura Publishing Company, Inc., ©1998.

synthesis. We demonstrated that hypoxia induces a fivefold increase in TH messenger ribonucleic acid (mRNA) steady state levels in carotid body cells.[6] We also found that DA metabolism is regulated by oxygen in the pheochromocytoma-derived cell line, PC12. During hypoxia, PC12 cells depolarize and release DA (see Chapter 15).[7,8] Hypoxia induces TH gene expression[9-12] and leads to augmentation of TH protein content and its enzymatic activity in PC12 cells,[8] in a manner similar to that measured in the carotid body type I cells.[6]

The molecular mechanism by which oxygen-sensitive cells sense a reduction in Po_2 and transduce this signal into regulation of gene expression is not well understood (see Chapter 7). Recently, novel and interesting evidence has indicated that a physiologic byproduct of oxidative metabolism, hydrogen peroxide (H_2O_2), participates in the oxygen-sensing pathway in various oxygen-sensitive cells. In this respect, Acker and coworkers[13,14] proposed that the oxygen sensor is represented by a membrane-bound multisubunit protein, similar to the leukocytes nicotinamide adenine dinucleotide phosphate (NAD(P)H) oxidase. The oxygen sensor includes a cytochrome b-like hemeprotein that modifies its conformation in response to alteration in environmental Po_2 . This affects activity of an associated oxidase, generating H_2O_2. The conformational change in cytochrome b during hypoxia decreases the activity of the oxidase and leads to a decrease in H_2O_2 formation. This, in turn, shifts glutathione (GSH) and protein sulfhydryl groups toward reduced forms. This hypothesis is particularly attractive for the regulation of gene expression, because a number of regulatory DNA and RNA-binding proteins are redox sensitive and bind to nucleic acids only in either reduced or oxidized forms. The regulatory function of H_2O_2 in regulation of gene expression by oxidative stress has been shown in the case of activation of the transcription factor NF-kB[15] and stimulation of the binding of iron regulatory protein (IRP) to iron responsive elements (IRE).[16] Moreover, hypoxic induction of the erythropoietin gene also involves changes in H_2O_2 concentration.[17] In the present study, we wanted to determine whether hypoxia actually leads to reduction in H_2O_2 levels in oxygen-sensitive PC12 cells, and whether changes in the H_2O_2 are involved in the signal transduction pathway that mediates the observed increase in tyrosine hydroxylase mRNA during hypoxia.

Experimental Procedures

Rat PC12 cells American Type Culture Collection (ATCC) were grown in DMEM/F12 medium with 10% fetal calf serum as previously described.[9-11] Immediately before each experiment (50% confluent cells), the regular medium was replaced by serum-free RPMI 1640 medium (iron free). This change did not affect viability of cells for at least 24 hours. Exposures of cells to gas mixtures were performed as described.[9-11] For each drug treatment, the concentrations and time course are given in the *Results* section. The doses of drugs used in the experiments did not affect viability of cells, as determined by trypan blue exclusion. Northern blot analysis was performed as described previously.[9]

Hydrogen Peroxide Measurements

H_2O_2 was measured using 2′7′-dichlorofluorescin diacetate (DCFDA, Molecular Probes, Eugene, OR).[18,19] DCFDA penetrates easily into the cells where it is cleaved to 2′7′-dichlorofluorescin (DCF) and reacts with H_2O_2 forming fluorescent 2′7′-dichlorofluoroscein, that is detected using spectrofluorometry. This assay is chemically specific for hydroperoxides. Since H_2O_2 is the major peroxide in the cells, it is generally accepted that DCF fluorescence is proportional to H_2O_2 concentration. Cells were plated at a density of 2.5×10^6 cells per well in 12-well tissue culture plates and treated with normoxia, hypoxia, or different drugs in serum-free RPMI 1640 medium for indicated periods of time. At the end of each experiment, cells were washed in loading buffer (150 mM NaCl, 5 mM KCl, 1 mM $MgSO_4$, 1 mM NaH_2PO_4, 20 mM Hepes, 1.8 mM $CaCl_2$, 10 mM glucose, pH 7.4), then loaded with 10 μM DCFDA in the same buffer for 5 minutes at 37° C. At this time, DCFDA containing buffer was promptly removed, cells washed with loading buffer and processed for spectrofluorometric measurements with the excitation wavelength 485 nm and the emission wavelength 530 nm. Emission from samples of cells that were not loaded with DCFDA was the same as from the loading buffer.

Hydrogen Peroxide Level in PC12 Cells is Modulated by Hypoxia and Reducing Agents

Analysis of H_2O_2 levels in PC12 cells using DCF fluorescence revealed that PC12 cells have readily detectable amounts of H_2O_2 during normoxia. Figure 1 shows that this constitutive presence of H_2O_2, measured as DCF fluorescence, was significantly reduced when PC12 cells were exposed to

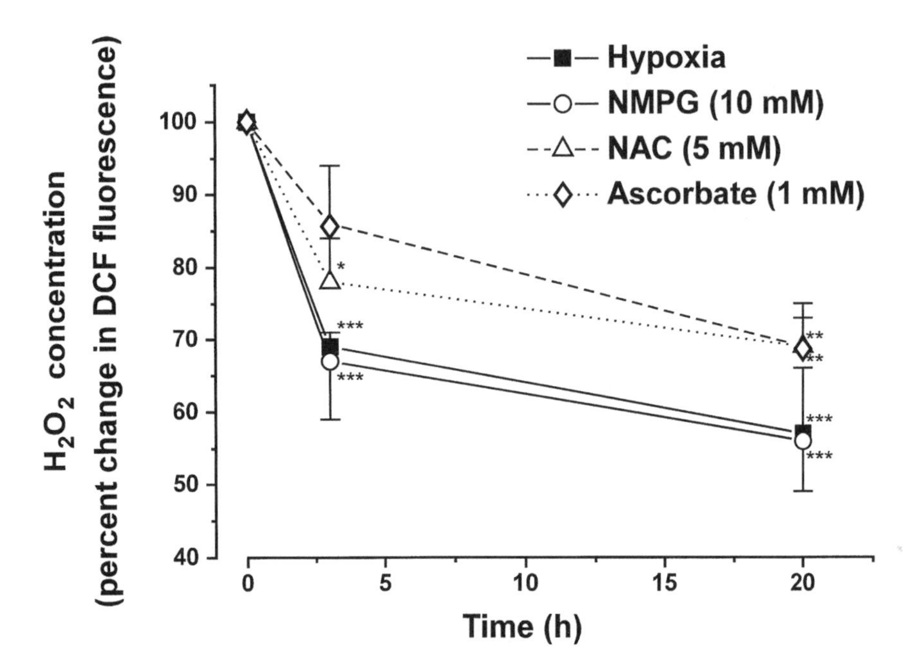

Figure 1. Effects of hypoxia and reducing agents on hydrogen peroxide (H_2O_2) concentration measured by dichlorofluorescin (DCF) fluorescence. Results are presented as percent change from the DCF fluorescence measured in cells exposed to normoxia (control − 100%). Hypoxia (**solid squares**) led to prompt and significant decrease in H_2O_2. N-methylpropionylglycine (NMPG) (**open circles**) decreased H_2O_2 similarly to hypoxia, while N-acetylcysteine (NAC) (**open triangles**) and L-ascorbate (**open diamonds**) were less effective. Each experiment was performed four times in duplicate or triplicate.

5% oxygen for up to 20 hours (the longest time studied). This decrease in DCF fluorescence was easily detected, despite the fact that the cells were washed and loaded with DCFDA (up to 30 minutes) in room air, i.e., under reoxygenating conditions. In two cases, after 20 hours exposure to hypoxia, PC12 cells were equilibrated with room air for 3 hours. Under these circumstances, we failed to measure a decrease in DCF fluorescence between control and treated cells. Simultaneous addition of 50 mM aminotriazole (ATZ), a catalase inhibitor, and 20 μM H_2O_2 prevented the reduction in H_2O_2 (not shown).

We next examined whether drugs that have antioxidant activity, i.e., that scavenge reactive oxygen intermediates, could reduce H_2O_2 content in PC12 cells. Figure 1 shows the effects of N-methylpropionylglycine (NMPG), N-acetylcysteine (NAC), and L-ascorbate on DCF fluorescence in PC12 cells. All these drugs are reducing agents that increase the amount of reduced thiol groups on GSH and proteins. NMPG showed the highest level of similarity with hypoxia as far as magnitude and time course of reducing H_2O_2. Two other reducing agents, NAC and L-ascorbate, were less effective, although they also lowered H_2O_2. In all three cases, the decrease in H_2O_2 was progressive over time and was larger after 20 hours than after 3 hours of treatment.

Hyodrgen Peroxide Production and Tyrosine Hydroxylase mRNA Expression

The expression of TH mRNA correlated with intracellular concentrations of H_2O_2. Figure 2 shows how changes in the levels of H_2O_2 affect TH mRNA expression. Hypoxia induced TH mRNA in a similar manner as previously described[9] (Figure 2Ab). The hypoxic induction of TH gene expression was abolished by simultaneous treatment of PC12 cells with 50 mM of the catalase inhibitor ATZ and 20 μM H_2O_2, which prevents a decrease in H_2O_2 during hypoxia (Figure 2Ac). Treatment of PC12 cells with catalase,[19] which decomposes H_2O_2 enzymatically, increased expression of TH mRNA in the absence of hypoxia (Figure 2B). Treatment of PC12 cells with NMPG, which decreases H_2O_2 (see above), caused a dose-dependent induction of TH mRNA that was identical in time course and magnitude to that measured under hypoxic conditions (Figure 2Cb & c). Moreover, the effects of NMPG could be completely counterbalanced (Figure 2Cd) by treatment of PC12 cells with 20 μM H_2O_2 and ATZ which resulted in recovery of H_2O_2 concentration to approximately 90% of the control value. NAC, at concentrations of 2 to 5 mM also induced TH mRNA levels, although less than hypoxia (not shown). L-ascorbate failed to induce TH mRNA up to 20 hours of treatment.

In view of the potential link between the heme-containing oxygen sensor and the activity of H_2O_2-generating oxidase (see *Introduction*), we examined whether pharmacologic treatments that are believed to affect function of hemeproteins and, thus, oxygen sensing,[20] would simultaneously affect H_2O_2 levels and TH gene expression. For this purpose, we have examined the effects of deferoxamine (DF), an iron chelator, and cobalt ion (Co^{2+}) on H_2O_2 levels and TH mRNA in PC12 cells.

Deferoxamine, by chelating iron, inhibits incorporation of iron into newly synthesized heme molecules, inhibiting heme synthesis. Thus, it was proposed that DF prevents resynthesis of the heme-containing oxygen sensor (assuming that the oxygen sensor has a turnover rate in the

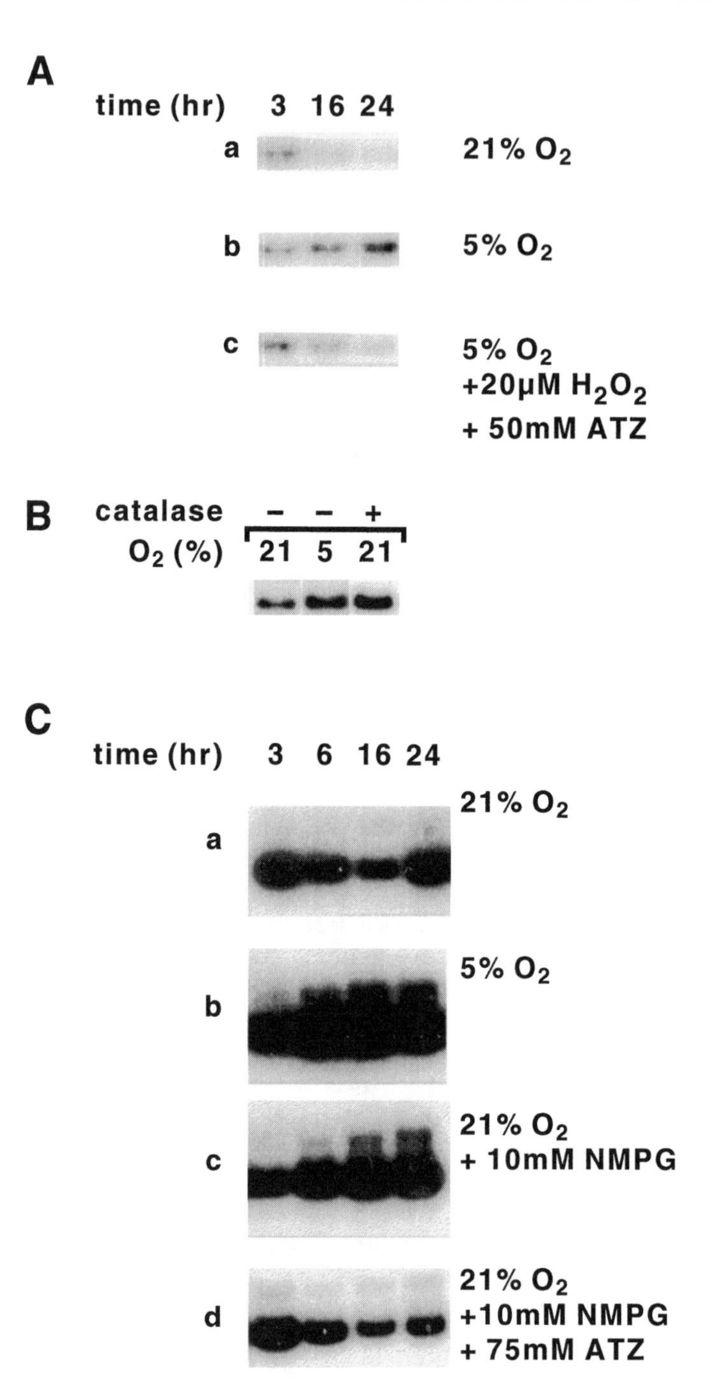
A
time (hr) 3 16 24
a
21% O2
b
5% O2
c
5% O2
+20μM H2O2
+ 50mM ATZ
B
catalase – – +
O2 (%) 21 5 21
C
time (hr) 3 6 16 24
a
21% O2
b
5% O2
c
21% O2
+ 10mM NMPG
d
21% O2
+10mM NMPG
+ 75mM ATZ

range of several hours).[20] DF mediated "removal" of the oxygen sensor from the associated H_2O_2-generating oxidase should, therefore, cause a decrease in constitutive levels of H_2O_2 and increase TH mRNA levels during normoxia. The "removal" of the oxygen sensor should also result in the failure of hypoxia to decrease H_2O_2 and prevent the hypoxia-induced increase in TH mRNA. In all experiments reported below, DF (100 μM) was added to serum and iron-free RPMI 1640 medium. DF failed to decrease H_2O_2 in PC12 cells at any time from 1 to 20 hours of treatment. It also failed to affect the hypoxia-mediated decrease in H_2O_2. Figure 3A shows the effects of DF treatment on TH mRNA. Treatment of the normoxic PC12 cells with DF for 6 and 24 hours caused a small induction of the TH mRNA (Figure 3A), with the larger increase at 24 hours. Simultaneous treatment with both hypoxia and DF resulted in augmentation of the hypoxia-induced increase in TH mRNA. When PC12 cells were treated with DF in the presence of serum, deferoxamine had an attenuating effect on hypoxic induction of TH mRNA and a very small stimulating effect on TH gene expression under normoxic conditions (not shown). In both cases, effects of DF on TH mRNA were less strong than the effects of hypoxia.

Cobalt ion (Co^{2+}) is believed to replace iron in newly synthesized oxygen-sensing heme protein, but because it does not bind oxygen it locks the putative oxygen sensor in the deoxy conformation, mimicking effects of hypoxia.[20] Thus, treatment with Co^{2+} should result in the decrease in H_2O_2 and induce TH mRNA similar to that caused by hypoxia. In addition, effects of Co^{2+} should be reversed by increasing concentration of iron, since increased iron availability shall prevent incorporation of Co^{2+} into the heme protein. Treatment of PC12 cells with Co^{2+} (100 μM) significantly decreased H_2O_2 to 60% $\pm$ 4% ($P < 0.001$) after 20 hours of treatment, but failed to affect H_2O_2 after 3 hours of treatment. Co^{2+} induced TH mRNA as early as after 3 hours with the peak at 6 hours of treatment. After 24 hours of Co^{2+} treatment, we failed to measure induction in TH

Figure 2. Effects of hydrogen peroxide (H_2O_2) on tyrosine hydroxylase (TH) messenger ribonucleic acid (mRNA). **A.** Induction of TH mRNA by hypoxia (b) can be abolished by simultaneous treatment with aminotriazole (ATZ), catalase inhibitor, and H_2O_2 (c). **B.** Inducing effect of hypoxia on TH mRNA can be mimicked by treatment of PC12 cells with catalase (4 mg/mL). **C.** Effects of hypoxia (b) on TH mRNA can be mimicked by treatment of PC12 cells with N-methylpropionylglycine (NMPG) (c), sulfhydryl reducing agent. Effects of NMPG on TH mRNA are also abolished by simultaneous treatment with ATZ and H_2O_2 (d), indicating involvement of H_2O_2 in the pathway.

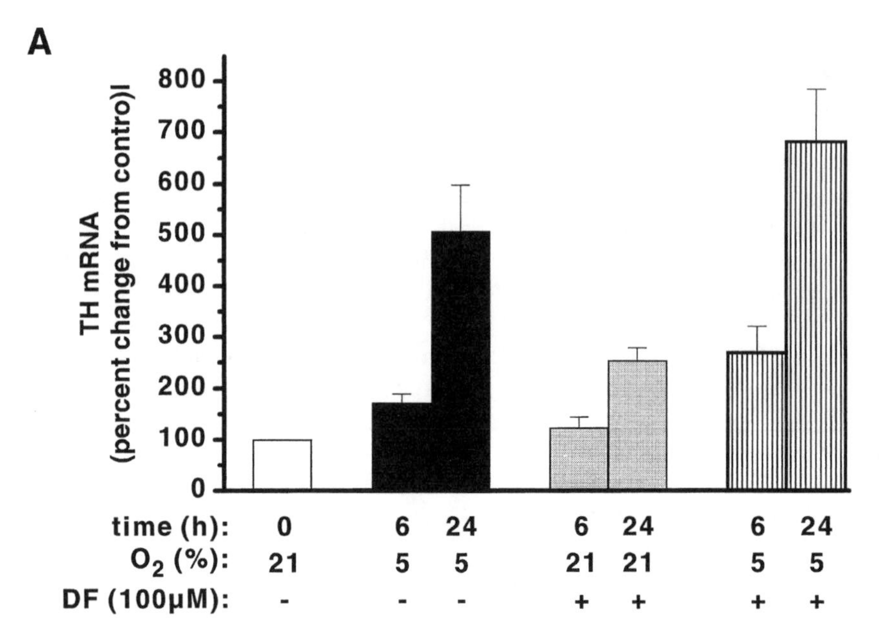
A
TH mRNA
(percent change from control)
800
700
600
500
400
300
200
100
0
time (h): 0 6 24 6 24 6 24
O_2 (%): 21 5 5 21 21 5 5
DF (100μM): - - - + + + +

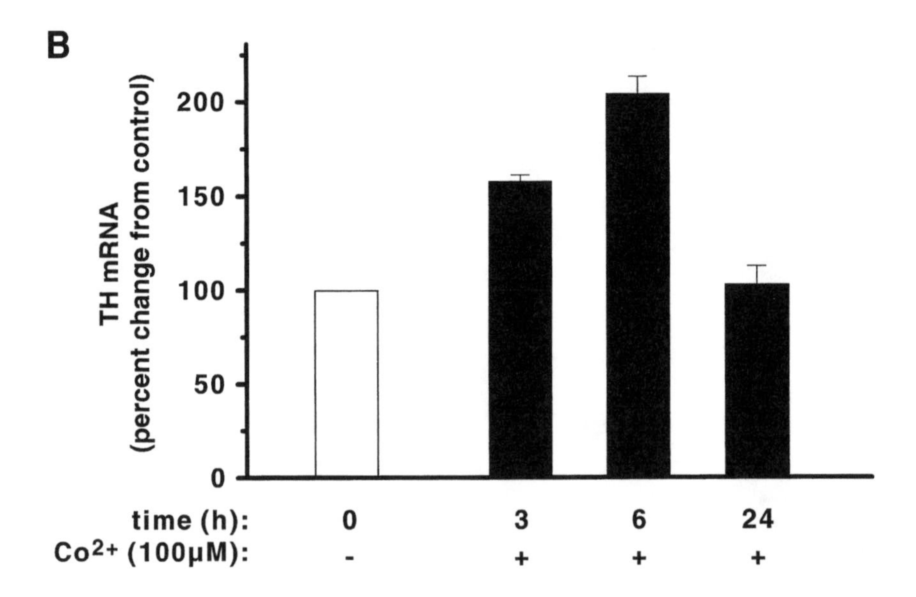
B
TH mRNA
(percent change from control)
200
150
100
50
0
time (h): 0 3 6 24
Co^{2+} (100μM): - + + +

mRNA (Figure 3B). Increasing the concentration of iron from 0 to 3 mM completely inhibited Co^{2+}-mediated induction of TH mRNA (not shown).

Hydrogen Peroxide as a Signal Transduction Molecule in the Oxygen-Dependent Regulation of Tyrosine and Hydroxylase Gene Expression

In this study, we have shown that hypoxia decreases concentrations of H_2O_2 in PC12 cells. We have also shown that oxygen-dependent regulation of TH gene expression correlates well with the levels of H_2O_2. The decrease in the concentration of H_2O_2 was readily measured after 1 hour of exposure of PC12 cells to hypoxia, despite reoxygenation that occurred during the procedure of loading PC12 cells with DCFDA (up to 30 to 40 minutes). On the other hand, reoxygenation lasting a few hours abolished the hypoxia-induced decrease in H_2O_2. This observation indicates that hypoxia-mediated decrease in H_2O_2 results from the decreased activity of an H_2O_2-generating enzyme or increased activity of an H_2O_2-scavenging system in a long-term (hours) manner. The source of the H_2O_2 that is affected by hypoxia is presently not known. H_2O_2 is generated by a number of enzymatic reactions, including the respiratory chain, microsomal cytochrome system, lipooxygenases and cyclooxygenases, xanthine oxidase, glucose oxidase, and monoaminooxidases.[21] However, inhibition of these oxidases using specific pharmacologic blockers failed to decrease H_2O_2 levels. Inhibition of the NAD(P)H oxidase with a specific inhibitor, diphenylene iodonium[22] (DPI, 0.1-10 μM), also failed to reduce H_2O_2 levels in PC12 cells, and did not affect expression of TH mRNA during either normoxia or hypoxia. Thus, the decrease in H_2O_2 measured during hypoxia may result from inhibited activity of a different oxidase system.

The decrease in H_2O_2 during hypoxia may also result from increased scavenging of H_2O_2, either by catalase, glutathione peroxidase (GPO), or by reactions with the small molecule antioxidants. Catalase is present predominantly in peroxisomes and catalyzes decomposition of H_2O_2 to

Figure 3. Effects of deferoxamine and cobalt on tyrosine hydroxylase (TH) messenger ribonucleic acid (mRNA) in PC12 cells. Results are presented as percent change from control. **A.** Deferoxamine (DF) induced TH mRNA during normoxia and hypoxia. Effects of DF and hypoxia were augmenting one another. The responses were larger after 24 hours of treatment than after 6 hours of treatment. **B.** Cobalt caused an early induction of TH mRNA (3-6 hours) and after 24 hours, the effect disappeared.

water and molecular oxygen.[23] GPO decomposes H_2O_2 using reduced GSH as the hydrogen donor. The reaction is absolutely specific for GSH, causing oxidation of the GSH into the GSSG form.[23] The activities of GPO or catalase have not been specifically measured in the PC12 cells during hypoxia; however, exposure of rats to 10% oxygen in the environment substantially augmented activity of the selen-containing GPO and catalase in the rats lung.[24] H_2O_2 may be also scavenged nonenzymatically by small molecule antioxidants, such as sulfhydryl-containing compounds, ascorbic acid, uric acid, thioethers, and others.[23] Cellular proteins contain sulfhydryl and thioether residues that may also react with the H_2O_2. Increased direct scavenging of H_2O_2 by sulfhydryl groups is the major mechanism by which NMPG and other reducing agents reduce H_2O_2 in PC12 cells. The high efficiency of NMPG in reducing H_2O_2 and inducing TH mRNA results from very good cell permeability of this drug, in contrast to NAC.

The molecular mechanism by which decreased H_2O_2 causes an increase in TH gene expression remains to be studied. Hypoxia-mediated increase in TH mRNA involves an increased rate of TH gene transcription and increased stability of TH mRNA.[9] Our laboratory is in the process of studying whether both TH gene transcription and TH mRNA stability are regulated by changes in the H_2O_2 in parallel to the changes measured in total TH mRNA. Increase in TH gene transcription results from increased binding of c-fos and jun-B transcription factors to the AP1 site and possibly hypoxia inducible factor-1 (HIF-1) transcription factor to the HIF-1 if binding site within the TH gene promoter.[12] Binding of these transcription factors to the DNA is redox dependent[25] and single cysteines were identified in the *fos* and *jun* proteins that were required to be in the reduced form in order to allow for protein binding to the nucleic acid.[26] Nuclear extracts of most cells contain a reducing protein, called redox factor-1 (Ref-1), that has the capability to reduce different transcription factors.[26] The activity of Ref-1 is redox dependent, and oxidation inhibits while reduction activates its redox activity.[27] Similarly, activation of the HIF-1 transcription factor results from redox-sensitive stabilization of its α subunit.[28] Increase in TH mRNA stability is due to increased binding of an hypoxia-inducible protein factor to the pyrimidine-rich region within the 3′ untranslated region of the TH mRNA.[10,11] Binding of this protein factor to the RNA, similarly to many other RNA-binding proteins, is redox sensitive. Protein binds only in the reduced form and does not bind in the oxidized form (unpublished results). Thus, it is tempting to suggest that hypoxia-induced decrease in the H_2O_2 leads to the shift in the state of the regulatory proteins toward more reducing forms that, in turn, results in quantitative induction of the protein binding or in the increased affinity of the protein binding to the nucleic acids.

There are at least two possible, nonexcluding mechanisms by which H_2O_2 may affect the protein redox state. First, decreased H_2O_2 generation during hypoxia may result in higher concentration of reduced GSH. This may, in turn, shift the equilibrium of the protein thiols remaining in the mixed protein-GSH disulfides toward more reduced forms, and enhance their binding to nucleic acids. This hypothesis is in accordance with the hypothesis proposed by Acker et al.[13,14,22] This hypothesis requires, however, intracellular subcompartmentalization of the oxygen-sensitive H_2O_2 generation, its reaction with reduced GSH and, finally, reaction of reduced GSH with regulatory nucleic acid binding proteins. GSH-related redox state is compartmentalized within cells with the ratio of GSSG/GSH higher within the endoplasmic reticulum where it serves in formation of protein disulfide bridges during protein synthesis than in cytosol.[29] The cytosolic and nuclear fractions contain the highest concentrations of the reduced GSH.[30]

The other possibility is that during normoxia, H_2O_2 generates hydroxyl radical (OH·) in the Fenton reaction catalyzed by intracellular iron. Hydroxyl radical could, in turn, react with protein thiol groups oxidizing them. This reaction would be inhibited during decreased concentrations of H_2O_2 (hypoxia), and also by administration of iron chelators, such as DF. In that case, DF should induce TH mRNA similarly to hypoxia. Indeed, in the absence of serum, DF induced TH mRNA, enhanced effects of hypoxia on TH mRNA, and the two effects were potentiating. Since DF did not affect H_2O_2 production, the result expected if it inhibits resynthesis of the heme-containing oxygen sensor, it is possible that effects of DF on TH mRNA result from inhibition of the OH· formation. Although it is not certain why DF effects vary depending on the presence or absence of serum in the cell culture media, it is likely that this difference results from the presence of iron ions in the serum.

The hypothesis suggesting the role of hydroxyl radicals in regulation of TH gene expression during hypoxia is potentially supported by the results of our experiments with cobalt. Although the initial hypothesis was that Co^{2+} locks oxygen sensor in the deoxy-conformation and in this mechanism decreases H_2O_2 production, it is clear from our experiments that cobalt stimulates TH gene expression before it affects H_2O_2 concentration. Thus, effects of cobalt on TH gene expression result from a different mechanism. Co^{2+}, similar to iron, is a transition metal catalyzing in vitro formation of OH· from H_2O_2 in the Fenton reaction. However, at physiologic pH values, Co^{2+} is actually unable to catalyze classic Fenton reaction in either the chemical or microsomal systems.[31] Moreover, under these conditions, Co^{2+} catalyzes production of superoxide rather than OH·.[31] Thus, under physiologic conditions, Co^{2+} may compete with iron in the Fenton reaction and, under sufficiently high concentrations of Co^{2+}, the superoxide ion is generated from the H_2O_2 rather than OH·. Thus, iron-dependent OH· formation is decreased leading to induction of TH gene expression. This hypothesis is supported by the observation that increasing concentrations of iron abolish Co^{2+}-dependent induction of TH mRNA. Again, subcompartmentalization of H_2O_2 generation, its involvement in Fenton reactions, and reaction between hydroxyl radicals and protein thiols must occur. Our results do not exclude the possibility that Co^{2+} and DF treatments regulate TH gene expression in a mechanism affecting resynthesis of the heme-containing oxygen sensor. However, they imply that both substances, as well as hypoxia, may affect TH gene expression in a mechanism that involves reactive oxygen intermediates (ROIs). Our laboratory continues work to identify the molecular mechanisms that regulate TH gene expression by the ROIs and redox state.

Acknowledgments

This work was supported by the NIH grant HL51078 HL58687 (MFC-K), American Heart Association Grant-in-Aid 9750110N (MFC-K), and NARSAD Young Investigator Award (MFC-K). SLK and WRP are supported by the NIH Training Grant HL 07571.

References

1. Fidone S, Gonzalez C, Yoshizaki K: Effects of low oxygen on the release of dopamine from the rabbit carotid body in vitro. *J Physiol* 333:93-110, 1982.
2. Fishman MC, Greene WL, Platika D: Oxygen chemoreception by carotid body cells in culture. *Proc Natl Acad Sci USA* 82:1448-1450, 1985.
3. Fidone S, Gonzalez C, Yoshizaki K: Effects of hypoxia on catecholamine synthesis in rabbit carotid body in vitro. *J Physiol* 333:81-91, 1982.
4. Hanbauer I, Lovenberg W, Costa E: Induction of tyrosine 3-monooxigenase in carotid body of rats exposed to hypoxic conditions. *Neuropharmacology* 16: 277-282, 1977.
5. Gonzalez C, Kwok Y, Gibb J, Fidone S: Effects of hypoxia on tyrosine hydroxylase activity in rat carotid body. *J Neurochem* 33:713-719, 1979.
6. Czyzyk-Krzeska MF, Bayliss DA, Lawson EE, Millhorn DE: Regulation of tyrosine hydroxylase gene expression in the rat carotid body by hypoxia. *J Neurochem* 58:1538-1546, 1992.
7. Zhu WH, Conforti L, Czyzyk-Krzeska MF, Millhorn DE: Hypoxia modulates excitation and dopamine secretion in PC12 cells through an O_2-sensitive K^+ current. *Am J Physiol* 271:C658-C665, 1996.

8. Feinsilver SH, Wong R, Rayabin DM: Adaptation of neurotransmitter synthesis to chronic hypoxia in cell culture. *Biochem Biophys Acta* 928:56-62, 1987.
9. Czyzyk-Krzeska MF, Furnari BA, Lawson EE, Millhorn DE: Hypoxia increases rate of transcription and stability of tyrosine hydroxylase mRNA in pheochromocytoma (PC12) cells. *J Biol Chem* 269:760-764, 1994.
10. Czyzyk-Krzeska MF, Dominski Z, Kole R, Millhorn DE: Hypoxia stimulates binding of a cytoplasmic protein to a pyrimidine rich sequence in the 3′-untranslated region of rat tyrosine hydroxylase mRNA. *J Biol Chem* 269:9940-9945, 1994.
11. Czyzyk-Krzeska MF, Beresh JE: Characterization of the hypoxia inducible protein binding site within the pyrimidine rich tract in the 3′ untranslated region of the tyrosine hydroxylase mRNA. *J Biol Chem* 271:3293-3299, 1996.
12. Norris ML, Millhorn DE: Hypoxia-induced protein binding to O_2-responsive sequences on the tyrosine hydroxylase gene. *J Biol Chem* 270:23774-23779, 1996.
13. Acker H, Boelling B, Delpiano MA, et al: The meaning of H_2O_2 generation in carotid body cells for Po_2 chemoreception. *J Autonom Nerv Sys* 41:41-52, 1992.
14. Acker H: Mechanisms and meaning of cellular oxygen sensing in the organism. *Resp Physiol* 95:1-10, 1994.
15. Meyer M, Schreck R, Baeuerle PA: H_2O_2 and antioxidants have opposite effects on activation of NF-kB and AP-1 in intact cells: AP-1 as secondary antioxidant-responsive factor. *EMBO J* 12:2005-2015, 1993.
16. Pantopoulos K, Hentze MW: Rapid responses to oxidative stress mediated by iron regulated protein. *EMBO J* 14:2917-2924, 1995.
17. Fandrey J, Frede S, Jelkman W: Role of hydrogen peroxide in hypoxia-induced erythropoietin production. *Biochem J* 303:507-510, 1994.
18. Cathcart R, Schwiers E, Ames BN: Detection of picomole levels of hydroperoxides using a fluorescent dichlorofluorescein assay. *Anal Biochem* 134:111-116, 1983.
19. Behl C, Davis JB, Lesley R, Schubert D: Hydrogen peroxide mediates amyloid β protein toxicity. *Cell* 77:817-827, 1994.
20. Goldberg MA, Dunning SP, Bunn HF: Regulation of the erythropoietin gene: evidence that the oxygen sensor is a heme protein. *Science* 242:1412-1415, 1988.
21. Grisham MB: *Reactive Metabolites of Oxygen and Nitrogen in Biology and Medicine.* Austin, TX: RG Landes Company; 20-28, 1992.
22. Acker H, Dufau E, Huber J, Sylvester D: Indications to an NADPH oxidase as a possible pO_2 sensor in the rat carotid body. *FEBS Lett* 256:75-78, 1989.
23. Grisham MB: *Reactive Metabolites of Oxygen and Nitrogen in Biology and Medicine.* Austin, TX: RG Landes Company; 47-55, 1992.
24. White CW, Jackson JH, McMurtry IF, Repine JE: Hypoxia increases glutathione redox cycle and protects lungs against oxidants. *J Appl Physiol* 65:2607-2615, 1988.
25. Abate C, Patel L, Rauschner III FJ, Curran T: Redox regulation of *fos* and *jun* DNA-binding activity in vitro. *Science* 249:1157-1161, 1990.
26. Abate C, Luk D, Gentz R, Rauschner III FJ, Curran T: Expression and purification of the leucine zipper and DNA-binding domains of fos and jun: both *fos* and *jun* contact DNA directly. *PNAS USA* 87:1032-1036, 1990.
27. Xanthoudakis S, Miao G, Wang R, et al: Redox activation of *fos-jun* DNA binding activity is mediated by a DNA repair enzyme. *EMBO J* 11:3323-3335, 1992.
28. Huang LE, Arany Z, Livingstone DM, Bunn HF: Activation of hypoxia inducible

transcription factor depends primarily upon redox sensitive stabilization of its α subunit. *J Biol Chem* 271:32253–32259, 1996.
29. Hwang C, Sinskey A, Lodish HF: Oxidized redox state of glutathione in the endoplasmic reticulum. *Science* 257:1496-1502, 1992.
30. Isaacs J, Binkley F: Glutathione dependent control of protein disulfide-sulfhydryl content by subcellular fractions of hepatic tissue. *Biochem Biophys Acta* 497: 192-204, 1977.
31. Kadiiska MB, Maples KR, Mason RP: A comparison of cobalt(II) and iron(II) hydroxyl and superoxide free radical formation. *Archiv Biochem Biophys* 275: 98-111, 1989.

Section 4

ION CHANNELS AND FUNCTIONAL RESPONSES TO HYPOXIA

Part 1

NEUROSECRETORY MECHANISMS

Chapter 11

Oxygen-Regulated Ion Channels:
Functional Roles and Mechanisms

José López-Barneo
Rafael Montoro
Patricia Ortegá-Sáenz
Juan Ureña

Introduction

Oxygen is a fundamental element on which most life forms depend. Provision of sufficient oxygen to the tissues and the protection of cells against damage due to the lack of oxygen are fundamental physiologic challenges. From bacteria to higher animals, there exists the capability of generating adaptive responses to hypoxia which help to minimize the deleterious effects of oxygen deficiency. Protracted hypoxia alters the cellular expression of genes encoding enzymes, hormones, and growth factors, constituting a widely operating system that, with a time course of hours or days, regulates the nonoxidative synthesis of adenosine triphosphate (ATP) and the utilization of oxygen, as well as its availability in the cell's immediate environment[1] (see Chapters 7-10). However, the survival of higher animals, and particularly of mammals, in acute hypoxia requires fast respiratory and cardiocirculatory adjustments that in the course of a few seconds restore or improve oxygen delivery to the most critical organs, such as the heart or the brain. Among these changes are, for example, hyperventilation and systemic arterial vasodilatation.

Although the systemic physiologic adaptations to hypoxic environments are well characterized, the molecular mechanisms underlying oxy-

From: López-Barneo, J and Weir, EK: *Oxygen Regulation of Ion Channels and Gene Expression.* Armonk, NY: Futura Publishing Company, Inc., ©1998.

gen sensing and how the variations of oxygen tension are translated into modifications of cellular excitability, secretory activity, or vascular contractility are poorly understood. In the past few years, it has become established that the activity of various types of ion channels can be regulated by oxygen tension in a time range of seconds.[2-4] Oxygen-regulated ion channels are believed to participate in the fast functional adjustments to low oxygen partial pressure (PO_2) and might be also involved in the sequence of events linking ambient oxygen tension and gene expression. In this chapter, we first review the role of ion channels in fast adaptations to low PO_2, with special emphasis in the cellular mechanisms underlying the transduction of the hypoxic stimulus in the arterial chemoreceptors. In the second part of this chapter, we discuss the possible mechanisms involved in oxygen sensing.

Oxygen-Sensitive Ion Channels and Stimulus-Secretion Coupling in Arterial Chemoreceptor Cells

The carotid bodies, the major arterial chemoreceptors, are among the best characterized oxygen-sensitive systems. These bilateral organs are capable of sensing arterial PO_2 and activating the brainstem respiratory centers to produce hyperventilation in response to low PO_2.[5,6] Research on the cellular mechanisms underlying arterial chemoreception has significantly progressed in the past few years following the discovery that the dopamine-containing glomus cells of the carotid body are electrically excitable[7,8] and have oxygen-regulated potassium (K^+) channels.[8-13] Since glomus cells were known to form afferent synapses with nerve fibers terminating in the petrosal ganglion, these electrophysiologic observations gave strong support to a model of chemotransduction that considers the carotid body to be a secondary sensory receptor with a sensory element (the glomus cell) interposed between the physiologic stimulus (the decrease of arterial PO_2) and the afferent nerve fibers.[14] As indicated below, more recent experiments in dispersed glomus cells of several mammalian species have demonstrated that they can behave as presynaptic-like elements where hypoxia induces a calcium (Ca^{2+})-dependent neurosecretory response.[14-17]

The major oxygen-dependent properties of isolated rabbit glomus cells are illustrated in Figure 1. Part A shows the current recorded from a membrane patch containing two functional oxygen-sensitive K^+ channels activated by membrane depolarization. Note that the open probability and the time that the channels are open decrease during exposure to hypoxia, although the single-channel current amplitude is unaffected. Inhibition of the K^+ conductance by low Po_2 leads to the increase of cellular excitability, which is manifested in current-clamped cells as an augmentation of the action potential firing frequency (Figure 1B). Because the large action potentials of rabbit glomus cells are due to the activation of sodium (Na^+) and Ca^{2+} channels,[8,18] increase in the cell's firing frequency is expected to produce a rise of cytosolic [Ca^{2+}]. Figure 1C shows in a unclamped cell loaded with the Ca^{2+} indicator Fura 2 that hypoxia produces a dose-dependent elevation of cytosolic [Ca^{2+}]. The relationship between the maximal cytosolic [Ca^{2+}] and the Po_2 level is plotted in Figure 1D. This relationship has a hyperbole-like shape that resembles the curve describing the Po_2 dependence of the discharge rate of the afferent nerve fibers in preparations of the entire carotid body.[5] The inset on panel 1D in Figure 1 shows that the hypoxia-induced rise of cytosolic [Ca^{2+}] is completely abolished upon removal of external Ca^{2+}. The neurosecretory response to hypoxia of a single, Fura 2-loaded, glomus cell is illustrated in Figure 2. Low Po_2 produces the typical rise of cytosolic [Ca^{2+}] that after reaching a threshold level of 150 nM triggers the release of dopamine. In this experiment, dopamine release was detected by amperometry and each spike in the recording represents the fusion of a single secretory vesicle.[15,17] Thus, the responses to low Po_2 in a single glomus cell are very similar to those observed in the entire carotid body and, therefore, it can be suggested that the oxygen-sensitive properties of glomus cells have an important role in the function of the entire organ.

Although the presynaptic-like secretory behavior of glomus cells can explain many features of sensory transduction in the carotid body, it must be kept in mind that other oxygen-sensitive mechanisms may also contribute to the detection of the changes in Po_2. Some authors have proposed the mitochondria as oxygen sensors in glomus cells,[19] capable of releasing the Ca^{2+} necessary for the secretory response to hypoxia.[20] In contrast with this proposal, it has been shown that the hypoxia-induced rise of Ca^{2+} in glomus cells depends almost exclusively on Ca^{2+} entry through voltage-gated channels[14-17] (Figure 1). However, a possible participation of mitochondria in chemotransduction is still compatible with the electrophysiologic observations, since these organella are known to contribute to the generation of oxygen radicals which could regulate membrane ionic permeability (see below). Other considerations relevant to the understanding of arterial chemotransduction are the variability of the electrophysiologic properties of glomus cells among the various species studied. This indicates that, although following a similar general scheme, some aspects of oxygen sensing may change in different animals. Most rabbit glomus cells have a high density of Na^+ channels and can generate action potentials of large amplitude repetitively.[18] In these same cells, low Po_2

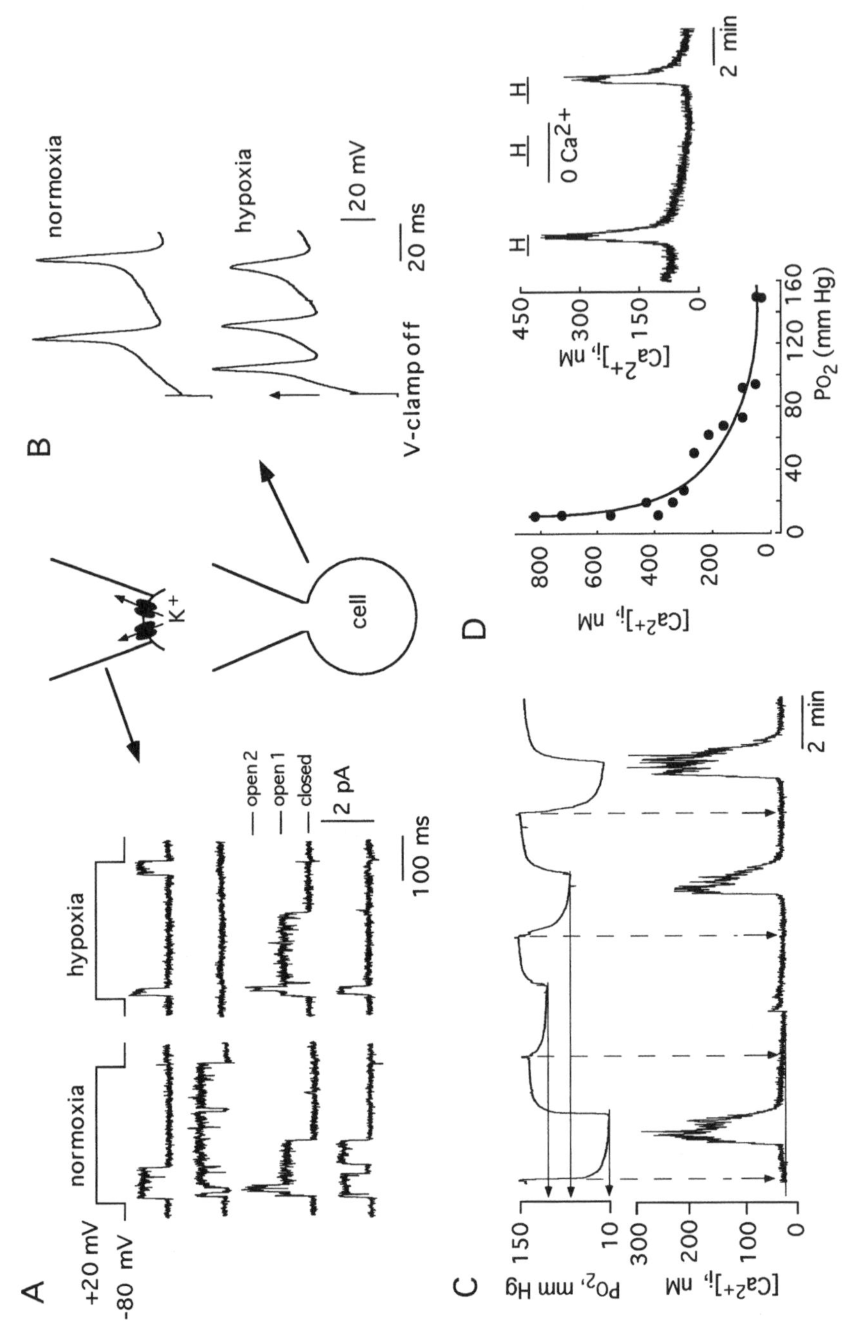
A
+20 mV
-80 mV
normoxia
hypoxia
open 2
open 1
closed
2 pA
100 ms
K+
cell
B
normoxia
hypoxia
20 mV
20 ms
V-clamp off
C
PO2, mm Hg
150
10
[Ca2+]i, nM
300
200
100
0
2 min
D
[Ca2+]i, nM
800
600
400
200
0
0
40
80
120
160
PO2 (mm Hg)
[Ca2+]i, nM
450
300
150
0
H
H
H
0 Ca2+
2 min

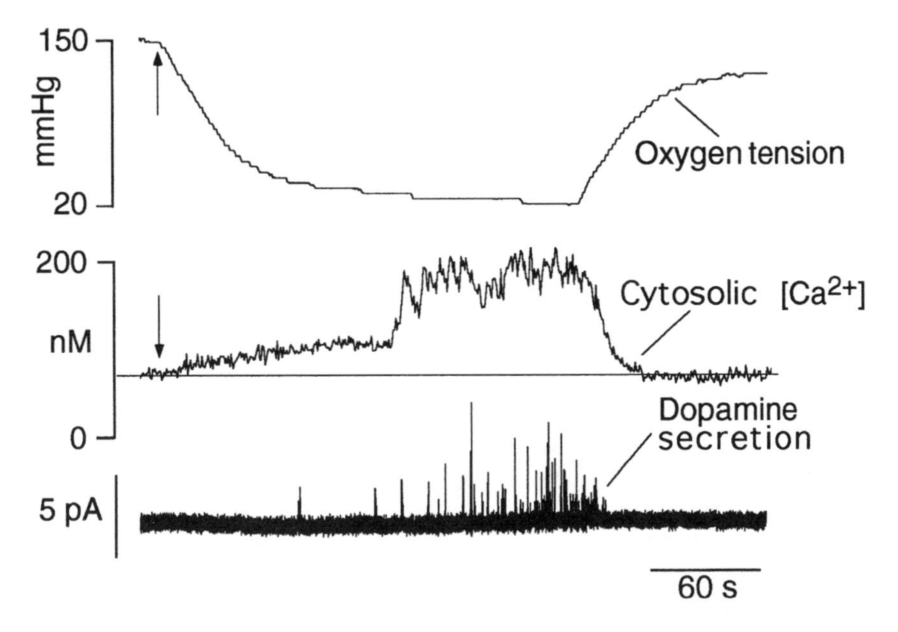

Figure 2. Neurosecretory response to hypoxia of a single glomus cell. The recordings illustrate the parallel changes of oxygen tension, cytosolic Ca^{2+}, and dopamine release. (Modified with permission from Reference 17.)

seems to inhibit the calcium channels at membrane potentials near threshold.[17] Since the most common oxygen-sensitive K^+ channels in rabbit glomus cells are voltage dependent, it is likely that, in situ, the cells which are spontaneously active in normoxic conditions are those most capable of converting reductions of Po_2 into the corresponding increases in firing frequency.[3] In fact, it is well known from previous work done in cats and rabbits that in normoxic, or even hyperoxic, conditions most sensory fibers of the sinus nerve exhibit a tonic resting firing, which is increased upon

Figure 1. Major oxygen-dependent cellular variables in rabbit glomus cells. **A.** Inhibition of oxygen-sensitive delayed rectifier K^+ channels by low Po_2. Recordings from a patch containing two active channels. **B.** Increase of action potential firing frequency in response to low Po_2 in a current-clamped glomus cell. Switching from voltage- to current-clamp is indicated by the **vertical arrow**. **C.** Rise of cytosolic Ca^{2+} in a Fura 2-loaded glomus cell exposed to various levels of hypoxia. The relationship between cytosolic $[Ca^{2+}]$ and Po_2 is indicated in **D.** The **inset** shows that the hypoxia (H)-induced rise of cytosolic Ca^{2+} depends on extracellular Ca^{2+}. (Modified with permission from References 15, 17, 18, and 47.)

exposure to low Po_2. We have explored whether, besides the delayed rectifier channels, there are other oxygen-sensitive K^+ channels in rabbit glomus cells, with negative or inconclusive results. In contrast with these properties of rabbit cells, rat glomus cells appear to lack Na^+ channels, do not seem to fire fast-action potentials spontaneously, and contain oxygen-sensitive Ca^{2+}-activated K^+ channels.[9,10] In these cells, hypoxia seems to produce a membrane depolarization, or "receptor" potential, which causes the opening of voltage-gated Ca^{2+} channels.[16] An oxygen-sensitive "resting" K^+ conductance, whose inhibition in low Po_2 could produce this receptor potential, has recently been described in rat glomus cells (see Chapter 12).[21] Finally, it must also be remembered that the carotid body has a highly sophisticated structure[5] and, therefore, its behavior surely depends, in addition to the oxygen-sensitive mechanisms, on autocrine and paracrine interactions between its various cellular constituents. Dopamine, one of the major transmitters stored in glomus cell granules, can inhibit the hypoxic response of carotid bodies,[22] which can be explained by the existence of autoreceptors that inhibit the calcium channels.[23] Thus, it seems that dopamine exerts an autocrine inhibition that imposes a limit to the hypoxic secretory response of glomus cells. Other aspects of carotid body physiology, such as the nature of the transmitter that activates the afferent sensory fibers or the properties of the glomus cell-afferent fiber synapse, are practically unexplored.

Ion Channels and Fast Cellular Responses to Hypoxia

Since oxygen-sensitive K^+ channels were found in carotid body glomus cells, other oxygen-regulated K^+, Ca^{2+}, or Na^+ conductances have been observed in several tissues. The various types of oxygen-sensitive ionic conductances described so far are summarized in the Table. ATP-regulated K^+ channels, existing in smooth and heart muscle as well as in other cells, although under indirect control of oxygen tension, are not included in the table (see Chapter 20). In most of the studies, the oxygen-sensitive ionic conductances were characterized in voltage- and current-clamped cells, including, in some cases, analysis at the single-channel level. In some preparations,[14-17,27,31,33] the electrophysiologic effects of low Po_2 have been complemented by the measurement of intracellular $[Ca^{2+}]$. Note that low Po_2 can either inhibit or potentiate channel activity. The bidirectional regulation of channel activity is possibly advantageous because it adds versatility to the electrophysiologic mechanisms that the various cell types may use in their strategies to adapt or respond to low

Table

O_2-Sensitive Ionic Conductances in Mammalian Cells. Effects of Low P_{O_2}.

1. **Carotid body glomus cells**
   - Adult rabbit
     - Delayed rectifier K^+ (inhibition)[8,9,11,13]
     - High voltage activated Ca^{2+} (inhibition at negative Vm)[17]
   - Adult rat
     - Ca^{2+}-activated K^+ (inhibition)[10]
     - Delayed rectifier K^+ in chronically hypoxic animals (inhibition)[24]
     - Resting or "leaky" K^+ (inhibition)[21]
2. **Cells in neuroepithelial bodies of lungs**
   - Delayed rectifier K^+, rat (inhibition)[25]
3. **Chromaffin cells**
   - Delayed rectifier K^+ in fetal adrenal medulla (inhibition), membrane depolarization[26]
   - Delayed rectifier K^+ in pheochromocytoma cells (PC12) (inhibition)[27]
4. **Vascular smooth muscle**
   - Lung arterial tree
     - Delayed rectifier K^+, canine and cat resistance myocytes (inhibition)[4,28–30]
     - L-type Ca^{2+}, rabbit resistance myocytes (potentiation at negative Vm)[31]
     - L-type Ca^{2+}, rabbit conduit and resistance myocytes (inhibition at negative Vm)[31]
     - Ca^{2+}-activated K^+, sheep fetus, lung pulmonary artery (inhibition)[32]
   - Systemic myocytes
     - L-type Ca^{2+}, rabbit (inhibition at negative Vm)[33]
     - Ca^{2+}, rat (inhibition)[34]
   - Ductus arteriosus
     - Delayed rectifier K^+, in sheep fetus (potentiation)[35]
5. **Heart muscle**
   - Non-inactivating Na^+, rat (potentiation)[36]
   - Recombinant α_{1c} cardiac L-type calcium channel, HEK cells (inhibition)[37]
6. **Central neurons**
   - Ca^{2+} and ATP-dependent K^+, rat neocortex and substantia nigra (inhibition)[38]
   - Voltage-dependent Na^+, rat neocortex (inhibition)[39]

P_{O_2}. Therefore, it seems clear that oxygen sensing by ion channels is a widely operating mechanism participating in many fast cellular adaptive responses to hypoxia. Besides the participation in arterial chemotransduction discussed above, oxygen-sensitive ion channels appear to be also involved in several cardiocirculatory and respiratory responses to low P_{O_2} in fetal and adult life, as well as during adaptation to air breathing in the newborn.[25-35] Furthermore, oxygen-sensitive ion channels may participate in the pathophysiology of abnormal states such as hypertension, cardiac arrhythmias, or ischemic neuronal damage[3,4,36,38,39] (see Chapters 13-19).

Mechanisms of Oxygen Sensing by Ion Channels

As pointed out in the preceding section, the progress in research on oxygen-regulated ion channels has yielded a collection of observations describing new oxygen-sensitive channels and/or cellular phenomena where they may play a role. However, the molecular nature of the mechanisms underlying oxygen sensing and how the change of Po_2 modifies channel activity are questions that appear to be rather elusive and remain essentially unknown. Our own experience with carotid body and vascular smooth muscle cells indicates that the oxygen sensors are rather labile and easily altered by cell dissociation procedures. Moreover, the oxygen-sensing processes may depend on subtle physico-chemical changes difficult to detect and characterize, or to distinguish from other alterations induced by the experimental protocol. This may also be the reason why the oxygen sensors that regulate the expression of erythropoietin and other mammalian genes, although intensively investigated, have not been yet identified.[1] The only well-characterized oxygen-sensor molecule is the heme protein Fix L which mediates the expression of the nitrogen fixation genes in bacteria grown in hypoxic environments[1,40] (see Chapter 4). In what follows, we discuss the possible mechanisms whereby changes of oxygen tension may be coupled to ion channel gating.

Redox Modulation of K^+ Channel Gating

An attractive hypothesis is that the modifications of oxygen tension are linked to channel activity through variations in the concentration of oxidants or reductants which modify the redox state of thiol groups in the channel molecule. In fact, the possible participation of hydrogen peroxide (H_2O_2) and other oxygen metabolites in the regulation of membrane cationic permeabilities was already postulated a long time ago.[41] More recently, it has been proposed that redox-based mechanisms participate in oxygen sensing by carotid body[42] or pulmonary smooth muscle[43] cells (see Chapter 16). In accord with these ideas, it has been shown in both carotid body cells[44] and pulmonary arterial myocytes[45,46] that reductants, such as reduced glutathione (GSH) or dithiothreitol (DTT), can mimic the effect of hypoxia on the oxygen-regulated K^+ channels. The redox regulation of a single oxygen-sensitive K^+ channel recorded in a glomus cell membrane patch is illustrated in Figure 3. Application of GSH to the internal face of the membrane produces a reversible reduction of channel open probability due to the increase in the number of records without openings and the decrease in the number of bursts per trace (Figure 3A). The mean burst duration (≈ 22 ms at +20 mV, not shown) or the single-channel conductance (≈ 20 pS in standard K^+ concentrations) is unaltered by GSH. Figure 3B shows that addition of GSH also results in a marked increase in the first latency of channel opening (indicated by the vertical arrows in the figure). This effect is further illustrated in Figure 3C with a cumulative first latency histogram. These alterations of the single-channel parameters can explain the decrease of macroscopic K^+ currents by GSH or DTT in glomus cells.[44] Interestingly, internally applied GSH has an effect very similar to hypoxia in these same channels[47]: increase in the number of blank records and first latency and decrease in the number of bursts in each trace. Both hypoxia and reductants leave the single-channel conductance unaltered. Figure 4 shows macroscopic K^+ currents recorded from two patch-clamped glomus cells and the alterations induced by external application of a reductant (DTT) and an oxidant (DTNB) (Figure 4A). These agents produce a reversible reduction or increase of current amplitude, respectively, even with 2 mM DTT added to the internal solution to buffer the intracellular redox state (Figure 4B). Therefore, the K^+ channels can be regulated by redox agents acting from either the external or the internal faces of the membrane.

Most voltage-dependent ion channels contain amino acid residues, particularly cysteine, susceptible of redox modification which are accessible to oxidants or reductants in the bulk of the solutions. In some recombinant K^+ channels, the redox state of cysteines in the amino-terminal of the α subunits or in some auxiliary β subunits regulates inactivation[48,49] (see Chapter 3). Hence, it was thought that redox regulation could be a particular property of some channels related with the sensitivity to Po_2.[44,50] However, it has recently been shown that generation of oxygen radicals can influence the activity of a broad spectrum of K^+ channels.[51] In addition, we have observed that *Shaker B* channels, which are representative of the Kv1 family of voltage-dependent K^+ channels, are also regulated by the redox state. In *Shaker B* channels with deletions of the amino-terminal (*Shaker B Δ6-46*) expressed in carbohydrate (CHO) cells, application of GSH (0.5 to 2 mM) at the internal face of the membrane produces a decrease of the size of the current and a marked deceleration of activation time course (Figure 5A). In these same channels, H_2O_2 has the opposite effect: increase of current amplitude and acceleration of activation time course (Figure 5B). As illustrated in Figure 5C, each α subunit of the *Shaker B Δ6-46* channels contain seven cysteine residues which could be the target

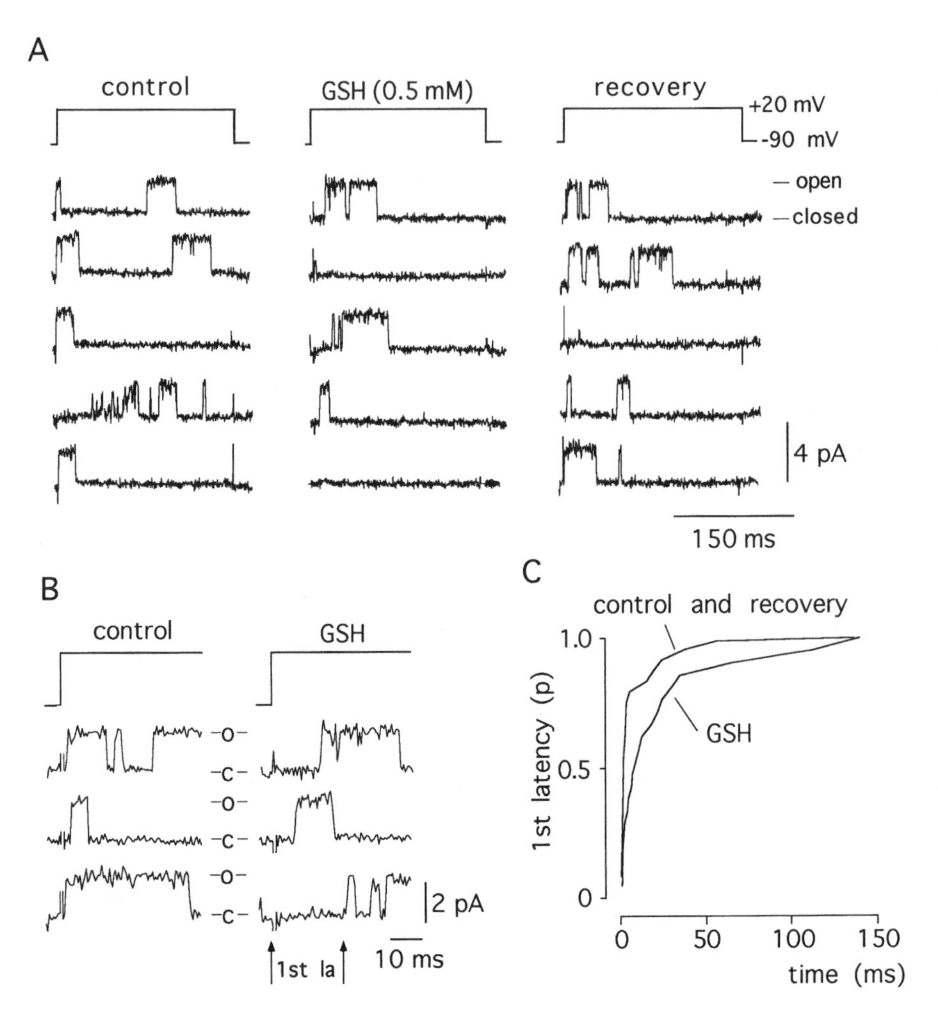

Figure 3. Modulation of a single oxygen-regulated K^+ channel by the application of reduced glutathione (GSH, 0.5 mM) to the internal face of the membrane. **A.** Representative recordings obtained by membrane depolarization to +20 mV. **B.** Modification of the activation latency (first latency) by GSH. **C.** Cumulative histogram of first latency showing the effect of GSH. Blank records are not considered. **Ordinate** represents the probability that the first latency value is ≤ t in the abscissa. The median first latency (2.5 ms in the standard experimental conditions) increased to 7.5 ms upon exposure to GSH. The concentrations of K^+ were 2.7 mM and 140 mM in the external and internal solutions, respectively.

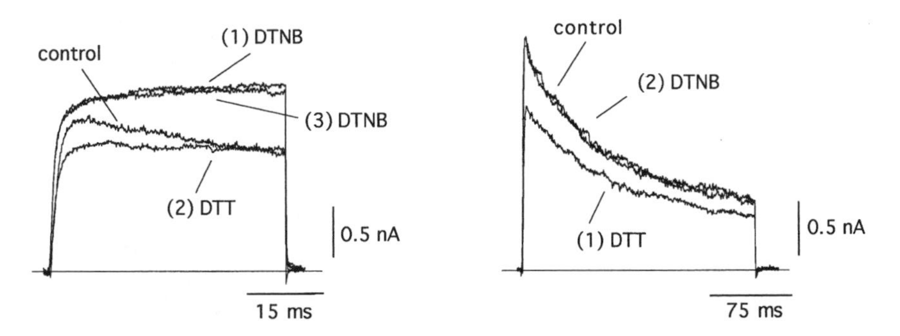

Figure 4. Redox regulation of the macroscopic K^+ currents of rabbit glomus cells. **A.** Currents recorded during depolarizing pulses to +20 mV in the standard solution (control) and after addition of dithiothreitiol (DTT, 2 mM) or 5-5′dithiobis (2-nitrobenzoic acid) (DTNB, 0.1 mM) to the bath. **B.** Recordings from a different cell where 2 mM DTT was added to the internal solution. The **numbers between parentheses** indicate in each case the order of application of the solutions. The concentrations of K^+ were 2.7 mM and 140 mM in the external and internal solutions, respectively. Holding potential, −80 mV.

of redox modification. Our preliminary experiments done with mutated *Shaker B* channels indicate that the sulfhydryl groups of cysteines mediate, at least in part, the redox regulation of the channels. Therefore, the changes produced by redox reagents in *Shaker* and the native oxygen-regulated K^+ channels are similar to those observed upon exposure of glomus cells to hypoxia. Hence, it is plausible that some of the Po_2-dependent effects observed in the various oxygen-sensitive K^+ channels studied are due to changes in the production of oxygen radicals which modify the redox state of the channel protein (see below).

Recapitulation of Mechanisms and Alternatives

Regulation Through Intermediate Oxygen Radicals

If the concentration of oxygen radicals mediates the effect of variations of Po_2 on the ion channels, the questions that arise are: Where the radicals are produced and how do they interact with specific channel types. A general mechanism possibly operating in all cells is the produc-

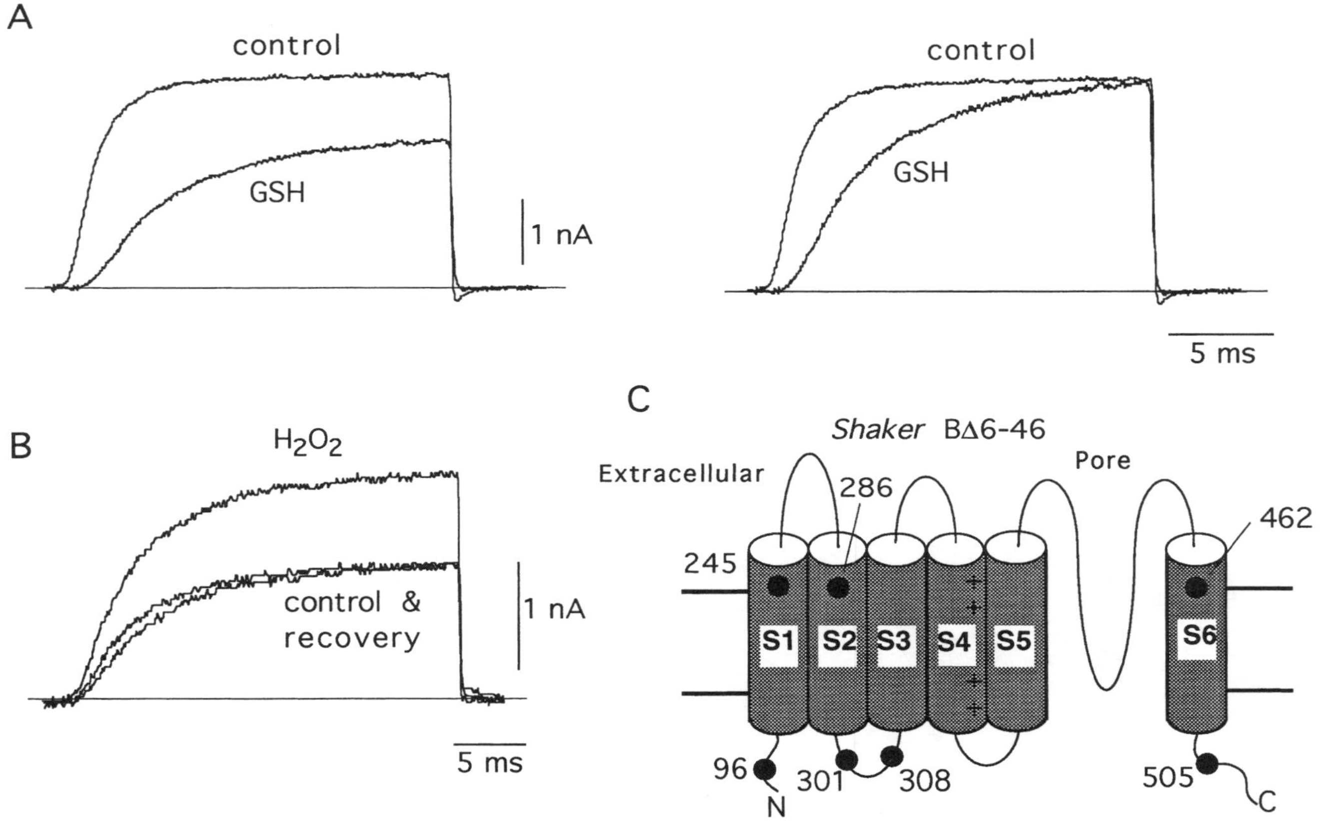
A
control
GSH
1 nA
control
GSH
5 ms
B
H_2O_2
control & recovery
1 nA
5 ms
C
Shaker BΔ6-46
Extracellular
Pore
286
462
245
S1
S2
S3
S4
S5
S6
96
N
301
308
505
C

tion of radicals in cytosolic organella, such as mitochondria or peroxisomes, which can interact with ion channels and other proteins. However, in the cell types that exhibit a special sensitivity to Po_2 changes (for instance glomus and neuroepithelial cells or pulmonary arterial smooth muscle), the existence of specific membrane-bound oxidases associated with the ion channels and capable of generating the reactive species in the vicinity of the target residues has been postulated. Among the proposed candidates are cytochrome b oxidases similar to the nicotinamide adenine dinucleotide phosphate (NADPH) oxidase of neutrophils[25,42,52] or the family of cytochrome P-450 oxidases.[53] The putative oxygen-sensing oxidase could be coexpressed with the main pore-forming α subunit as an auxiliary subunit, thus, conferring oxygen sensitivity on the channels[42] (see Chapter 2). In fact, the K^+ channel β subunits already cloned have about 30% to 40% sequence identity with a broad family of oxido-reductases which suggests that they may share a common ancestral origin.[54]

In favor of the critical role of oxido-reductases in the regulation of the oxygen-sensitive cellular functions are the pharmacologic effects of diphenylene iodonium (DPI), which is a potent inhibitor of a variety of flavoproteins, that can also inhibit the response to hypoxia of carotid body and neuroepithelial cells as well as the induction of erythropoietin and other genes.[25,42,55] We have also recently observed that DPI mimics the effect of hypoxia, increasing cytosolic Ca^{2+} in glomus cells in a manner that is dependent on external Ca^{2+}. However, there are doubts regarding the specificity of the effect of DPI on the various cell types. DPI reduces the amplitude of Ca^{2+} and K^+ currents in pulmonary smooth muscle and neonatal rat glomus cells[56,57] and can also reversibly inhibit the activity of recombinant *Shaker B* channels expressed in CHO cells (Ortega-Sáenz and López-Barneo, unpublished results).

◄———

Figure 5. Redox regulation of recombinant *Shaker* B Δ6-46 K^+ channels expressed in Chinese hamster ovary (CHO) cells. **A.** Superposition of representative recordings of K^+ currents obtained during depolarization to +20 mV with the standard internal solution and with 2.5 mM glutathione (GSH) added. The scaled currents in the **panel at right** indicate that besides the reduction of current amplitude, GSH produces a marked deceleration of activation kinetics. At this voltage, the time to reach half maximal activation (≈ 2 ms in the control solutions) increased to 4.1 ms in the presence of GSH. **B.** In a different cell application of hydrogen peroxide (H_2O_2) (0.1%) produced a reversible increase in current amplitude. Pulses were applied to −10 mV from a holding potential of −80 mV. The concentrations of K^+ were 2.7 mM and 140 mM in the external and internal solutions, respectively. **C.** Proposed secondary structure of K^+ channel α subunits with indication of the position of cysteine residues in *Shaker* B channels.

Allosteric Regulation

The reversible regulation of ion channel activity by P_{O_2} appears to be resistant to intracellular dialysis and in some preparations, it can be also observed in excised membrane patches.[12,38] These facts suggest that the interaction of oxygen with the channels is a membrane delimited mechanism. The redox-based sensors require as substrates regenerating redox pairs, such as NAD(P)/NAD(P)H, that unless they are concentrated somewhere near the membrane should be washed out during the whole-cell patch-clamp experiments. It is, therefore, conceivable that independent of the redox modulation of channel activity, there are oxygen sensors associated with the ion channels capable of undergoing conformational changes during oxygenation and deoxygenation and, thus, modifying allosterically the channel's kinetic properties.[2] The best candidates for this kind of regulation are membrane-bound heme proteins, such as the cloned oxygen sensor of *Rhizobium meliloti* (Fix L), that can change catalytic activity according to its oxygenated state.[1,40] Interestingly, the oxygenation state of hemoglobin, associated with the internal face of the membrane, is also known to alter the ion transport properties of erythrocytes.[58]

Direct Oxygen Sensing by the Pore-Forming Channel Subunits

Another possibility to consider is the existence of structural domains in some of the main pore-forming channel subunits that can bind reversibly molecular oxygen.[2] We have tested this hypothesis with various recombinant K^+ channel α subunits expressed in CHO cells and obtained conflicting results. In preliminary experiments, we observed that hypoxia could reversibly reduce the amplitude of the macroscopic K^+ currents. However, the variability of the results lead us to realize that, besides oxygen tension, other variables might also be altered during the experimental protocol. For instance, a nonuniform bubbling of the solutions can produce small fluctuations of their osmolarity causing appreciable changes in the amplitude and kinetics of the currents. In the context of this discussion, a recent paper describing that the activity of recombinant L-type Ca^{2+} channels, resulting from the stable expression of the cardiac α_{1c} subunit in HEK cells can be reversibly inhibited by lowering P_{O_2} appears to be of special interest.[37] These findings are of particular relevance because they suggest that the oxygen-sensing domain could be in the channel-forming subunit. In addition, the stably transfected HEK cells may represent an ideal preparation where molecular biology and electrophysiologic techniques can be combined to investigate the physico-chemical processes underlying oxygen sensing by ion channels.[59]

In conclusion, oxygen-regulated ion channels are involved in the fast cellular responses to hypoxia. These channels appear to be regulated by oxygen tension; however, the oxygen-sensing mechanisms and how oxygen influences channel activity remain unknown. Several possible forms of interaction of oxygen with the ion channels, which may well act in parallel, are discussed. Oxygen sensing by ion channels and the oxygen-dependent regulation of gene expression are possibly related phenomena, acting in different time ranges, that may share similar basic principles and mechanisms.

Acknowledgments

The work in our laboratory is supported by the Dirección General de Investigación Científica y Técnica (DGICYT) of the Spanish Ministry of Science and Education and the Andalusian Government.

References

1. Bunn HF, Poyton RO: Oxygen sensing and molecular adaptations to hypoxia. *Physiol Rev* 76:839-885, 1996.
2. López-Barneo J: Oxygen-sensitive ion channels: how ubiquitous are they? *Trends Neurosci* 17:133-135, 1994.
3. López-Barneo J: Oxygen-sensing by ion channels and the regulation of cellular functions. *Trends Neurosci* 19:435-440, 1996.
4. Weir EK, Archer SL: The mechanism of acute hypoxic pulmonary vasoconstriction: the tale of two channels. *FASEB J* 9:183-189, 1995.
5. Gonzalez C, Almaraz L, Obeso A, et al: Carotid body chemoreceptors: from natural stimuli to sensory discharges. *Physiol Rev* 74:829-898, 1994.
6. Peers C: O_2 sensing by the carotid body. *Prim Sensory Neuron* 1:197-208, 1996.
7. Duchen MR, Caddy KWT, Kirby GC, et al: Biophysical studies of the cellular elements of the rabbit carotid body. *Neuroscience* 26:291-311, 1988.
8. López-Barneo J, López-López JR, Ureña J, et al: Chemotransduction in the carotid body: K^+ current modulated by Po_2 in type I chemoreceptor cells. *Science* 242: 580-582, 1988.
9. Delpiano MA, Hescheler J: Evidence for a Po_2-sensitive K^+ channel in the type I cell of the carotid body. *FEBS Lett* 249:195-198, 1989.
10. Peers C: Hypoxic supression of K^+ currents in type I carotid body cells: selective effect on the Ca^{2+}-activated K^+ current. *Neurosci Lett* 119:253-256, 1990.
11. Stea A, Nurse CA: Whole-cell and perforated patch recordings from O_2-sensitive rat carotid body cells grown in short- and long-term culture. *Pflügers Arch* 418: 93-101, 1991.
12. Ganfornina MD, López-Barneo J: Single K^+ channels in membrane patches of

arterial chemoreceptor cells are modulated by O_2 tension. *Proc Natl Acad Sci USA* 88:2927-2930, 1991.
13. Ganfornina MD, López-Barneo J: Potassium channel types in arterial chemoreceptor cells and their selective modulation by oxygen. *J Gen Physiol* 100:401-426, 1992.
14. López-Barneo J, Benot AR, Ureña J: Oxygen sensing and the electrophysiology of arterial chemoreceptor cells. *News Physiol Sci* 8:191-195, 1993.
15. Ureña J, Fernández-Chacón R, Benot AR, et al: Hypoxia induces voltage-dependent Ca^{2+} entry and quantal dopamine secretion in carotid body glomus cells. *Proc Natl Acad Sci USA* 91:10208-10211, 1994.
16. Buckler KJ, Vaughan-Jones RD: Effects of hypoxia on membrane potential and intracellular calcium in rat neonatal carotid body type I cells. *J Physiol* 476:423-428, 1994.
17. Montoro RJ, Ureña, J, Fernández-Chacón R, et al: Oxygen sensing by ion channels and chemoreception in single glomus cell. *J Gen Physiol* 107:133-143, 1996.
18. López-López JR, González C, Ureña J, et al: Low Po_2 selectively inhibits K channel activity in chemoreceptor cells of the mammalian carotid body. *J Gen Physiol* 93:1001-1015, 1989.
19. Lahiri S: Chromophores in O_2 chemoreception: the carotid body model. *News Physiol Sci* 9:161-165, 1994.
20. Biscoe TJ, Duchen MR: Responses of type I cells dissociated from the rabbit carotid body to hypoxia. *J Physiol* 428:39-59, 1990.
21. Buckler KJ: A novel oxygen-sensitive potassium current in rat carotid body type I cells. *J Physiol* 498:649-662, 1997.
22. Donnelly DF, Smith EJ, Dutton RE: Neural response of carotid body chemoreceptors following dopamine blockade. *J Appl Physiol* 50:172-177, 1981.
23. Benot AR, López-Barneo J: Feedback inhibition of Ca^{2+} currents by dopamine in glomus cells of the carotid body. *Eur J Neurosci* 2:809-812, 1990.
24. Wyatt CN, Wright C, Bee D, et al: O_2-sensitive K^+ currents in carotid body chemoreceptor cells from normoxic and chronically hypoxic rats and their roles in hypoxic chemotransduction. *Proc Natl Acad Sci USA* 92:295-299, 1995.
25. Joungson C, Nurse C, Yeger H, et al: Oxygen sensing in airway chemoreceptors. *Nature* 365:153-155, 1993.
26. Thompson RJ, Jackson A, Nurse CA: Developmental loss of hypoxic chemosensitivity in rat adrenomedullary chromaffin cells. *J Physiol* 498:503-510, 1997.
27. Zhu WH, Conforti L, Czyzyk-Krzeska MF, et al: Membrane depolarization in PC-12 cells during hypoxia is regulated by an O_2-sensitive K^+ current. *Am J Physiol* 271:C658-C665, 1996.
28. Post JM, Hume JR, Archer SL, et al: Direct role for potassium channel inhibition in hypoxic pulmonary vasoconstriction. *Am J Physiol* 262:C882-C890, 1992.
29. Yuan X, Goldman WF, Tod ML, et al: Hypoxia reduces potassium currents in cultured rat pulmonary but not mesenteric arterial myocytes. *Am J Physiol* 264: L116-L123, 1993.
30. Archer SL, Huang JMC, Reeve HL, et al: Differential distribution of electrophysiologically distinct myocytes in conduit and resistance arteries determines their response to nitric oxide and hypoxia. *Circ Res* 78:431-442, 1996.
31. Franco-Obregón A, López-Barneo J: Differential oxygen sensitivity of calcium channels in rabbit smooth muscle cells of conduit and resistance pulmonary arteries. *J Physiol* 491:511-518, 1996.

32. Cornfield DN, Reeve HL, Tolarova S, et al: Oxygen causes fetal pulmonary vasodilation through activation of a calcium-dependent potassium channel. *Proc Natl Acad Sci USA* 93:8089-8094, 1996.
33. Franco-Obregón A, Ureña J, López-Barneo J: Oxygen-sensitive calcium channels in vascular smooth muscle and their possible role in hypoxic arterial relaxation. *Proc Natl Acad Sci USA* 92:4715-4719, 1995.
34. Soloviev AI, Stefanov AV, Baziliyk OV, et al: Changes in plasma membrane ionic permeability and related contractile responses in vascular smooth muscle at hypoxia. *Pathophysiology* 3:11-20, 1996.
35. Tristani-Firouzi M, Reeve HL, Tolarova S, et al: Oxygen-induced constriction of rabbit ductus arteriosus occurs via inhibition of a 4-aminopyridine-, voltage-sensitive potassium channel. *J Clin Invest* 98:1959-1965, 1996.
36. Ju Y-K, Saint DA, Gage PW: Hypoxia increases persistent sodium current in rat ventricular myocytes. *J Physiol* 497:337-347, 1996.
37. Fearon IM, Palmer ACV, Balmforth AJ, et al: Hypoxia inhibits the recombinant $\alpha 1$c subunit of the human cardiac L-type Ca^{2+} channel. *J Physiol* 500:551–556, 1997.
38. Jiang C, Haddad GH: A direct mechanism for sensing low oxygen levels in central neurons. *Proc Natl Acad Sci USA* 91:7198-7201, 1994.
39. Cummins TR, Jiang C, Haddad GG: Human neocortical excitability is decreased during anoxia via sodium channel modulation. *J Clin Invest* 91:608-615, 1993.
40. Gilles-González MA, Ditta S, Helinski DR: A hemprotein with kinase activity encoded by the oxygen sensor of *Rhizobium meliloti. Nature* 350:170-172, 1991.
41. Sies H: Peroxisomal enzymes and oxygen metabolism in liver. In: Reivich M, et al (eds). *Tissue Hypoxia and Ischemia.* New York: Plenum Publishing Corp.; 51-66, 1977.
42. Acker H, Huber D, Silvester D: Indications to an NAD(P)H oxidase as a possible PO_2 sensor in the rat carotid body. *FEBS Lett* 256:75-78, 1989.
43. Archer SL, Huang J, Henry T, et al: A redox-based O_2 sensor in rat pulmonary vasculature. *Circ Res* 73:1100-1112, 1993.
44. Benot A, Ganfornina MD, López-Barneo J: Potassium channel modulated by hypoxia and the redox status in glomus cells of the carotid body. In: Weir EK, et al (eds). *Ion Flux in Pulmonary Vascular Control.* New York: Plenum Publishing Corp.; 177-187, 1993.
45. Yuan X, Tod ML, Rubin LJ, et al: Deoxyglucose and reduced glutathione mimic the effect of hypoxia on K^+ and Ca^{2+} conductances in pulmonary artery cells. *Am J Physiol* 267:L52-L63, 1994.
46. Post JM, Weir EK, Archer SL, et al: Redox regulation of K^+ channels and hypoxic pulmonary vasoconstriction. In: Weir EK, et al (eds). *Ion Flux in Pulmonary Vascular Control.* New York: Plenum Publishing Corp.; 189-204, 1993.
47. Ganfornina D, López-Barneo J: Gating of O_2-sensitive K^+ channels of arterial chemoreceptor cells and kinetic modifications induced by low Po_2. *J Gen Physiol* 100:427-455, 1992.
48. Ruppersberg JP, Stocker M, Pongs O, et al: Regulation of fast inactivation of cloned mammalian IK(A) channels by cysteine oxydation. *Nature* 352:711-714, 1991.
49. Rettig J, Heinemann SH, Wunder F, et al: Inactivation properties of voltage-gated K^+ channels altered by presence of β subunit. *Nature* 369:289-294, 1994.

50. Vega-Saenz de Miera E, Rudy B: Modulation of K^+ channels by hydrogen peroxide. *Biochem Biophys Res Comm* 186:1681-1687, 1992.
51. Duprat F, Guillemare E, Romey G, et al: Susceptibility of cloned K^+ channels to reactive oxygen species. *Proc Natl Acad Sci USA* 92:11796-11800, 1995.
52. Wang D, Youngson C, Wong V, et al: NADPH-oxidase and a hydrogen peroxide sensitive K^+ channel may function as an oxygen sensor complex in airway chemoreceptors and small cell lung carcinoma cell lines. *Proc Natl Acad Sci USA* 93:13182-13187, 1996.
53. Yuan X, Tod ML, Rubin LJ, et al: Inhibition of cytochrome P-450 reduces voltage-gated K^+ currents in pulmonary arterial myocytes. *Am J Physiol* 268:C259-C270, 1995.
54. McCormack T, McCormack K: Shaker K^+ channel β subunits belong to an NADP(H)-dependent oxidoreductase superfamily. *Cell* 79:1133-1135, 1994.
55. Gleadle JM, Ebert BL, Ratcliffe PJ: Diphenylene iodonium inhibits the induction of erythropoietin and other mammalian genes by hypoxia. Implications for the mechanisms of oxygen sensing. *Eur J Biochem* 234:92-99, 1995.
56. Weir E, Wyatt C, Reeve H, et al: Diphenylene iodonium inhibits both potassium and calcium currents in isolated pulmonary artery smooth muscle cells. *J Appl Physiol* 76:2611-2615, 1994.
57. Wyatt C, Weir EK, Peers C: Diphenylene iodonium blocks K^+ and Ca^{2+} currents in type I cells isolated from the neonatal rat carotid body. *Neurosci Lett* 172: 63-66, 1994.
58. Motais R, García-Romeu F, Borgese F: The control of Na^+/H^+ exchange by molecular oxygen in trout erythrocytes. *J Gen Physiol* 90:197-207, 1987.
59. López-Barneo J: Perspectives in physiology. Recombinant Ca^{2+} channels get O_2-sensitive. *J Physiol* 500:1, 1997.

Chapter 12

Oxygen Sensing in Arterial Chemoreceptors:

Role of a Novel Oxygen-Dependent Potassium Channel

Keith J. Buckler

Introduction

The carotid body is the principal oxygen chemoreceptor involved in respiratory and cardiovascular control. The excitation of this receptor by hypoxia evokes both respiratory and cardiovascular reflexes, which promote compensatory changes in ventilation and cardiac output. Although the mechanisms of oxygen sensing are still poorly understood, there is growing evidence for the following model. The basic sensory unit is a primary receptor cell, the type I cell, which communicates with afferent nerve endings through reciprocal synapses. Although the pharmacology of synaptic transmission is ill defined, the type I cell secretes catecholamines (principally dopamine) in response to hypoxia.[1,2] Since this secretory response is very closely correlated with neural discharge,[2,3] it is thought to be central to chemotransduction. Catecholamine secretion proceeds via the exocytosis of dense core vesicles, the signal for which is a rise in intracellular calcium.[4] This chapter concerns the electrophysiologic mechanisms responsible for generating this calcium signal (see Chapters 11, 13-15).

From: López-Barneo, J and Weir, EK: *Oxygen Regulation of Ion Channels and Gene Expression*. Armonk, NY: Futura Publishing Company, Inc., ©1998.

Mechanism of the Hypoxic Rise in $[Ca^{2+}]_i$

Although it was originally proposed that hypoxia evoked calcium release from internal (mitochondrial) stores,[5] more recent studies have convincingly shown that Ca^{2+} influx is the primary cause of the hypoxic elevation of $[Ca^{2+}]_i$.[6,7] The observation that the Ca^{2+} response is partially inhibited by dihydropyridines indicates that the Ca^{2+} influx is mediated by L-type, and probably other, voltage-gated Ca^{2+} channels.[6,7]

In the rat type I cell, hypoxia evokes voltage-gated Ca entry through membrane depolarization (Figure 1). The resting membrane potential of isolated rat type I cells, measured using the perforated patch whole-cell recording technique, is normally about -50 mV[7,8] and is stable. Regular pacemaker-like electrical activity, as is proposed to occur in rabbit type I cells,[4,6] has not been reported in rat type I cells. In the presence of a hypoxic stimulus, there is a sustained decline in resting membrane potential (Figure 1 and Reference 7). In some cells, this receptor potential is accompanied by electrical activity. These action potentials usually have a slow upstroke velocity and often fail to overshoot 0 mV.[7] The properties of these action potentials reflect the paucity of voltage-gated Na channels in rat type I cells,[9] such that those action potentials which do occur are probably mediated by voltage-gated Ca channels. This proposal is reinforced by the observation of electrical activity in rat type I cells in the absence of extracellular sodium.[8]

In current-clamp recordings, the above electrical events are accompanied by a rapid rise in $[Ca^{2+}]_i$. If the cells are voltage clamped close to their normal resting membrane potential, however, the hypoxic $[Ca^{2+}]_i$ response is greatly attenuated[7] (Figure 1). This observation confirms the importance of voltage-gated Ca^{2+} entry in mediating the hypoxic rise in $[Ca^{2+}]_i$.

Voltage-gated Ca^{2+} entry probably occurs both as a result of the initiation of electrical activity and as a consequence of the receptor potential itself, since an increase in $[Ca^{2+}]_i$ is seen in cells which do not show significant electrical activity. In the rat type I cell, under voltage-clamp conditions, $[Ca^{2+}]_i$ increases dramatically with membrane depolarization positive to about -40 mV,[8] coinciding with the threshold for activation of voltage-gated Ca^{2+} currents. Under current-clamp conditions, the resting membrane potential in hypoxia/anoxia is frequently positive to -40 mV. In addition, irrespective of whether well-defined action potentials are present, there is often a marked increase in voltage noise in hypoxia (spontaneous variation in the resting membrane potential; e.g., Figure 1). This

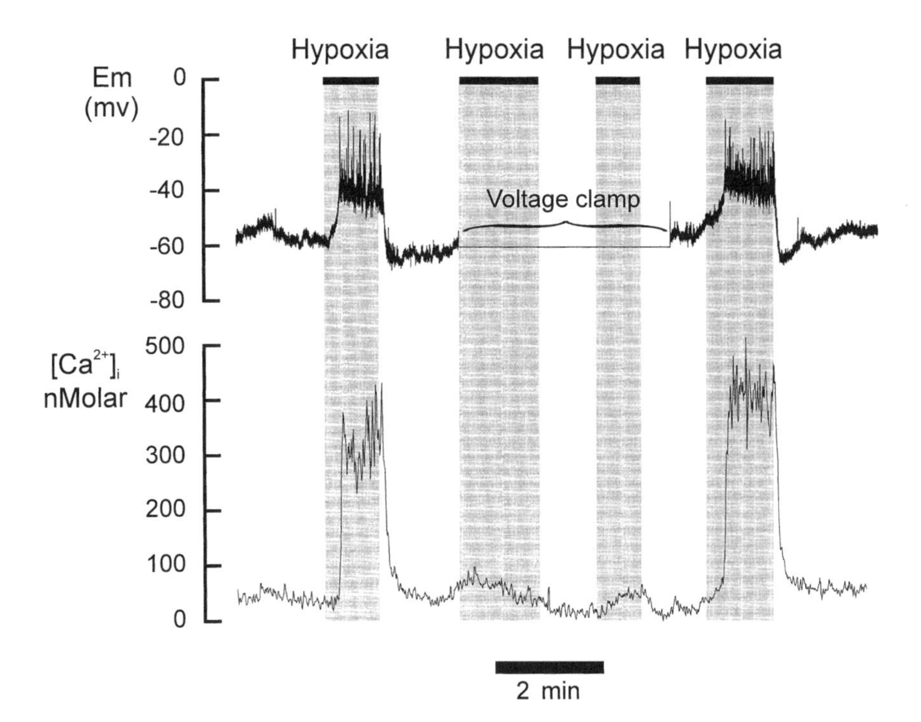

Figure 1. Hypoxia causes membrane depolarization and voltage-gated Ca^{2+} entry. Simultaneous recording of membrane potential and $[Ca^{2+}]_i$ in a neonatal rat type I cell. Note that hypoxia (5% CO_2 /95% N_2,, Po_2 approximately 10 Torr) causes a substantive membrane depolarization and coincident rise in $[Ca^{2+}]_i$ under current-clamp conditions (1st and 3rd hypoxic challenges), but when the cell is voltage clamped (2nd hypoxic challenge) the rise in $[Ca^{2+}]_i$ is greatly reduced. Electrophysiologic measurements were performed using the perforated patch (amphotericin B) whole-cell recording technique. Cell calcium was measured using Indo-1. Experiment performed at 37° C in bicarbonate buffered saline equilibrated with 5% CO_2/95% air (control).

voltage noise means that significant activation of voltage-gated Ca^{2+} channels may also occur at *average* membrane potentials negative to -40 mV. Thus, although weak action potentials are seen in many cells, they are not absolutely necessary to evoke a $[Ca^{2+}]_i$ response as the receptor potential alone is often sufficient to cause a significant rise in $[Ca^{2+}]_i$.

With respect to $[Ca^{2+}]_i$ signaling, it should also be noted that there are both caffeine[8] and probably IP_3-sensitive Ca^{2+} stores in rat type I cells.[10] It is, therefore, possible that Ca^{2+} stores may contribute to the hypoxic rise of $[Ca^{2+}]_i$ by participating in Ca^{2+} influx-induced Ca^{2+} release. In addition, if type I cells release acetylcholine upon stimulation,[11] this could further augment the Ca^{2+} response by acting through both nicotinic and muscarinic receptors on the same or neighboring cells to cause further depolarization, calcium influx, and calcium release from internal stores.[10] All of these events, however, would be secondary to an initial Ca^{2+} influx. The depolarizing receptor potential (and any accompanying electrical activity) is, therefore, the primary cause of the rise in $[Ca^{2+}]_i$ and so is thought to be a key stage in the chemotransduction process.

At this point, it is of interest to note that the response of type I cells to hypoxia, i.e., membrane depolarization followed by voltage-gated Ca^{2+} influx, is similar to that reported for other chemostimuli, including hypercapnic acidosis[8] and the mitochondrial uncoupler (and potent chemostimulus) 2,4-dinitrophenol.[12] Thus, the pathways for transducing various stimuli, acid, hypoxia, and inhibitors of oxidative phosphorylation appear to converge on, or possibly even before, the regulation of membrane potential and type I cell excitability. It should also be noted that the same individual cells respond to both forms of natural stimuli.

Role of Voltage-Gated K Channels

It has been proposed that the depolarization observed in hypoxia might be due to the inhibition of voltage/calcium-activated potassium channels. Indeed, the above model for stimulus (hypoxia) secretion coupling was originally based on the observation that hypoxia, anoxia, and histotoxic hypoxia (CN^-) inhibit voltage-gated K^+ currents in isolated type I cells.[4,13-17] Subsequently, similar observations have been made in pulmonary vascular smooth muscle[18] and neuroendothelial bodies in the lung.[19] This suggests that the inhibition of K^+ channels might be a common mechanism for hypoxic excitation of oxygen-sensitive tissues.

To date, two main types of oxygen-sensitive K channels have been characterized in carotid body type I cells. These are: 1) a high conductance (190 pS) calcium-activated potassium channel (BK_{Ca}) found in rat type I cells[19] sensitive to inhibition by both external TEA and charybdotoxin[14,16,20]; and 2) a medium conductance (40 pS) voltage-gated, calcium-insensitive potassium channel found in rabbit type I cells and referred to as the Ko_2 channel.[21] This channel is inhibited by both 5 mM TEA and 1 mM 4-AP.[13,21-24] Other oxygen-sensitive K currents have also been reported, including an inward rectifier in fetal rabbit type I cells [25] and a calcium-insensitive, voltage-gated K channel in chronically hypoxic rat type I cells.[26,27]

Although the effects of hypoxia upon BK_{Ca} and K_{O2} are well substantiated, their role in hypoxic chemotransduction is uncertain. Both BK_{Ca} and K_{O_2} are essentially voltage gated with activation thresholds of around -40 to -30 mV. Moreover, there are a number of publications reporting that pharmacologic inhibitors of these K channels have little effect upon neural discharge in the intact carotid body. For example, Donnelly [27,28] reported that both TEA and charybdotoxin (Ctx) had no effect upon neural discharge in the isolated superfused rat carotid body. Pepper et al[29] similarly noted that Ctx had little effect on neural discharge under control conditions, but did slightly augment the response to hypoxia. Thus, it would seem that the inhibition of BK_{Ca} channels by hypoxia cannot fully account for the oxygen-sensing properties of the intact carotid body.

Recent studies on the effects of K^+ channel blockers in isolated type I cells have given similar results.[30] The effects of several K channel inhibitors have been tested on cells which responded to either hypoxia or anoxia with a large, rapid rise in $[Ca^{2+}]_i$. These included 20 nM Ctx, an inhibitor of BK_{Ca} channels, 10 mM TEA, a potent inhibitor of BK_{Ca}, K_{O_2}, and other K channels; 1 and 5 mM 4-AP, an inhibitor of K_{O_2} and other K channels. None of these inhibitors evoked a significant rise in $[Ca^{2+}]_i$ (Figure 2).

These observations indicate that the inhibition of maxi-K^+, and other voltage-gated K^+ channels, may be unable to evoke a significant depolarization of type I cells. Indeed, in a separate series of experiments, a combination of 10 mM TEA and 5 mM 4-AP failed to depolarize resting membrane potential (control = -58 mV, plus TEA & 4-AP = -60).[30] Thus, neither BK_{Ca} channels nor any other TEA or 4-AP sensitive K^+ channels appear to make a significant contribution to the control of the resting membrane potential under normoxic conditions. Consequently, inhibition of any such channels cannot account for the depolarization seen in hypoxia.

Effects of Hypoxia Upon Electrical Properties of Type I Cells

Under normal recording conditions (standard bicarbonate buffered media), anoxia evokes a small inward shift in holding current of a few pA in type I cells voltage clamped to their normal resting potential.[7] Given the high input resistance of type I cells,[7,32] this current is sufficient to cause a significant depolarization. Anoxia also reduces the resting membrane conductance of type I cells substantially[30] (from around 300 pS to about 130 pS (Figure 3B). These observations indicate that the depolarizing receptor potential results from the inhibition of an outward current. Again,

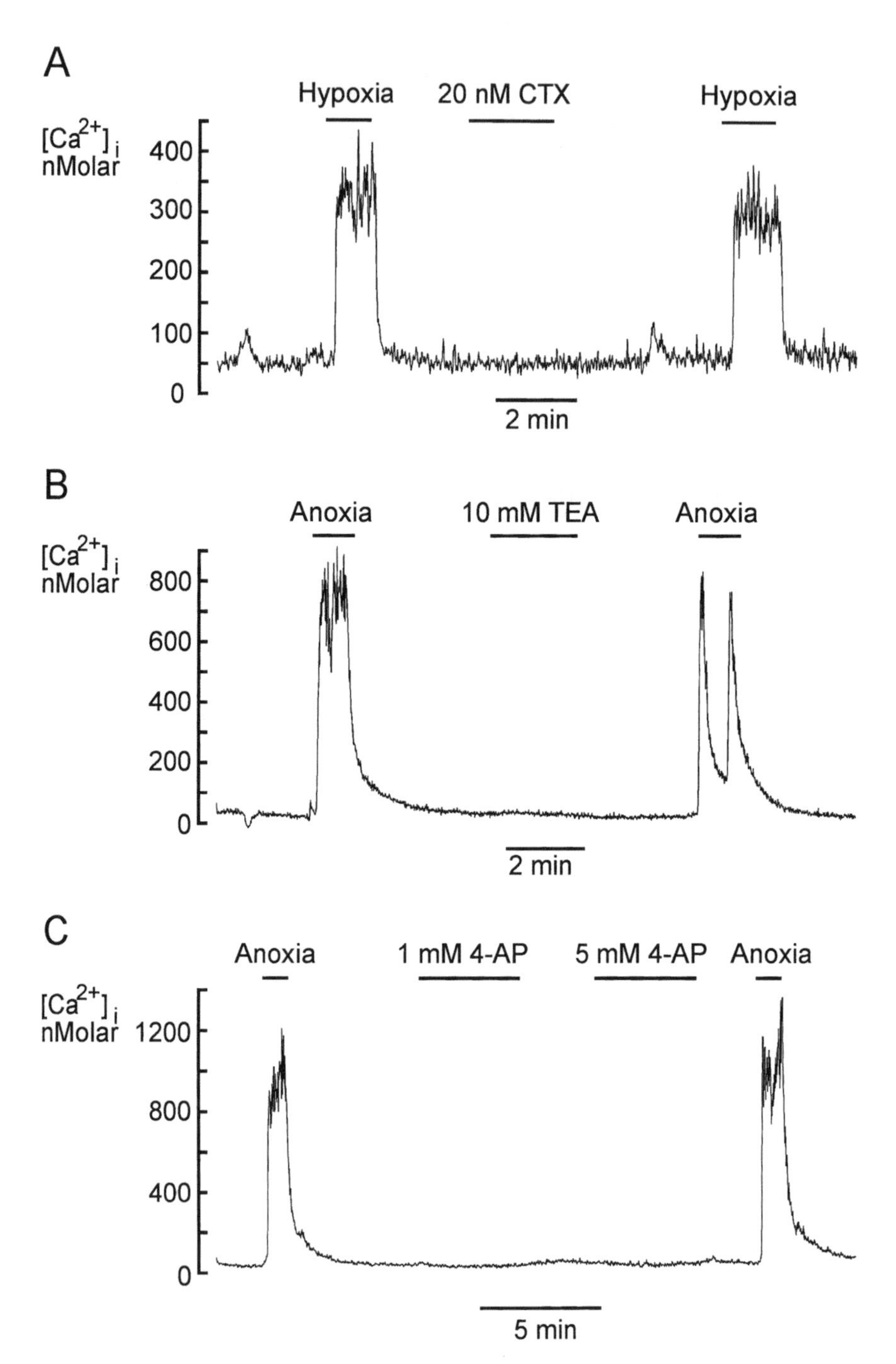
A
Hypoxia
20 nM CTX
Hypoxia
[Ca2+]i nMolar
400
300
200
100
0
2 min
B
Anoxia
10 mM TEA
Anoxia
[Ca2+]i nMolar
800
600
400
200
0
2 min
C
Anoxia
1 mM 4-AP
5 mM 4-AP
Anoxia
[Ca2+]i nMolar
1200
800
400
0
5 min

it is of interest to note that other chemostimuli also decrease resting membrane conductance.[8]

The current voltage relation of this oxygen-sensitive current was determined over a limited range of potentials from −100 to −30 mV (chosen to isolate small currents active around the resting membrane potential from large voltage-gated currents). Although the oxygen-sensitive current is only a few pA, in the region of the resting potential (Figure 3C, trace a-b), its inhibition does account for a marked decrease in resting membrane conductance and a dramatic shift in the cells, zero current potential (compare trace a and b in Figure 3B; see also Reference 30). This oxygen-sensitive current typically reversed around −90 mV (Figure 3C) suggesting that it resulted from the inhibition of a potassium current. This was confirmed by repeating the experiment in high extracellular K^+. Under these conditions, the current-voltage relation of the oxygen-sensitive current was dramatically right-shifted along the voltage axis with a concomitant large shift in the reversal potential (compare Figure 3C, traces a-b and c-d). Thus, the oxygen-sensitive current is carried principally by potassium ions.

This oxygen-sensitive K^+ current is, however, resistant to inhibition by both TEA (10 mM) and 4-AP (5 mM).[30] It is, therefore, clearly distinct from any other oxygen-sensitive K^+ current previously reported in the carotid body.

Further studies have revealed that this new oxygen-sensitive K^+ current shows little voltage sensitivity, even over a wide range of potentials (−90 – +30 mV). It also shows no time-dependent activation or inactivation during depolarizing or hyperpolarizing voltage-clamp pulses of up to 300 ms duration in the range −100 to −20 mV.[30] This current results, therefore, from what is generally referred to as a background or leak conductance; that is, a small conductance active at all potentials with little or no voltage sensitivity.

Despite the fact that this is a very small conductance (approximately 200 pS), compared to the voltage-activated currents in this cell, it contrib-

Figure 2. Effects of potassium channel inhibitors on $[Ca^{2+}]_i$ in type I cells. **A.** Effects of 20 nM charybdotoxin (Ctx) compared with hypoxia (Po_2 10-15 Torr). Similar results obtained in five other experiments. **B.** Effects of 10 mM TEA compared to anoxia. Similar results obtained in seven other experiments. **C.** Effects of 1 and 5 mM 4-AP; similar results obtained in 4 and 6 other experiments (see results). Note that unlike hypoxia/anoxia, none of these K channel inhibitors evoked a rise in $[Ca^{2+}]_i$. (Reproduced with permission from Reference 30.)

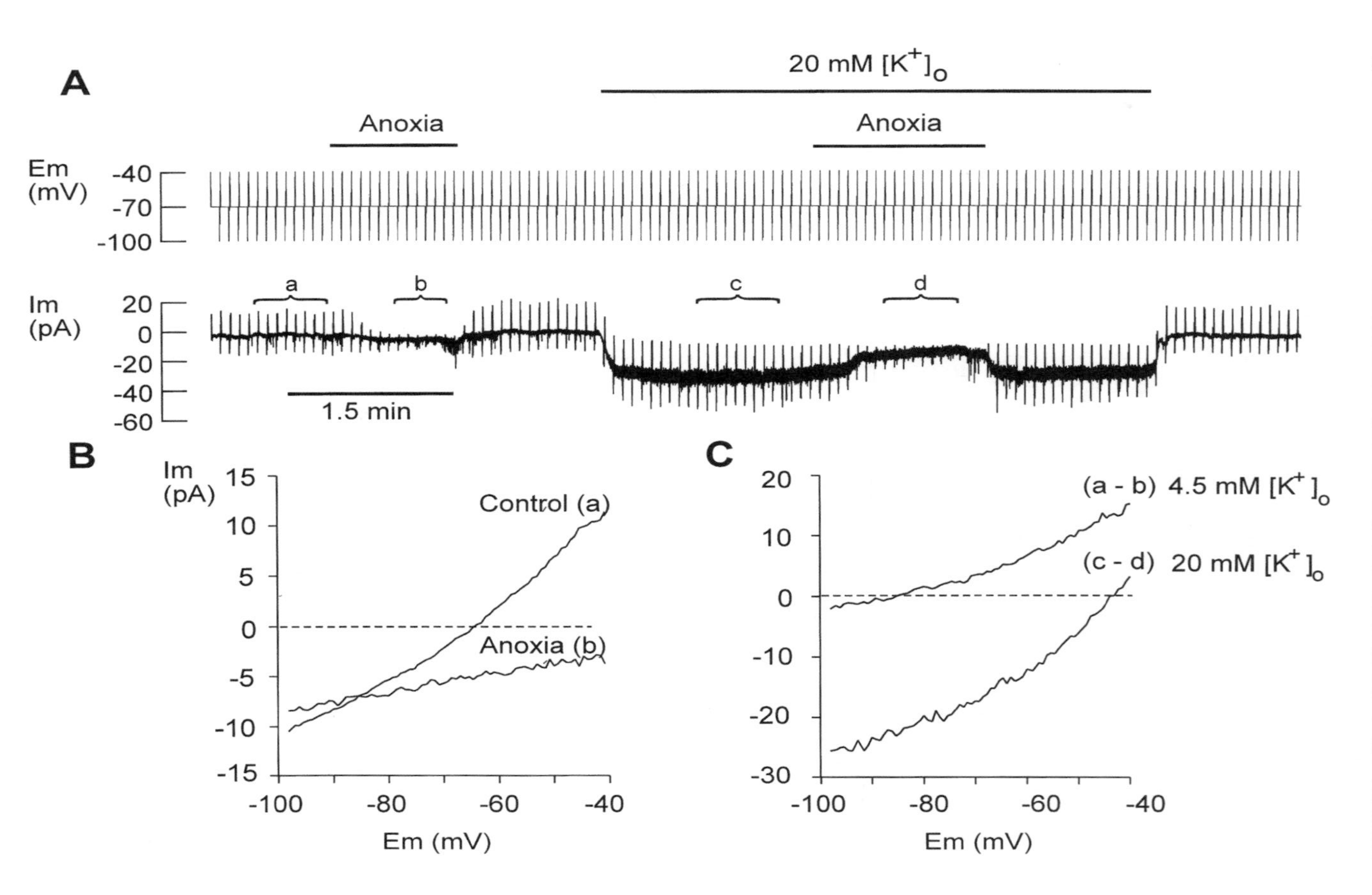
A
20 mM [K+]o
Anoxia
Anoxia
Em (mV)
-40
-70
-100
Im (pA)
20
0
-20
-40
-60
a
b
c
d
1.5 min
B
Im (pA)
15
10
5
0
-5
-10
-15
Control (a)
Anoxia (b)
-100
-80
-60
-40
Em (mV)
C
20
10
0
-10
-20
-30
(a - b) 4.5 mM [K+]o
(c - d) 20 mM [K+]o
-100
-80
-60
-40
Em (mV)

utes 50% to 80% of the total membrane K^+ conductance around the resting potential.[30] Its inhibition by hypoxia is, therefore, of major importance in generating the receptor potential.

In summary, these investigations have shed new light on the role of K channels in oxygen chemoreception in that it is now clear that the response to hypoxia cannot be explained by the inhibition of large voltage-gated K^+ conductances alone. Instead, it is proposed that the initial depolarization, or receptor potential, is mediated via the inhibition of a small, voltage-insensitive, resting K^+-conductance. This will probably serve to initiate electrical activity and Ca^{2+} influx, which could then be further controlled by the modulation of voltage-gated/Ca^{2+}-dependent channels. Although such a role for BK^+_{Ca} channels remains to be formally proven in these cells, it has recently been reported that Ctx, although not excitatory under normoxic conditions, can potentiate the effects of moderate hypoxia.[29] In any event, since the receptor potential is primarily responsible for initiating Ca influx which then causes secretion, it is apparent that the oxygen-sensitive resting K^+ current plays a major role in oxygen chemoreception in these cells.

Figure 3. Anoxia inhibits a background K^+ conductance. **A.** Cells were voltage clamped at a holding potential of −70 mV and subject to a 500 ms voltage ramp from −100 to −40 mV every 5 seconds. The experiment starts in normal extracellular $[K^+]_o$ (4.5 mM). Under these conditions, anoxia causes a slight inward shift in holding current and a substantial decline in the amplitude of the ramp current. Partway through the experiment, $[K^+]_o$ is increased to 20 mM (K^+ substituted for Na^+) causing a large inward shift in holding current. In 20 mM $[K^+]_o$, anoxia again reduces the ramp current, but now causes an outward shift in holding current. **B.** The current voltage relation obtained under normoxic and anoxic conditions and normal $[K^+]_o$. Under normoxic conditions, the cells' I/V relation shows a zero current potential of −65 mV (this corresponds to what the cells' resting potential would be were it not voltage-clamped). Under anoxic conditions, however, the current-voltage relation is markedly flattened (i,e., there is a substantial decrease in membrane conductance) and there is no zero current potential within the range of potentials tested (i.e., under anoxic conditions, the cells' resting potential probably lies positive to −30 mV). **C.** Current voltage relations of difference currents (control − anoxia) derived from the voltage ramps in A. a−b = I/V relation of oxygen-sensitive current in 4.5 mM $[K]_o$ and c−d = I/V relation of oxygen-sensitive current in 20 mM $[K^+]_o$. Note large positive shift in reversal potential of the oxygen-sensitive current in 20 mM $[K^+]_o$ (from approximately −85 mV in 4.5 mM $[K^+]_o$ to −45 mV in 20 mM $[K^+]_o$; approximate values for E_K are −93 and −54 mV). (Figure adapted with permission from Reference 30.)

References

1. Fidone S, Gonzalez C, Yoshizaki K: Effects of hypoxia on catecholamine synthesis in rabbit carotid body in vitro. *J Physiol* 333:93-110, 1982.
2. Rigual R, Gonzalez E, Gonzalez C, et al: Synthesis and release of catecholamines by the cat carotid body in vitro: effects of hypoxic stimulation. *Brain Res* 374: 101-109, 1986.
3. Gonzalez C, Almaraz L, Obeso A, et al: Carotid body chemoreceptors: from natural stimuli to sensory discharges. *Physiol Rev* 74:829-898, 1994.
4. Montoro RJ, Urena J, Fernandez-Chacon R, et al: Oxygen sensing by ion channels and chemotransduction in single glomus cells. *J Gen Physiol* 91:10208-10211, 1996.
5. Biscoe TJ, Duchen MR: Cellular basis of transduction in carotid chemoreceptors. *Am J Physiol* 258:L271-L278, 1990.
6. Lopez-Barneo J, Benot AR, Urena J: Oxygen sensing and the electrophysiology of arterial chemoreceptor cells. *NIPS* 8:191-195, 1993.
7. Buckler KJ, Vaughan-Jones RD: Effects of hypoxia on membrane potential and intracellular calcium in rat neonatal carotid body type I cells. *J Physiol* 476:423-428, 1994.
8. Buckler KJ, Vaughan-Jones RD: Effects of hypercapnia on membrane potential and intracellular calcium in rat carotid body type I cells. *J Physiol* 478:157-171, 1994.
9. Peers C, Buckler KJ: Transduction of chemostimuli by the type-I carotid body cell. *J Memb Biol* 144:1-9, 1995.
10. Dasso LLT, Buckler KJ, Vaughan-Jones RD: Muscarinic and nicotinic receptors raise intracellular Ca^{2+} levels in rat carotid body type I cells. *J Physiol* 498: 327–338, 1997.
11. Eyzaguirre C, Zapata P: Perspectives in carotid body research. *J Appl Physiol* 57:931-957, 1984.
12. Buckler KJ, Vaughan-Jones RD: Effects of the metabolic uncoupler DNP on intracellular pH and Ca^{2+} in enzymatically isolated neonatal rat carotid body type I cells. *J Physiol* 459:345P, 1993.
13. Lopez-Barneo J, Lopez-Lopez JR, Urena J, et al: Chemotransduction in the carotid body: K^+ current modulated by Po_2 in type I chemoreceptor cells. *Science* 241: 580-582, 1988.
14. Peers C, O'Donnell J: Potassium currents recorded in type I carotid body cells from the neonatal rat and their modulation by chemoexcitatory agents. *Brain Res* 522:259-266, 1990.
15. Hescheler J, Delpiano MA, Acker H, et al: Ionic currents of type I cells of the rabbit carotid body measured by voltage clamp experiments and the effect of hypoxia. *Brain Res* 486:79-88, 1989.
16. Peers, C: Hypoxic suppression of K^+-currents in type I carotid body cells: selective effect on the Ca^{2+}-activated K^+-current. *Neurosci Lett* 119:253-256, 1990.
17. Stea A, Nurse CA: Whole-cell and perforated-patch recordings from O_2-sensitive rat carotid body cells grown in short- and long-term culture. *Pflugers Arch* 418: 93-101, 1991.
18. Post JM, Hume JR, Archer SL, et al: Direct role for potassium channel inhibition in hypoxic pulmonary vasoconstriction. *Am J Physiol* 262:C882-C890, 1992.
19. Youngson C, Nurse C, Yeger H, et al: Oxygen sensing in airway chemoreceptors. *Nature* 365:153-155, 1993.

20. Wyatt CN, Peers C: Ca^{2+}-activated K^+-channels in isolated type I cells of the neonatal rat carotid body. *J Physiol* 483:559-565, 1995.
21. Ganfornina MD, Lopez-Barneo J: Single K^+-channels in membrane patches of arterial chemoreceptor cells are modulated by O_2 tension. *Proc Natl Acad Sci USA* 88:2927-2930, 1991.
22. Lopez-Lopez J, Gonzalez C, Urena J, et al: Low Po_2 selectively inhibits K channel activity in chemoreceptor cells of the mammalian carotid body. *J Gen Physiol* 93:1001-1015, 1989.
23. Ganfornina MD, Lopez-Barneo J: Potassium channel types in arterial chemoreceptor cells and their selective modulation by hypoxia. *J Gen Physiol* 100:401-426, 1992.
24. Lopez-Lopez JR, De Luis DA, Gonzalez C: Properties of a transient K^+ current in chemoreceptor cells of rabbit carotid body. *J Physiol* 460:15-32, 1993.
25. Delpiano MA, Hescheler J: Evidence for a P_{O2} sensitive K^+ channel in the type-I cell of the rabbit carotid body. *FEBS Lett* 249:195-198, 1989.
26. Wyatt CN, Wright C, Bee D, et al: O_2-sensitive K^+-currents in carotid body chemoreceptor cells from normoxic and chronically hypoxic rats and their roles in hypoxic chemotransduction. *Proc Natl Acad Sci USA* 92:295-299, 1995.
27. Doyle TP, Donnelly DF: Effects of Na^+ and K^+ channel blockade on hypoxia induced catecholamine release from rat carotid body in vitro. *J Appl Physiol* 77:2606-2611, 1994.
28. Cheng PM, Donnelly DF: Relationship between changes of glomus cell current and neural response of rat carotid body. *J Neurophys* 74:2077-2086, 1995.
29. Pepper DR, Landauer RC, Kumar P: Effect of charybdotoxin on hypoxic chemosensitivity in the adult rat carotid body in vitro. *J Physiol* 487:177P, 1995.
30. Buckler KJ: A novel oxygen-sensitive potassium current in rat carotid body type I cells. *J Physiol* 498:649-662, 1997.
31. Duchen MR, Caddy KW, Kirby GC, et al: Biophysical studies of the cellular elements of the rabbit carotid body. *Neuroscience* 26:291-311, 1988.

Chapter 13

Potassium Channels in Carotid Body Type I Cells and Their Sensitivity to Hypoxia: Studies in Chronically Hypoxic and Developing Rats

Chris Peers

Introduction

Regulation of potassium (K^+) channels by oxygen tension was first demonstrated in rabbit type I carotid body cells in 1988.[1] Since that first study, numerous reports have appeared in the literature describing the inhibitory actions of hypoxia on K^+ currents in a variety of tissue types, including pulmonary vascular smooth muscle,[2,3] neuroepithelial bodies,[4] central neurones,[5] and, most recently, in the clonal rat pheochromocytoma cell line, PC12.[6] There is also an emerging awareness that hypoxia can regulate voltage-gated calcium (Ca^{2+}) channels in type I cells[7] and vascular smooth muscle cells.[8] Although our understanding of the mechanisms underlying ion channel regulation by hypoxia is in its infancy, it is increasingly clear that this is a widespread phenomenon of great physiologic importance, and, in different tissue types, hypoxic inhibition of channels serves to mediate different cellular functions (see Chapter 11). For exam-

From: López-Barneo, J and Weir, EK: *Oxygen Regulation of Ion Channels and Gene Expression.* Armonk, NY: Futura Publishing Company, Inc., ©1998.

ple, in pulmonary vascular smooth muscle cells, hypoxic inhibition of K^+ channels can account for hypoxic pulmonary vasoconstriction by causing cell depolarization and, hence, triggering Ca^{2+} influx.[9] In the systemic circulation, hypoxic inhibition of Ca^{2+} channels may lower intracellular $[Ca^{2+}]$ and so contribute to hypoxic vasodilation (see Chapters 16-19).[8]

A Central Role for Oxygen-Sensitive K^+ Channels in Type I Carotid Body Cells

In the carotid body, hypoxic inhibition of K^+ currents has been reported in type I cells isolated from embryonic and adult rabbits, and neonatal rats.[10] Perhaps in part because of the diversity of species and ages chosen for study, there are important contrasting results obtained in different laboratories. In rabbit embryonic type I cells, hypoxia inhibits an inwardly rectifying K^+ channel of approximately 140 pS conductance.[11] Reduced opening of this channel leads to profound cell depolarization, although the exact Po_2 versus channel open probability relationship has not been determined. These findings contrast with those found in adult rabbit type I cells. In these physiologically mature cells, hypoxia selectively inhibits a specific voltage-gated K^+ current of 42 pS conductance which has been termed the Ko_2 channel.[12,13] Inhibition of this channel can be demonstrated in excised membrane patches which are washed free of cell constituents,[12,13] indicating that oxygen regulation of this channel type is a tightly coupled mechanism, although whether the channel itself acts as the oxygen sensor, or it is coupled to a membrane-bound sensor, remains to be demonstrated. Inhibition of the Ko_2 channel leads to increased excitability of type I cells, thus, causing increased Ca^{2+} influx and, hence, increased neurotransmitter release.[14] The Po_2 versus channel open probability correlates well with earlier studies comparing Po_2 with whole-cell K^+ current amplitude[15] but, for some time, this relationship was puzzling, since maximal channel inhibition was observed at oxygen levels which would not excite the intact organ. This finding has recently been accounted for by the observation that Ca^{2+} channels in adult rabbit cells are themselves inhibited by hypoxia.[7] This inhibition is strongly voltage dependent, such that at low activating potentials, inhibition is greatest, while at higher potentials, inhibition by hypoxia is lost. Thus, adult rabbit type I cells can undergo considerable depolarization at relatively high Po_2 levels, but rises of intracellular Ca^{2+} are suppressed owing to Ca^{2+} channel inhibition. However, when stimulus intensity increases (i.e., when Po_2 levels decrease further), the cells depolarize to a greater extent and hypoxic inhibition of Ca^{2+} channels is relieved, allowing sufficient Ca^{2+}

influx to trigger transmitter release at more physiologically appropriate Po_2 levels.[7,14]

Electrophysiologic studies of type I cells from rats have largely been confined to neonates (approximately 10 days old) to date.[10,16,17] These cells also have oxygen-sensitive K^+ channels, but their properties differ markedly from those seen in adult rabbit cells. Whole-cell recordings originally revealed that hypoxia selectively inhibited Ca^{2+}-sensitive K^+ (K_{Ca}) channels,[17] although there is now also evidence to suggest that a low conductance, oxygen-sensitive K^+ "leak" channel is present in these cells.[18] Rat type I cells do not appear to fire action potentials spontaneously, but in hypoxia they depolarize[19,20] and increased electrical excitability is seen,[20] leading to a rise of intracellular [Ca^{2+}] and, hence, presumably, neurosecretion. Hypoxia does not inhibit K_{Ca} channels in excised patches,[19] but single-channel inhibition has been demonstrated using perforated vesicle recordings, indicating that a cytosolic factor mediates hypoxic inhibition of channels in these cells.[19] At present, this mediator remains to be identified, but the possible involvement of cyclic nucleotides has recently been discounted.[21] Instead, there is pharmacologic evidence for the involvement of cytochrome P450,[22] as has been suggested in pulmonary vascular smooth muscle.[23]

While differences in results between laboratories remain to be clarified, it is impossible to ignore the central role that oxygen-sensitive K^+ channels play in carotid body chemotransduction and, therefore, the role they play in influencing ventilation. Some of our recent studies have focused on the electrophysiologic properties of type I cells isolated from either rats born and reared in chronically hypoxic (CH) conditions,[24] or rats of different ages reared normoxically.[25] These animals have been of interest since ventilatory responses to acutely inspired hypoxic gas mixtures are markedly different in CH rats,[26] and are also known to undergo postnatal maturation.[27] In this chapter, results from these different studies are compared in order to examine how electrophysiologic changes in type I cells from these different animals might account for known alterations in ventilatory responses of corresponding intact animals.

Postnatal Maturation of the Carotid Body and the Effects of Chronic Hypoxia

The oxygen sensitivity of the carotid body is well known to undergo postnatal maturation, although the rate of maturation is species dependent.[27] In rat, this process has been demonstrated in vitro using intact carotid bodies and measurements of carotid sinus nerve discharge.[28-30] Donnelly and Doyle simultaneously monitored nerve discharge and catecholamine levels (the latter with a polarized carbon fiber electrode inserted into the organ), and demonstrated that the increase in afferent chemosensory discharge and released catecholamines elicited by exposure to hypoxic superfusate both increased with age, particularly for organs isolated from animals between 2 and 10 days old (differences between 10-day-olds and adults were far less marked).[29] These age-related changes parallel the well-documented increased ventilatory response to acutely inspired hypoxic gas mixtures as animals and individuals mature postnatally.

The ventilatory response to inspired hypoxic gas mixtures is blunted or even absent in animals born and reared under CH conditions.[26] This has also been reported to be the case in adult animals exposed to CH conditions,[31] and in high altitude residents.[32] Such blunting of oxygen sensitivity is reminiscent of the immature response seen in very young, normoxically reared animals.[27] The effects of CH are also associated with hypertrophy and hyperplasia of type I cells,[33,34] but little is known of the functioning of these cells in isolation. Given the central role that K^+ channels play in transduction of hypoxic stimuli (see above), we have, therefore, investigated whether there might be age-dependent changes in the properties of K^+ channels in isolated type I cells, and whether these might compare with differences seen in K^+ channels in type I cells isolated from rats born and reared under CH (10% oxygen) conditions.[24]

A Comparison of K^+ Currents in Chronically Hypoxic and Immature Normoxic Type I Cells

We have recently isolated cells from rats aged 4 days, 10 days, and adult (170 g, at least 5 weeks old) and used conventional whole-cell patch-clamp recordings to characterize K^+ currents[25] (recording details are documented elsewhere[21,22]). We noted a marked increase in K^+ current density with increasing age, i.e., K^+ current amplitude divided by cell membrane capacitance (Table), the latter indicative of cell size, as illustrated in Figure 1A. The age-related changes in K^+ current density were reminiscent of the effects of CH; Figure 1B plots current density relationships in type I cells of young rats (approximately 10 days old) reared normoxically or in a hypoxic (10% oxygen) chamber. As can be seen, there are striking similarities between the effects of CH and the effects of age, i.e., current densities seen in 4-day-olds (Figure 1A) are significantly smaller than

Table
A Comparison of K^+ Currents in Type I Cells Isolated from Normoxically Reared Rats of Different Ages and Chronically Hypoxic Rats

	Membrane Capacitance (pF)	*K^+ Current Density (pA/pF)*	*% of K^+ Current Due to IK_{Ca}*	*% Inhibition by Hypoxia*
4-day old	3.6 ± 0.2	121 ± 11	20.7 ± 3.6	12.1 ± 3.9
10-day old	2.9 ± 0.1	188 ± 19	38.1 ± 3.9	25.9 ± 2.8
adult	3.0 ± 0.2	260 ± 28	40.8 ± 3.1	28.9 ± 3.0
10-day old, chronically hypoxic	6.3 ± 0.3	72.2 ± 6.5	<15*	24.7 ± 2.9

All values quoted are means ± s.e.m. (except *, which is estimated) taken from between 17 and 47 cells from each age group or from chronically hypoxic type I cells. All values concerning K^+ current amplitude, density or degree of inhibition caused by hypoxia (Po_2 approximately 20 mm Hg) are based on measurements of currents obtained by step depolarizations to +20 mV from a holding potential of −70 mV.

those of older animals, and current density in CH type I cells are significantly reduced as compared with age-matched, normoxically reared cells (Figure 1B). On the basis of these initial findings, it was tempting to speculate that conditions of postnatal CH in some way preserve the type I cells in an immature state. Indeed, this may also be true morphologically since the mean membrane capacitance was significantly greater in CH type I cells as compared with age-matched controls, and was also greater in 4-day-old cells as compared with cells isolated from older animals (Table 1).

Previous studies in young rat type I cells have indicated that whole-cell K^+ currents arise due to the activation of at least two K^+ channel types: K_{Ca} channel (sensitive to blockade by charybdotoxin), and a voltage-gated, Ca^{2+}-insensitive K^+ channel.[35] To investigate whether changes in K^+ current density were due to a generalized increase in K^+ channel expression or a selective action on either subtype of channel, the proportion of K^+ current attributable to activation of K_{Ca} channels was estimated by changing the superfusate to one containing raised [Mg^{2+}] (6 mM) and lowered [Ca^{2+}] (0.1 mM). This alteration has previously been shown to inhibit IK_{Ca} by preventing significant Ca^{2+} influx during step depolarizations.[36] The fraction of whole-cell K^+ current inhibited was significantly less in 4-day-old cells as compared with 10-day-olds and adults, whereas these latter two age groups showed similar degrees of inhibition (Table). For CH type I cells, the amount of whole-cell K^+ current attributable to IK_{Ca} was estimated by examining the effects of 20 nM charybdotoxin to

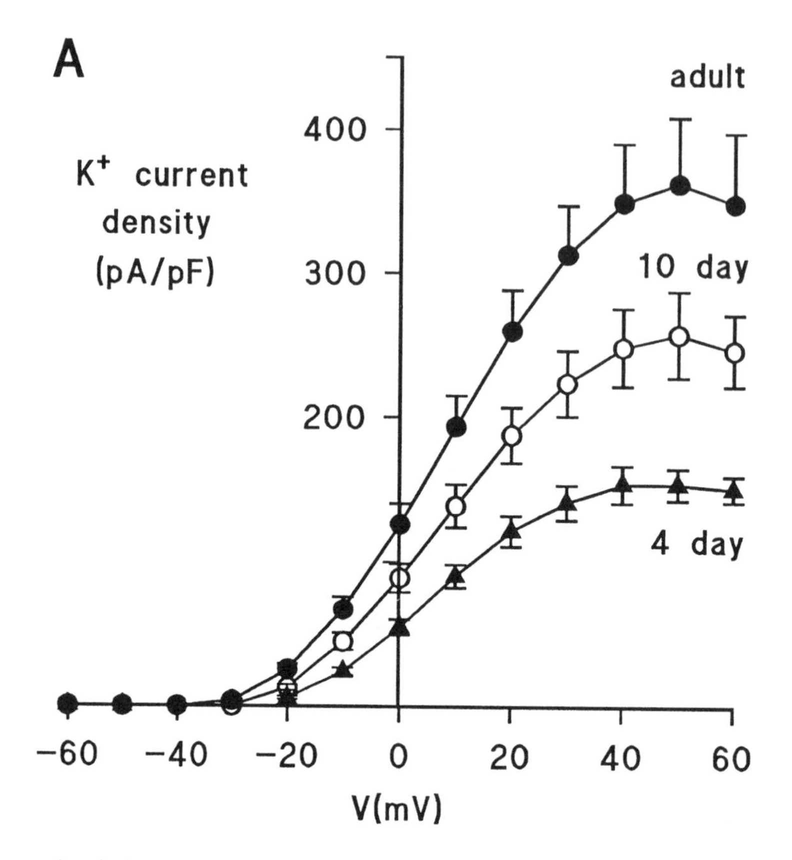

Figure 1. **A.** Mean (± s.e.m.) current density-voltage relationships in type I cells isolated from normoxically reared adult (**filled circles**, n = 46 cells), 10-day-old (**open circles**, n = 47) and 4-day-old (**filled triangles**, n = 40) rats. Data obtained from measurement of current amplitudes evoked by the various test potentials shown from a holding potential of −70 mV. For each cell, current amplitudes were then divided by that cell's membrane capacitance. **B.** Mean (± s.e.m.) current density-voltage relationships in type I cells isolated from rats aged approximately 10 days and reared either normoxically (**filled circles**, n = 17) or in a chronically hypoxic (CH) environment (10% oxygen, **open circles**, n = 20). Data obtained as in A. (Reproduced with permission from Reference 24.)

reduce whole-cell K^+ current amplitudes.[24] As for 4-day-old cells, functional expression of K_{Ca} was significantly less in CH type I cells (Table 1).

A lowering of perfusate P_{O_2} has previously been shown to inhibit selectively K_{Ca} channels in 10-day-old rat type I cells (see above), and our most recent observations suggest that this is true in cells of all ages stud-

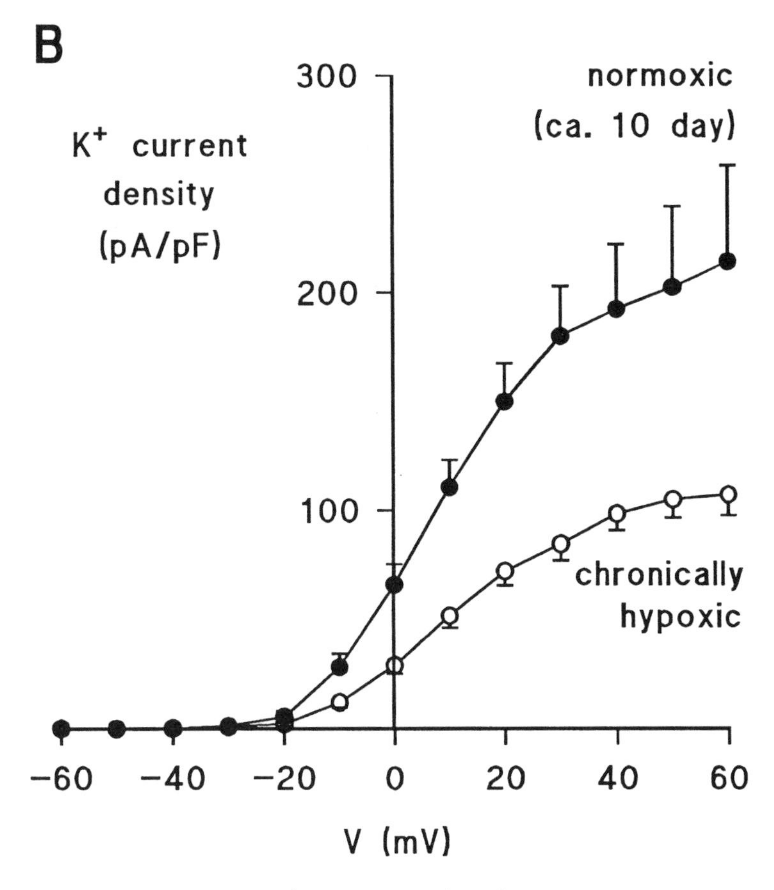

Figure 1. *(continued)*

ied, since hypoxia was without significant effect on residual currents recorded in raised [Mg^{2+}] (6 mM), lowered [Ca^{2+}] (0.1 mM) solutions in cells of any age examined (unpublished observations). Figure 2 (A-C) illustrates that the degree of inhibition of K^+ currents caused by hypoxia (Po_2 approximately 20 mm Hg) increases with increasing age (Table). These findings are in marked contrast to results obtained in CH type I cells. As illustrated in Figure 2D, hypoxia caused reversible inhibitions of K^+ current amplitudes which were not significantly different in magnitude as compared with cells of age-matched, normoxically reared animals. Given that CH type I cells express relatively few functional K_{Ca} channels, this indicates that in CH type I cells acute hypoxia inhibits a K^+ current which is not attributable to K_{Ca} channels.

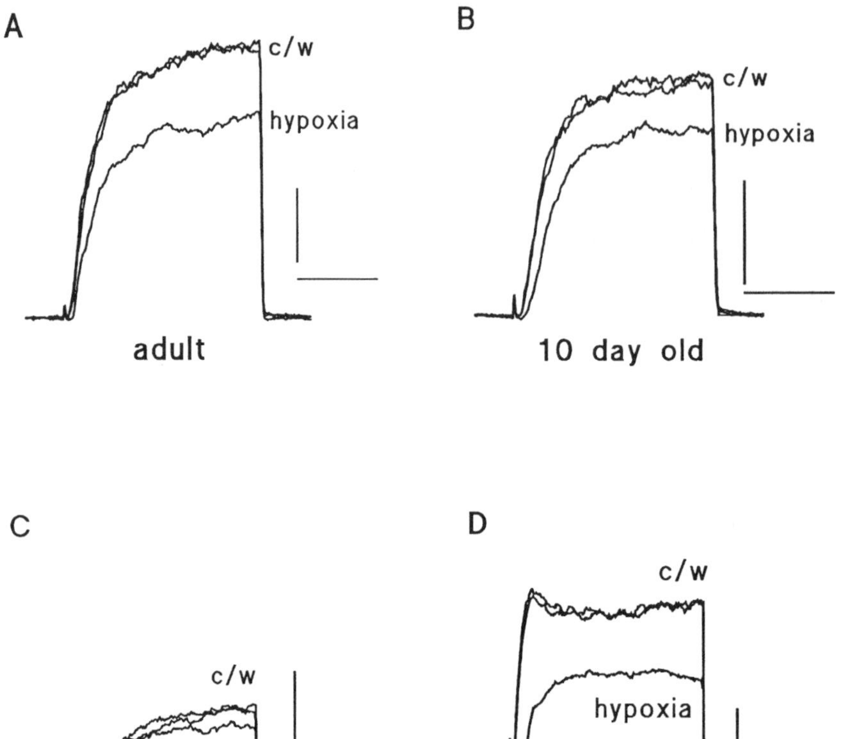

Figure 2. Effects of hypoxia (Po_2 approximately 20 mm Hg) on whole-cell K^+ currents recorded in rat type I cells. Cells were isolated from normoxically reared rats of different ages, as indicated (**A-C**), and from chronically hypoxic (CH) rats ages approximately 10 days (**D**). In all traces, currents were evoked by 50 ms step depolarizations from −70 mV to +20 mV. **Calibration bars**: vertical, 250 pA; horizontal, 20 ms. This applies to all traces.

These comparisons make unlikely the possibility that exposure to CH preserves the carotid body type I cell in an immature state. When comparing CH type I cells of 10-day-olds to normoxically reared, immature (4-day-old) cells, there are notable similarities (Table); in both cases, cells are enlarged as compared with older cells, and K^+ current density is markedly reduced. Furthermore, the proportion of K^+ current attributable to activation of K_{Ca} channels is far less than in older cells. However, in the response to acute hypoxia, the two cell types differ importantly; in cells from 4-day-old rats, hypoxia has only a small effect on K^+ currents, and this is selective for K_{Ca} channels. By contrast, K^+ currents in CH type I cells show a larger inhibition in response to acute hypoxia, comparable to those seen in age-matched controls.[24] Thus while K^+ channel expression might be considered retarded in CH, there still appears to be oxygen-sensing mechanisms (which in the absence of K_{Ca} channels couple to another channel type). In immature cells, hypoxic responses are far less pronounced.

The physiologic consequences of developmental changes and adaptive changes to CH remain to be fully elucidated, but we have shown previously that, while normoxically reared, 10-day-old rat type I cells depolarize in hypoxia, CH type I cells do not.[24] We speculate that the K^+ channel inhibited by hypoxia is, therefore, not contributing to the setting of resting membrane potential. It will be of interest to see whether K_{Ca} channels of immature (4-day-old) type I cells are present in sufficient density to significantly affect resting membrane potential. Until then, all discussion concerning how developmental changes in K^+ currents contribute to the maturation of the intact organ must remain speculative, but the studies reported here suggest that K^+ channel expression could be a major determinant in both postnatal maturation and adaptation to CH.

Acknowledgments

This work is based on results obtained in my laboratory primarily by Chris Hatton, Liz Carpenter, and Chris Wyatt, whose skills, hard work, and enthusiasm are always greatly appreciated. I am also extremely grateful for the collaborative efforts of Dr. Denise Bee (Sheffield University), and Drs. Prem Kumar and David Pepper (Birmingham University) without whose input these studies could not have been carried out. This work was generously supported by The Wellcome Trust and the British Heart Foundation.

References

1. Lopez-Barneo J, Lopez-Lopez JR, Urena J, et al: Chemotransduction in the carotid body: K^+ current modulated by Po_2 in type I chemoreceptor cells. *Science* 241: 580-582, 1988.

2. Post JM, Hume JR, Archer SL, et al: Direct role for potassium channel inhibition in hypoxic pulmonary vasoconstriction. *Am J Physiol* 262:C882-C890, 1992.
3. Yuan X-J, Goldman WF, Tod ML, et al: Hypoxia reduces potassium currents in cultured rat pulmonary but not mesenteric arterial myocytes. *Am J Physiol* 264: L116-L123, 1993.
4. Youngson C, Nurse CA, Yeger H, et al: Oxygen sensing in airway chemoreceptors. *Nature* 365:153-155, 1993.
5. Jiang C, Haddad GG: Oxygen deprivation inhibits a K^+ channel independently of cytosolic factors in rat central neurons. *J Physiol* 481:15-26, 1994.
6. Zhu WH, Conforti L, Czyzyk-Krzeska MF, et al: Membrane depolarization in PC12 cells during hypoxia is regulated by an O_2-sensitive K^+ current. *Am J Physiol* 271:C658-C665, 1996.
7. Montoro RJ, Urena J, Fernandez-Chacon R, et al: Oxygen sensing by ion channels and chemotransduction in single glomus cells. *J Gen Physiol* 107:133-143, 1996.
8. Franco-Obregon A, Urena J, Lopez-Barneo J: Oxygen-sensitive calcium channels in vascular smooth muscle and their possible roles in hypoxic arterial relaxation. *Proc Natl Acad Sci USA* 92:4715-4719, 1995.
9. Weir EK, Archer SL: The mechanism of acute hypoxic pulmonary vasoconstriction: the tale of two channels. *FASEB J* 9:183-189, 1995.
10. Peers C, Buckler KJ: Transduction of chemostimuli by the type I carotid body cell. *J Memb Biol* 144:1-9, 1995.
11. Delpiano MA, Hescheler J: Evidence for a Po_2-sensitive K^+ channel in the type-I cell of the rabbit carotid body. *FEBS Lett* 249:195-198, 1989.
12. Ganfornina MD, Lopez-Barneo J: Single K^+ channels in membrane patches of arterial chemoreceptor cells are modulated by O_2 tension. *Proc Natl Acad Sci USA* 88:2927-2930, 1991.
13. Ganfornina MD, Lopez-Barneo J: Gating of O_2-sensitive K^+ channels of arterial chemoreceptor cells and kinetic modulation induced by low Po_2. *J Gen Physiol* 100:427-455, 1992.
14. Urena J, Fernandez-Chacon R, Benot AR, et al: Hypoxia induces voltage-dependent Ca^{2+} entry and quantal dopamine secretion in carotid body glomus cells. *Proc Natl Acad Sci USA* 91:10208-10211, 1994.
15. Lopez-Lopez J, Gonzalez C, Urena J, et al: Low Po_2 selectively inhibits K channel activity in chemoreceptor cells of the mammalian carotid body. *J Gen Physiol* 93:1001-1015, 1989.
16. Stea A, Nurse CA: Whole-cell and perforated patch recordings from O_2-sensitive rat carotid body cells grown in short- and long-term culture. *Pflügers Arch* 418: 93-101, 1991.
17. Peers C: Hypoxic suppression of K^+ currents in type I carotid body cells: selective effect on the Ca^{2+}-activated K^+ current. *Neurosci Lett* 119:253-256, 1990.
18. Buckler KJ: Effects of hypoxia on resting (leak) potassium conductance in carotid body type-I cells of the neonatal rat. *J Physiol* 489:56P, 1995.
19. Wyatt CN, Peers C: Ca^{2+}-activated K^+ channels in isolated type I cells of the neonatal rat carotid body. *J Physiol* 483:559-565, 1995.
20. Buckler KJ, Vaughan-Jones RD: Effects of hypoxia on membrane potential and intracellular calcium in rat neonatal carotid body type I cells. *J Physiol* 476:423-428, 1994.
21. Hatton CJ, Peers C: Hypoxic inhibition of K^+ currents in isolated rat type I carotid body cells: evidence against the involvement of cyclic nucleotides. *Pflügers Arch* 433:129–135, 1996.

22. Hatton CJ, Peers C: Effects of cytochrome P450 inhibitors on ionic currents in isolated rat type I carotid body cells. *Am J Physiol* 271:C85-C92, 1996.
23. Yuan X-J, Tod ML, Rubin LJ, et al: Inhibition of cytochrome P450 reduces voltage-gated K^+ currents in pulmonary arterial myocytes. *Am J Physiol* 268:C259-C270, 1995.
24. Wyatt CN, Wright C, Bee D, et al: O_2-sensitive K^+ currents in carotid body chemoreceptor cells from normoxic and chronically hypoxic rats and their roles in hypoxic chemotransduction. *Proc Natl Acad Sci USA* 92:295-299, 1995.
25. Carpenter E, Hatton CJ, Pepper DR, et al: Developmental changes in isolated rat type I carotid body cell K^+ currents and their modulation by hypoxia. *J Physiol* 501:49–58, 1997.
26. Eden GJ, Hanson MA: Effects of chronic hypoxia from birth on the ventilatory response to acute hypoxia in the newborn rat. *J Physiol* 392:11-19, 1987.
27. Hanson M, Kumar P: Chemoreceptor function in the fetus and neonate. *Adv Exp Med Biol* 360:99-108, 1994.
28. Pepper DR, Landauer RC, Kumar P: Postnatal development of CO_2-O_2 interaction in the rat carotid body in vitro. *J Physiol* 485:531-541, 1995.
29. Donnelly DF, Doyle TP: Developmental changes in hypoxia-induced catecholamine release from rat carotid body. *J Physiol* 475:267-275, 1994.
30. Kholwadwala D, Donnelly DF: Maturation of carotid chemoreceptor sensitivity to hypoxia: in vitro studies in the newborn rat. *J Physiol* 453:461-473, 1992.
31. Wach RA, Bee D, Barer GR: Dopamine and ventilatory effects of hypoxia and almitrine in chronically hypoxic rats. *J Appl Physiol* 67:186-192, 1989.
32. Severinghaus JW, Bainton CR, Carcelen A: Respiratory insensitivity to hypoxia in chronically hypoxic man. *Respir Physiol* 1:308-334, 1966.
33. Dhillon DP, Barer GR, Walsh M: The enlarged carotid body of the chronically hypoxic and hypercapnic rat: a morphometric study. *Q J Exp Physiol* 69:301-317, 1984.
34. McGregor KH, Gil J, Lahiri S: A morphometric study of the carotid body in chronically hypoxic rats. *J Appl Physiol* 57:1430-1438, 1984.
35. Peers C: Selective effect of lowered extracellular pH on Ca^{2+}-dependent K^+ currents in type I cells isolated from the neonatal rat carotid body. *J Physiol* 422: 381-395, 1990.
36. Peers C: Effects of D600 on hypoxic suppression of K^+ currents in isolated type I carotid body cells of the neonatal rat. *FEBS Lett* 271:37-40, 1990.

Chapter 14

Oxygen Sensing by Rat Chromaffin Cells: Adrenal Medulla and Carotid Body Contrasted

Colin A. Nurse
Adele Jackson
Roger J. Thompson
H. Zhong

Introduction

The ability to sense oxygen and make appropriate respiratory and cardiovascular adjustments is crucial if animals are to survive hypoxia. In mammals, glomus or type I cells in the carotid body are the main oxygen sensors which regulate blood Po_2 via reflex control of ventilation.[1] Thus, in response to low Po_2, several groups have demonstrated that type I cells depolarize and/or increase action potential frequency via closure of potassium (K^+) channels.[2–6] The resulting entry of extracellular calcium is then thought to trigger release of excitatory neurotransmitter(s) from type I cells onto apposed sensory nerve endings, which relay afferent signals to the central nervous system (see Chapters 11-13).[1,2] Type I cells derive from the embryonic neural crest and express a chromaffin phenotype[7,8]; consistent with the latter property, they release catecholamines (mainly dopamine) following exposure to acute hypoxia.[1,9,10]

From: López-Barneo, J and Weir, EK: *Oxygen Regulation of Ion Channels and Gene Expression*. Armonk, NY: Futura Publishing Company, Inc., ©1998.

Whereas the carotid body plays a central role in oxygen sensing and blood Po_2 homeostasis in both neonatal and mature animals,[1] the fetus and newborn face particular challenges in surviving the transition to extrauterine life. In particular, the stresses of birth, which involve intermittent episodes of oxygen deprivation and asphyxia, are associated with a catecholamine surge that originates in the adrenal medulla and is essential for proper regulation of cardiovascular, respiratory, and metabolic responses in the neonate.[11,12] In the absence of this surge, there is a high risk of mortality which can be demonstrated during exposure of adrenalectomized newborn rat pups to hypoxic challenge.[11] Interestingly, this vital catecholamine surge still occurs in species, e.g., rat and man, where functional sympathetic innervation of the adrenal medulla is immature or absent at birth. Studies by Seidler and Slotkin showed that acute hypoxia reduces adrenal catecholamine levels in the rat by a "non-neurogenic" mechanism, which disappears after birth at a rate that parallels the development of a functional sympathetic innervation.[13,14]

The above observations raise the possibilty that adrenomedullary chromaffin cells (AMC) in the rat may express oxygen-sensing mechanisms. Using whole-cell recording techniques and measurements of catecholamine release by High Performance Liquid Chromatography (HPLC), we show that, unlike the CB, oxygen sensing by AMC is restricted to the perinatal period.[15]

Experimental Procedures

Cultures

Primary cultures enriched in dissociated rat AMCs were prepared using a modification of the method of Doupe et al,[16] and described in detail elsewhere.[15] Dissociated rat CB cultures were prepared as previously described.[5,17,18] The cultures were grown at 37° C in a humidified atmosphere of 95% air : 5% carbon dioxide for 1 to 3 days before they were used in the patch-clamp experiments, or for determination of catecholamine (CA) release.

Electrophysiology

Voltage- and current-clamp recordings were carried out using either conventional whole-cell or nystatin perforated-patch techniques as previously described.[5,15] For membrane potential measurements in current-clamp mode, the perforated-patch method was used. Junction potentials (2–10 mV) were cancelled at the beginning of each experiment. Typically, voltage and current clamp recordings were obtained using an extracellular fluid with the following composition (mM): NaCl, 135; KCl, 5; $CaCl_2$, 2; $MgCl_2$, 2; glucose, 10; N-2-hydroxyethylpiperazine-N′-2-ethane sulfonic acid (HEPES), 10 at pH 7.4. The pipette solutions for conventional whole-cell and perforated-patch recordings were similar to those previously described.[5,15] Most recordings were obtained at room temperature (23° C) with the aid of an Axopatch-1D patch clamp amplifier equipped with a 1 GΩ headstage feedback resistor, an A-D converter, and pCLAMP software version 6.0 (Axon Instruments). Solutions were perfused under gravity and removed by suction. Hypoxic solutions were obtained by bubbling 100% nitrogen with or without the oxygen scavenger, 1 mM Na dithionite[4]; the Po_2 was measured with an oxygen electrode placed in the perfusion chamber.

Catecholamine Secretion

CA secretion from living cultures was determined by HPLC (Waters, model 510), according to procedures previously described.[15] Electrochemical detection was used to identify peaks corresponding to dopamine, norepinephrine, epinephrine, and the internal standard, di-3,4-hydroxybenzylamine hydrobromide (DHBA). Chromatograms were analyzed with a Waters 740 Data Module (Millipore, Milford, MA) and quantified by the peak area ratio method. To study CA release, cultures were first rinsed in DMEM/F12 medium before incubation for 15 minutes to 1 hour at 37° C in 100 μl bicarbonate-buffered salt solution (BBSS). Cultures were exposed to either a normoxic (Po_2 = 160 mm Hg) or hypoxic (Po_2 = 75 or 35 mm Hg) atmosphere in the presence of 5% carbon dioxide (pH = 7.4). At the end of some release experiments, cultures were processed for tyrosine hydroxylase (TH) immunofluorescence as previously described,[17,18] to obtain an absolute count of the number of AMCs present.

Hypoxia Suppresses Voltage-Dependent K^+ Currents in Both Neonatal Adrenomedullary and Glomus Cells

In electrophysiologic studies, cultures of dissociated rat CB cells or AMCs were studied with conventional whole-cell or nystatin perforated-

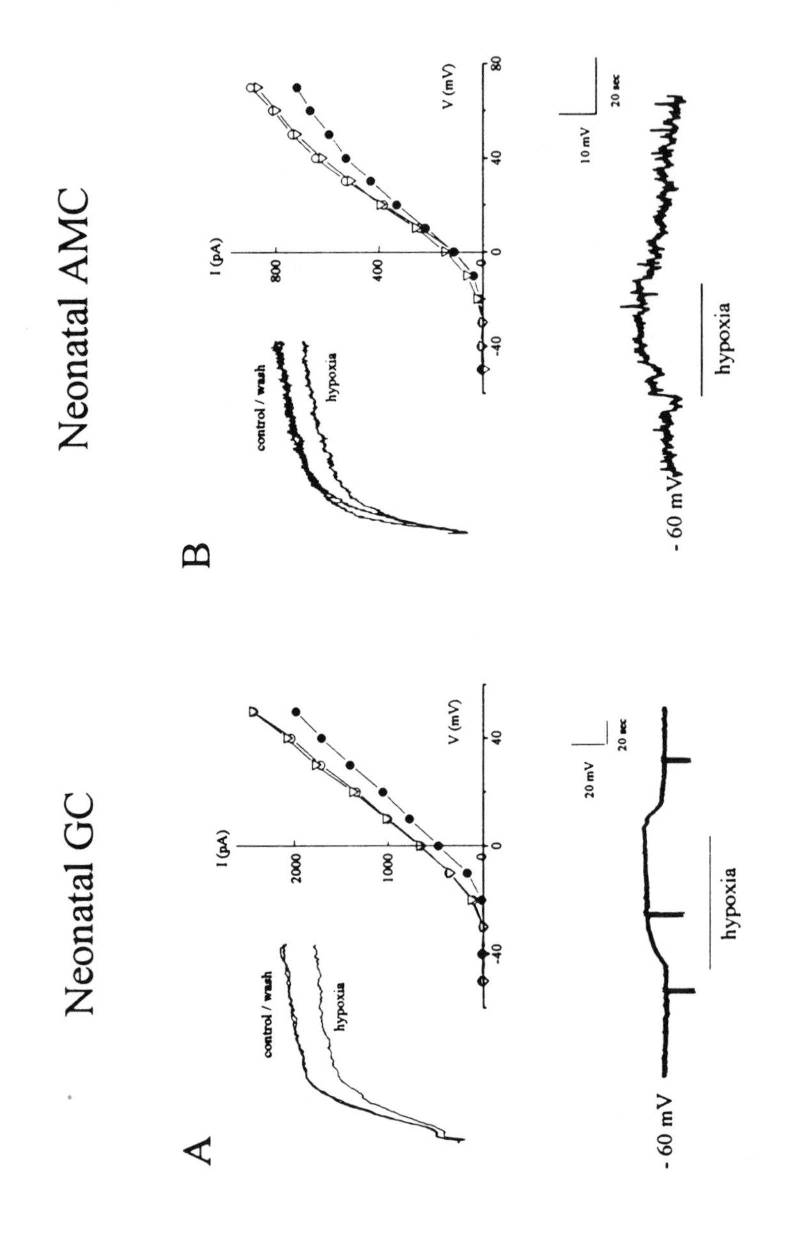
A
Neonatal GC
control / wash
hypoxia
I (pA)
2000
1000
-40
0
40
V (mV)
20 mV
20 sec
- 60 mV
hypoxia
B
Neonatal AMC
control / wash
hypoxia
I (pA)
800
400
-40
0
40
80
V (mV)
10 mV
20 sec
- 60 mV
hypoxia

patch techniques after 1 to 5 days in vitro. The majority of recordings from AMCs were done after 1 to 3 days in vitro.

As expected from previous voltage clamp studies on rat CB,[4,5] hypoxia reversibly suppressed outward K^+ current in *neonatal* glomus cells (GC). An example is illustrated in Figure 1A where hypoxia (Po_2 = ~30 Torr) suppressed K^+ current at depolarized voltages > −20 mV. The percent suppression varied from cell to cell and was typically in the range of 15% to 30%. A comparable level of hypoxia was also effective in suppressing the outward current in the majority (~70%) of *neonatal* AMC (n = 55) (Figure 1B). During voltage steps to +20 mV from a holding potential of −60 mV, the average K^+ suppression was 24% when the Po_2 was lowered from 160 Torr to ~40 Torr.[15] Previous studies in neonatal rat GC identified Ca^{2+}-dependent K^+ channels as the K^+ channel subtype that was closed by hypoxia,[4,20] although whether the same channel type mediates the hypoxic response in neonatal AMC is presently under investigation. Interestingly, in a recent study on PC12 cells, a cell line derived from the rat adrenal medulla, it was found that hypoxia suppressed a calcium- *insensitive*, delayed rectifier type K^+ current.[21]

Hypoxia Depolarizes both Neonatal Adrenomedullary and Glomus Cells

The effects of hypoxia on the membrane potential of *neonatal* AMC and GC were investigated with perforated-patch recording in current-clamp mode. In several experiments, hypoxia elicited a 10 to 15 mV depolarization in both cell types (Figures 1A and 1B; lower traces), and the depolarization was accompanied by a conductance *decrease*,[15] consistent with the closing of ion channels that were open at the resting potential. An example of this decrease in conductance is illustrated in Figure 1A

Figure 1. Comparison of the effects of acute hypoxia on outward K^+ currents and membrane potential in *neonatal* glomus (GC) and adrenomedullary chromaffin (AMC) cells. **A.** Under voltage clamp, hypoxia (Po_2 = 25–30 Torr) reversibly suppresses K^+ current in neonatal GC during voltage steps from −60 mV to +20 mV (**upper left traces**), or to various step potentials positive to + 30 mV (I-V plot; **closed circles**). In **lower trace**, hypoxia reversibly depolarizes a neonatal GC associated with a conductance *decrease*, indicated by passing brief constant hyperpolarizing current pulses (**downward deflections**). **B.** Similar records are shown for neonatal AMCs; they demonstrate that adrenal chromaffin cells in *neonatal* rats possess similar oxygen-sensing mechanisms as carotid body glomus cells. **Upper left traces** and **I-V plots** are leak subtracted.

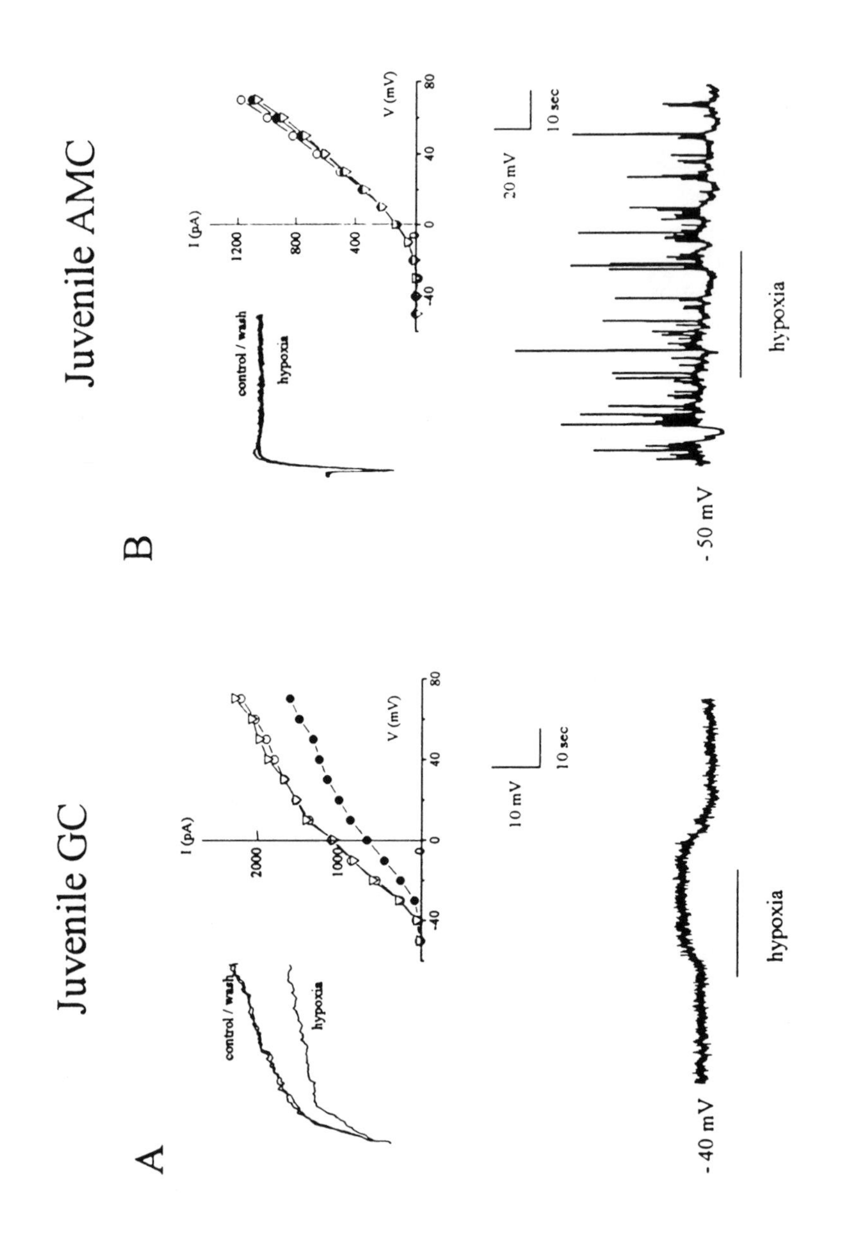
A
Juvenile GC
control / wash
hypoxia
I (pA)
2000
1000
0
-40
0
40
80
V (mV)
10 mV
10 sec
- 40 mV
hypoxia
B
Juvenile AMC
control / wash
hypoxia
I (pA)
1200
800
400
0
-40
0
40
80
V (mV)
20 mV
10 sec
- 50 mV
hypoxia

(lower trace) for a neonatal GC, by passing brief constant hyperpolarizing current pulses. The hypoxia-induced depolarization in neonatal rat GC is consistent with reports from other laboratories.[6,20] In neonatal AMC, the depolarization was sometimes sufficient to elicit action potentials even during recordings at room temperature.[15]

Differential Effects of Hypoxia on Membrane Properties of Juvenile Adrenomedullary and Glomus Cells

As was the case for neonates, GC obtained from juvenile (P14-P16) rats were also sensitive to hypoxia during whole-cell recordings. In eight cells studied under voltage clamp, there was a clear reversible suppression of the voltage-dependent K^+ current in seven cases (e.g., Figure 2A; upper traces); under current clamp, there was a membrane depolarization of 5 to 10 mV (n = 5; e.g., Figure 2A; lower traces). In marked contrast, >95% juvenile AMC (n = 27) obtained from animals of a comparable age were unresponsive to hypoxia in both voltage and current-clamp studies (e.g., Figure 2B). In Figure 2B (lower trace), the AMC was spontaneously active, but there was no obvious effect of hypoxia on spike frequency (see Reference 15). These results suggest that in the rat, the oxygen-sensing mechanism in AMCs is only transiently expressed in the perinatal period.

Hypoxia-Induced Catecholamine Release in Adrenomedullary and Carotid Body Cultures

In order to test whether the above contrasting membrane responses in AMC and GC during hypoxia correlate with their secretory activities, CA release was measured in AMC and CB cultures using HPLC. As ex-

Figure 2. Comparison of the effects of acute hypoxia on outward K^+ currents and membrane potential in *juvenile* glomus (GC) and adrenomedullary chromaffin (AMC) cells. Sequence of traces in **A** and **B** is similar to that described in Figure 1. In contrast to Figure 1, however, only juvenile GC are sensitive to hypoxia; juvenile AMC are *unresponsive* to hypoxia in both voltage (B; **upper records**) and current clamp (B; **lower record**) studies. Note in **B**, this juvenile AMC was spontaneously active, but hypoxia had no obvious effect on spike frequency. Age of juvenile rats varied from 13 to 21 days.

pected from previous studies on neonatal rat CB cultures,[9] hypoxia (Po_2 = ~75 Torr) caused almost a threefold increase in dopamine secretion relative to basal, during a 15-minute exposure (Figure 3A). Similar results were obtained in juvenile CB cultures (Figure 4A), supporting the main conclusion from our electrophysiologic studies that the oxygen-sensing mechanism is present in both neonatal and juvenile GCs. In these experiments, release samples were collected in two successive 15-minute intervals, in which the first sample represented basal release under normoxic (Po_2 = 160 Torr) conditions. The second release or test sample was collected after exposure to normoxia or hypoxia (Po_2 = 75 Torr) and the dopamine content expressed as a ratio, relative to the first sample (Figures 3A and 4A).

AMC cultures also secreted CA, although, in this case, epinephrine was the principal CA released.[15] As shown in Figure 3B, hypoxia was also effective in stimulating epinephrine secretion from neonatal AMC

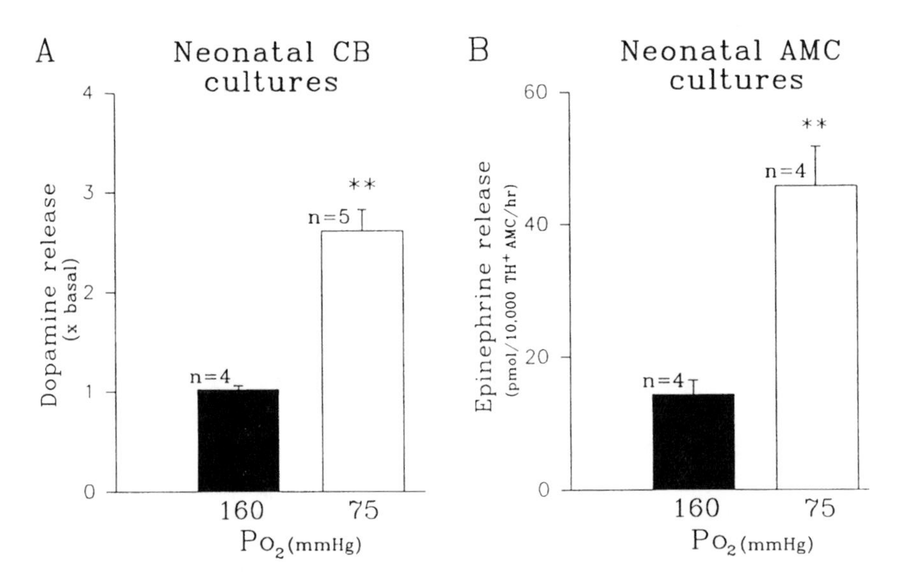

Figure 3. Comparison of the effects of Po_2 on catecholamine release in carotid body (CB) and adrenomedullary chromaffin cell (AMC) cultures derived from *neonatal* rats. Catecholamines (CA) were determined by High Performance Liquid Chromatography (HPLC) and only representative data from the main CA released, i.e., dopamine for CB cultures and epinephrine for AMC cultures, are presented; CA release was normalized to the number of tyrosine hydroxylase (TH +) cells (counted after immunofluorescent staining) present at the end of release experiments. In **A,B**. reducing Po_2 from 160 to 75 mm Hg caused a significant ($P<0.01$;**) increase in CA secretion, indicating the presence of oxygen-sensing mechanisms in both types of *neonatal* cultures.

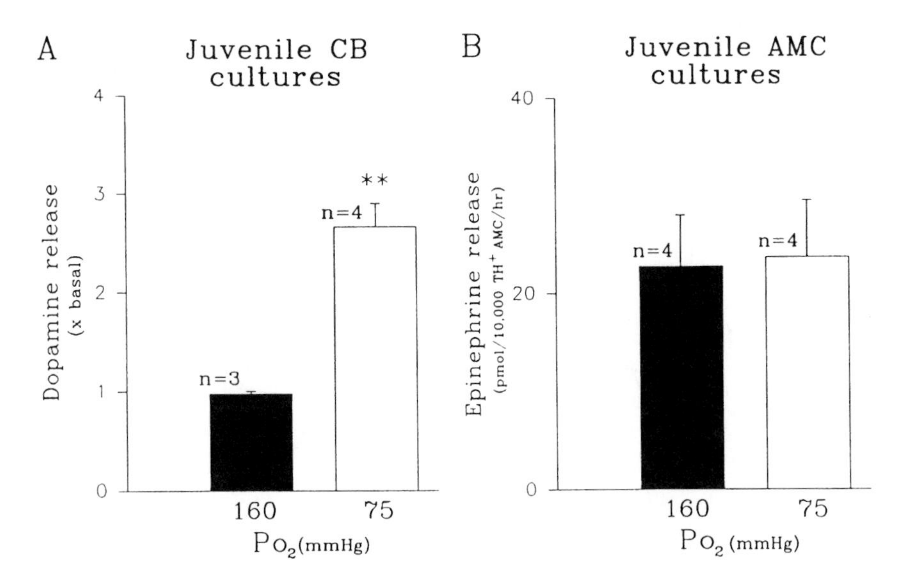

Figure 4. Comparison of the effects of Po_2 on catecholamine release in carotid body (CB) and adrenomedullary chromaffin cell (AMC) cultures derived from *juvenile* rats. Experimental details are similar to Figure 3. Note however, that whereas juvenile CB cultures continue to show Po_2-dependent catecholamine release (**A**), juvenile AMC cultures do not (**B**). Thus, reducing Po_2 from 160 to 75 mm Hg significantly ($P<0.01$) stimulated dopamine release in CB cultures, but had no significant effect on epinephrine release from AMC cultures.

cultures. In these studies, release was normalized to the number of TH-positive AMCs present in the culture at the end of each release experiment. Hypoxia also augmented release of the other CA in neonatal AMC cultures; the effect was dose-dependent and appeared to require entry of extracellular calcium since the hypoxia-induced release was abolished by the L-type calcium channel blocker, nifedipine (10 μM).[15] Notably, and in agreement with the electrophysiologic data, hypoxia failed to induce CA secretion in *juvenile* AMC cultures (Figure 4B), confirming that the mechanism for sensing oxygen in these cells was lost or downregulated during postnatal development.

Comparison of the Effects of Hypoxia on Adrenomedullary and Glomus Cells

In this study, we compared the effects of hypoxia on two related chromaffin cell types derived from the embryonic neural crest. One cell type, i.e., GC of the CB, has been well studied with respect to its oxygen-sensing mechanisms in both neonatal and mature animals.[1,2] While these mechanisms may undergo postnatal maturation, it is clear that GCs play an important role in the ability of mammals to respond appropriately to acute hypoxia. Thus, not surprisingly, we found that isolated GCs from both neonatal or juvenile rats were sensitive to hypoxia. In contrast, however, we found that AMCs from the rat adrenal medulla possessed similar oxygen-sensing properties, but these properties were lost with postnatal maturation. Thus, whereas acute hypoxia caused K^+ current suppression, membrane depolarization, and catecholamine secretion in AMCs from *newborn* rats, those from *juvenile* rats (aged 2–3 weeks) were unresponsive to hypoxia. It remains to be determined whether similar K^+ channel subtypes are involved in the hypoxic chemosensitivity of GCs and AMCs.

Although these cells share a similar embryonic origin, as well as some morphological and biochemical properties, their main innervation derives from different sources.[1,8,11] Whereas the major innervation of GCs is afferent, via dopaminergic sensory fibers in the carotid sinus nerve, AMCs receive principally an efferent innervation via preganglionic (autonomic) cholinergic fibers from the splanchnic nerve. These facts, together with the absence or immaturity of the innervation of rat AMCs at birth,[13,14] raise the interesting and testable hypothesis that the developing cholinergic innervation may regulate oxygen chemoreceptive properties in these cells.

In neonatal AMCs, the hypoxia-induced depolarization was accompanied by conductance *decrease*, as was the case for GCs. Although closure of K^+ channels provides a likely explanation for this initial depolarization, the question still remains whether more than one different K^+ channel subtype mediates oxygen-sensitive responses in AMCs. In the rat CB, at least two oxygen-sensitive K^+ channel types, i.e., a calcium-dependent, voltage-sensitive one,[4] and a calcium-independent, voltage-insensitive one (see Chapter 12), have been described. Since in rat AMCs, the hypoxia-sensitive, voltage-dependent K^+ current was activated at potentials positive to -30 mV, it is doubtful whether these channels mediate the initial depolarization at the observed resting potentials of -55 mV. Whether closure of a K^+-selective leak channel, similar to the one described in rat GCs (see Chapter 12), is involved requires further study.

Our results suggest a mechanism for adrenal CA release during hypoxic stress in the newborn rat, where sympathetic innervation is immature.[11,12] The hypoxic-sensing mechanism we have described in neonatal AMCs may well have evolved for the specific purpose of facilitating the animal's transition to extrauterine life.[11] However, since the oxygen-sensing mechanism in these cells appears to be developmentally regulated, the preparation should prove attractive for identifying the molecular determinants of oxygen chemosensitivity.

Acknowledgments

We thank Cathy Vollmer for expert technical assistance. In addition, we thank Dr. Min Zhang who took part in some of the electrophysiologic experiments. Dr. A. Jackson was supported by a Research Traineeship from the Heart and Stroke Foundation of Ontario. This work was supported by operating grants from Hospital for Sick Children Foundation (Toronto), Heart and Stroke Foundation of Ontario, and Medical Research Council of Canada. The HPLC apparatus was purchased with an equipment grant from the Natural Sciences and Engineering Research Council of Canada.

References

1. Gonzalez C, Almaraz L, Obeso A, et al: Carotid body chemoreceptors: from natural stimuli to sensory discharges. *Physiol Rev* 74:829–898, 1994.
2. Lopez-Barneo J: Oxygen-sensing by ion channels and the regulation of cellular functions. *Trends Neurosci* 19:435–440, 1996.
3. Delpiano MA, Hescheler J: Evidence for a Po_2-sensitive K^+ channel in the type-I cell of the rabbit carotid body. *FEBS Lett* 249:195–198, 1989.
4. Peers C: Hypoxic suppression of K^+-currents in type I carotid body cells: selective effect on the Ca^{2+}-activated K^+-current. *Neurosci Lett* 119:253–256, 1990.
5. Stea A, Nurse CA: Whole-cell and perforated-patch recordings from O_2-sensitive rat carotid body cells grown in short- and long-term culture. *Pflüg Arch* 418: 93–101, 1991.
6. Buckler KJ, Vaughan-Jones RD: Effects of hypoxia on membrane potential and intracellular calcium in rat neonatal carotid body type I cells. *J Physiol* 476: 423–428, 1994.
7. Pearse AGE, Polak JM, Rost FWD, et al: Demonstration of the neural crest origin of type I (APUD) cells in the avian carotid body, using a cytochemical marker system. *Histochemie* 34:191–203, 1973.
8. McDonald DM, Mitchell RA: The innervation of glomus cells, ganglion cells and blood vessels in the rat carotid body: a quantitative ultrastructural analysis. *J Neurocytol* 4:177–230, 1975.
9. Fishman MC, Greene WL, Platika D: Oxygen chemoreception by carotid body cells in culture. *Proc Natl Acad Sci USA* 82:1448–1450, 1985.
10. Montoro RJ, Urena J, Fernandez-Chacon R, et al: Oxygen sensing by ion channels and chemotransduction in single glomus cells. *J Gen Physiol* 107:133–143, 1996.
11. Lagercrantz H, Slotkin TA: The stress of being born. *Sci Amer* 254:100–107, 1986.
12. Slotkin TA, Seidler FJ: Adrenomedullary catecholamine release in the fetus and

newborn: secretory mechanisms and their role in stress and survival. *J Develop Physiol* 10:1–16, 1988.
13. Seidler FJ, Slotkin TA: Adrenomedullary function in the neonatal rat: responses to acute hypoxia. *J Physiol* 385:1–16, 1985.
14. Seidler FJ, Slotkin TA: Ontogeny of adrenomedullary responses to hypoxia and hypoglycaemia: role of splanchnic innervation. *Brain Res Bull* 16:11–14, 1986.
15. Thompson RJ, Jackson A, Nurse CA: Developmental loss of hypoxic chemosensitivity in rat adrenomedullary chromaffin cells. *J Physiol* 498.2:503–510, 1997.
16. Doupe AJ, Landis SC, Patterson PH: Environmental influences in the development of neural crest derivatives: glucocorticoids, growth factors, and chromaffin cell plasticity. *J Neurosci* 5:2119–2142, 1985.
17. Nurse CA: Carbonic anhydrase and neuronal enzymes in cultured glomus cells of the carotid body of the rat. *Cell Tiss Res* 261:65–71, 1990.
18. Jackson A, Nurse CA: Plasticity in cultured carotid body chemoreceptors: environmental modulation of GAP-43 and neurofilament. *J Neurobiol* 26(4): 485–496, 1995.
19. Stea A, Jackson A, Nurse CA: Hypoxia and N^6, $O^{2'}$-dibutryladenosine 3′,5′-cyclic monophosphate, but not nerve growth factor, induce Na^+ channels and hypertrophy in chromaffin-like arterial chemoreceptors. *Proc Natl Acad Sci USA* 89:9469–9473, 1992.
20. Wyatt CN, Wright C, Bee D, et al: O_2-sensitive K^+ currents in carotid body chemoreceptor cells from normoxic and chronically hypoxic rats and their roles in hypoxic chemotransduction. *Proc Natl Acad Sci USA* 92:295–299, 1995.
21. Zhu WH, Conforti L, Czyzyk-Krzeska MF, et al: Membrane depolarization in PC-12 cells during hypoxia is regulated by an O_2-sensitive K^+ current. *Am J Physiol* 40:C658–C665, 1996.

Chapter 15

Mechanisms of Oxygen Chemosensitivity in a Model Cell Line System

Laura Conforti
Wylie H. Zhu
Shuichi Kobayashi
David E. Millhorn

Introduction

Our laboratory has successfully demonstrated that PC12 cells can be used as a model system to study gene expression and signal transduction pathways that regulate transcription of the tyrosine hydroxylase (TH) gene during hypoxia.[1,2] TH is the rate-limiting enzyme in dopamine (DA) synthesis, a neurotransmitter released from both carotid body type I and PC12 cells during hypoxia.[3,4] Both carotid body type I cells[5] and PC12 cells originate from neural crest[6] and both are similar with respect to morphology and neurotransmitter phenotype. Based on these premises, we expected the PC12 cells to behave like carotid body type I cells or other oxygen-sensitive cells when exposed to sudden decrease of partial pressure of oxygen (Po_2). Oxygen-sensitive cells in most tissues are excitable and respond to hypoxia with the inhibition of an oxygen-sensitive K (Ko_2) channel, membrane depolarization, and an increase in cytosolic

From: López-Barneo, J and Weir, EK: *Oxygen Regulation of Ion Channels and Gene Expression.* Armonk, NY: Futura Publishing Company, Inc., ©1998.

calcium (see Chapter 11).[7] The advantage of an oxygen-sensitive cell line is the availability of a large number of homogeneous cells which provide an ideal substrate for electrophysiologic and molecular biological studies of the fundamental mechanisms of chemosensitivity. Here, we present evidence that PC12 cells respond to hypoxia in a manner that is similar to other oxygen-sensitive cells. PC12 cells express an oxygen-sensitive K channel that is similar to the Ko_2 channel recorded in rabbit carotid body type I cells[8] and pulmonary artery smooth muscle cells.[9] The Ko_2 channel in PC12 cells appears to belong to the *Shaker* subfamily of K channels. Inhibition of the Ko_2 channel in PC12 cells induces cell depolarization and an increase in intracellular Ca^{2+}.

Experimental Procedures

Cell Culture

Experiments were performed on rat PC12 cells in Dulbecco's Modified Eagle's/Ham's F-12 Medium (DMEM/F-12) supplemented with 10% fetal bovine serum, 15 mM HEPES, and penicillin/streptomycin (100 U/mL and 100 mg/mL, respectively). Cells were maintained in a normoxic incubator. PC12 were enzymatically dissociated (0.25% trypsin with 1 mM EDTA) and plated at low density (ca. 100,000/mL) for further experiments.

Electrophysiology

Macroscopic K^+ currents were recorded in whole-cell voltage-clamp configuration,[10] as previously described.[11] The cells were placed in a perfusion chamber that was situated on an inverted microscope. The cells were perfused constantly with external solution (2 mL/min perfusion rate). The volume of the medium in the chamber was maintained at 200 to 400 μL. Whole-cell patch pipettes had a 3 to 5 MΩ resistance when filled with the pipette solution. Current amplitude was measured at the end of the test pulse. Single-channel experiments were performed in cell-attached configuration.[10] Single-channel patch electrodes had a 10 to 15 MΩ resistance when filled with the pipette solution. Data were analyzed using pClamp 6.0.3 software. Values for open probability [N $\times$ Po (open probability)] were calculated dividing the time spent in the open state at each current level by the total duration of the recording.[9] All experiments were carried out at room temperature.

Experimental Solutions and Exposure of Cells to Hypoxia

The compositions of the external and pipette solutions for whole-cell experiments were (in mM): 140 NaCl, 2.8 KCl, 2 $CaCl_2$, 2 $MgCl_2$, 10 Hepes, 10 Glucose (pH 7.4) and 140 K-Gluconate, 1 $CaCl_2$, 11 EGTA, 2 $MgCl_2$, 3 ATP-sodium, and 10 Hepes (pH 7.2). For single-channel experiments, the bath and pipette solution compositions were (in mM): K-Gluconate 120, KCl 20, $MgCl_2$ 2, Hepes 10 and $CaCl_2$ 2, glucose 5, EGTA 5 (pH 7.4) and N-methyl-D-glucamine (NMG)-Gluconate 140, KCl 2.8, $MgCl_2$ 2, Hepes 10, and $CaCl_2$ 2 (pH 7.4).

Graded hypoxia was obtained by equilibrating the perfusion medium with air, 10% and 2% oxygen (balanced with N_2) and 100% N_2 with the oxygen chelator sodium dithionite (1 mM). The mean Po_2 was measured in the chamber using an oxygen-sensitive electrode. To study the effect of hypoxia on gene expression, cells were maintained for the entire course of an experiment (18 hours) in an incubator equipped with an oxygen sensor that regulates the mixing of N_2 with air to give the desired level of hypoxia (10% oxygen).

Measurement of Intracellular Ca^{2+}

Cells plated onto glass coverslips were exposed to 5 μM Fura 2 for 30 minutes (37° C). Cells were imaged using a Zeiss IM 35 fluorescence microscope equipped with a monochromator attached to a high resolution Hamamatsu SIT camera. The ratio of light intensity at the two wavelengths (340/380 nm) was calculated on-line and stored on the computer.

Reverse Transcriptase-Polymerase Chain Reaction (RT-PCR)

Total cellular ribonucleic acid (RNA) was isolated using TRI REAGENT™, as previously described.[1] Genomic deoxyribonucleic acid (DNA) was removed from total RNA with DNase treatment. RT-PCR was performed according to the protocol provided by Perkin-Elmer Cetus. Total RNA samples (1 μg) were reverse transcribed as indicated in the kit protocol. The PCR primers for the Kv genes were designed to the following regions of cDNAs: nucleotides 746 to 1153 of Kv1.2[12]; nucleotides 1375 to 1610 of Kv1.3[12]; nucleotides 2434 to 2991 of Kv2.1[13]; nucleotides 1165 to 1579 of Kv3.1;[14] and nucleotides 587 to 838 of Kv3.2c.[15] The

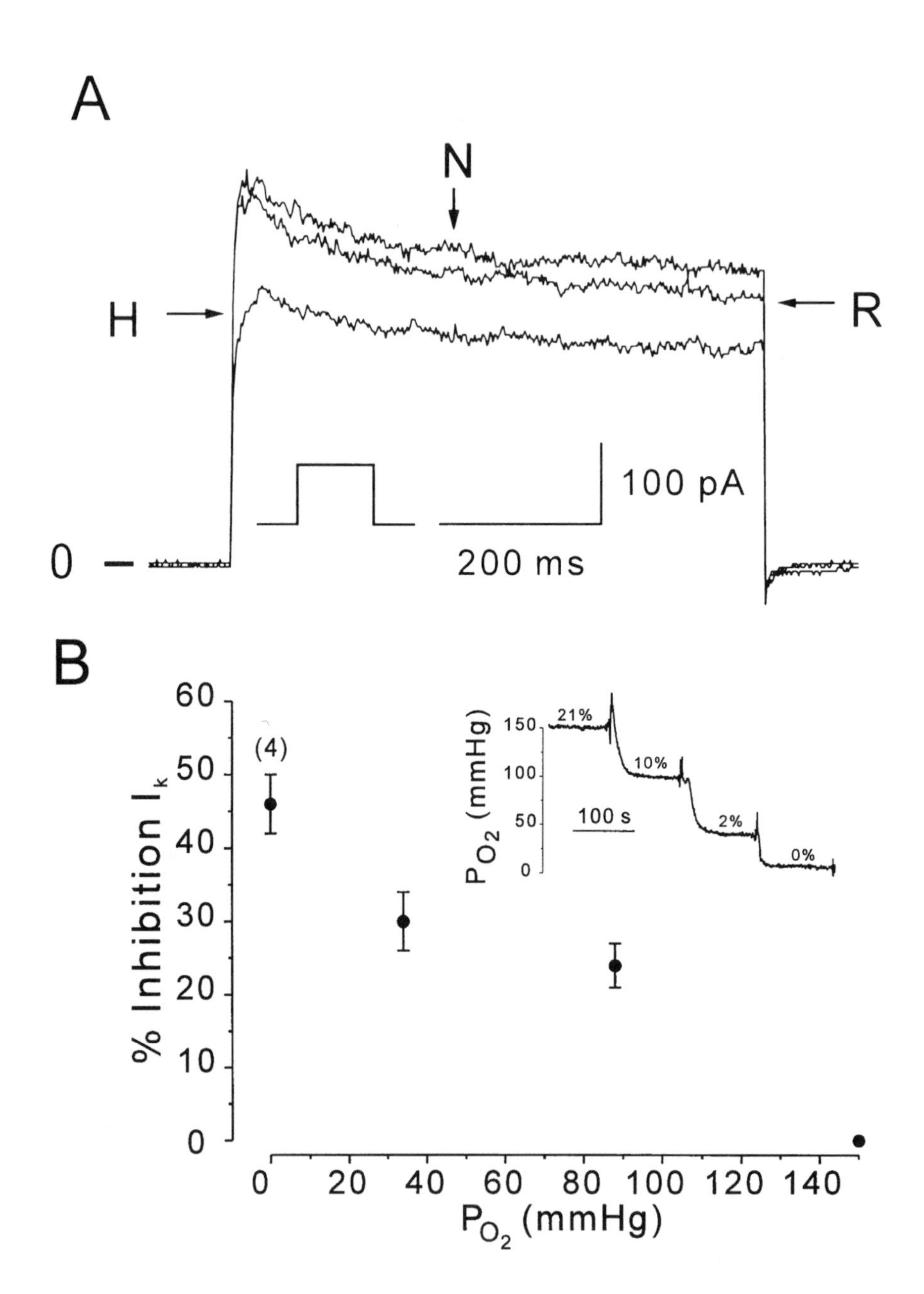
A
N
H
R
100 pA
200 ms
0
B
% Inhibition I_k
60
50
40
30
20
10
0
(4)
0 20 40 60 80 100 120 140
P_O2 (mmHg)
P_O2 (mmHg)
150
100
50
0
21%
10%
2%
0%
100 s

quantification of the change in K channel expression after prolonged exposure to hypoxia was performed by nonradioactive RT-PCR and image analysis.[16] Parallel experiments were performed for equal amounts (1 μg) of total RNA collected from cells grown in normoxic or hypoxic environments (see above). PCR products were collected at the number of cycles before reaching saturation (Kv1.2 at 35 cycles and the other genes at 25 cycles). The intensity of the ethidium bromide fluorescence was measured, and reported in arbitrary units with respect to that of the controls (set as 100). The PCR products were sequenced using an automated DNA sequencer.

Hypoxia Induces a Decrease of K^+ Current and a Rise of Cytosolic Ca^{2+} in PC12 Cells

PC12 cells express an oxygen-sensitive K current (IK_{O_2}) that is qualitatively and quantitatively similar to the K current (I_K) in rabbit type I cells[8] and pulmonary artery smooth muscle cells.[9] Figure 1A shows the inhibitory effect of hypoxia (0 mm Hg) on I_K measured in PC12 cells (22% $\pm$ 3% inhibition; n = 1). I_K was measured in whole-cell voltage clamp. The hypoxia-inhibitory response was reversed upon return to normoxia. This current, which was blocked with tetraethylammonium (TEA), a K channel blocker, did not show significant inactivation with maintained depolarization, was not sensitive to Ca^{2+}, and was independent of the holding voltage. These findings suggest that the K_{O_2} channel in PC12 cells belongs to the delayed rectifier family of K channels. We also found that the magnitude of hypoxia-induced I_K inhibition was dependent on the severity of hypoxia. Exposure to progressively lower P_{O_2} gradually reduced I_K, as shown in Figure 1B. Interestingly, continuous and progressive exposure to lower P_{O_2}-induced sensitization of IK_{O_2} resulting in a larger

Figure 1. Response to hypoxia of PC12 cells. **A.** Presence of an oxygen-sensitive K current in PC12 cells. Voltage-dependent outward K currents were recorded before (N, normoxia, 150 mm Hg), after steady-state inhibition by hypoxia (H, 0 mm Hg) and after returning to a normoxic conditions (**R**). Currents were elicited, in whole-cell patch voltage-clamp configuration, with step pulse depolarization to +50 mV from −90 mV HP (800 ms duration). **B.** P_{O_2}-dependent effect of hypoxia on I_K. Currents were elicited with same protocol as described above. Cells were exposed with progressively lower P_{O_2}, measured in the chamber by an oxygen-sensitive electrode. The actual P_{O_2} measurement is shown as an **inset**. Each **data point** represents the average of six independent cells.

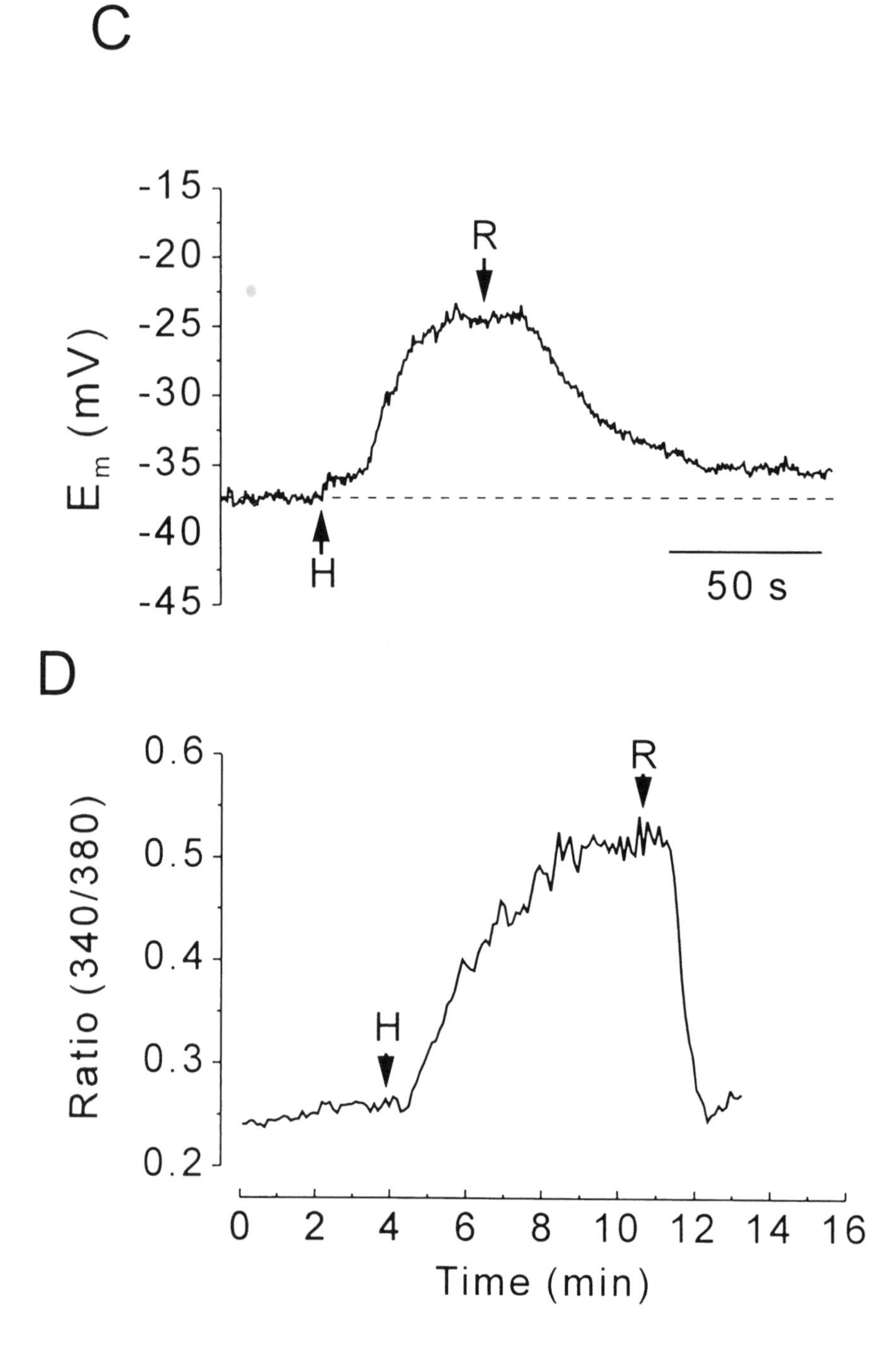
C
-15
-20
-25
-30
-35
-40
-45
E_m (mV)
R
H
50 s
D
0.6
0.5
0.4
0.3
0.2
Ratio (340/380)
R
H
0
2
4
6
8
10
12
14
16
Time (min)

current inhibition (ca. 45%; Figure 1B) than single exposure at the same Po_2 (ca. 20%; Figure 1A). This phenomenon might have physiologic relevance since, under most conditions, changes in Po_2 are often gradual and continuous. The role of the Ko_2 channel in oxygen chemosensitivity is not entirely clear. In carotid body cells, hypoxia induces depolarization followed by an increase in intracellular Ca^{2+} and eventual secretion of the neurotransmitter.[17] A similar function is mediated by the IKo_2 in PC12 cells. Figures 1C and 1D show the effect on hypoxia on PC12 cell function. Whole-cell current-clamp studies of membrane potential showed that hypoxia caused membrane depolarization (normal resting membrane potential in PC12 cells was -35 to -45 mV; Figure 1C). The amount of depolarization depended on the degree of the hypoxic stimulus (12 $\pm$ 1 mV, n = 6, Po_2 ca. 11 mm Hg; 19 $\pm$ 2 mV, n = 9, Po_2 0 mm Hg). Hypoxia also induced an increase in cytosolic Ca^{2+} in PC12 cells (Figure 1D).

Hypoxia Selectively Inhibits a Specific Type of K^+ Channel

The oxygen-sensitive Kh (Ko_2) channel was characterized in cell-attached configuration. Figure 2 shows representative recordings from a 20 pS Ko_2 channel. The slope conductance was determined with ramp pulse depolarization and reported as an inset (21 $\pm$ 3 pS; n = 4). Upon application of a step pulse depolarization, the channel opened early during the pulse depolarization and remained open for most of the pulse duration. Hypoxia led to an approximate 30% inhibition of the ensemble average current amplitude measured at the end of the pulse protocol (n = 3). The effect of hypoxia on this channel is due to a decrease in open probability ($N \times Po$), from 1.43 in normoxia to 0.62 during hypoxia. Other K channels are also present in PC12 cells: a 20 pS transient K channel, a small conductance K channel (14 pS), and a Ca^{2+}-activated K channel (102 pS). None of these channels was inhibited by hypoxia. Results from whole-cell as well as single-channel experiments indicate that the Ko_2 channel is a delayed rectifier type of K^+ channel (characterized by slow inactivation).

Figure 1. *(continued)* **C.** Hypoxia-induced membrane depolarization. Continuous recording of membrane voltage (E_m) was performed in current-clamp mode. **Dotted line** indicates the resting potential. **D.** Hypoxia increased cytosolic Ca^{2+}, measured with Fura-2. **Arrows** indicate the point of introduction of hypoxia (**H**) and return to normoxia (**R**).

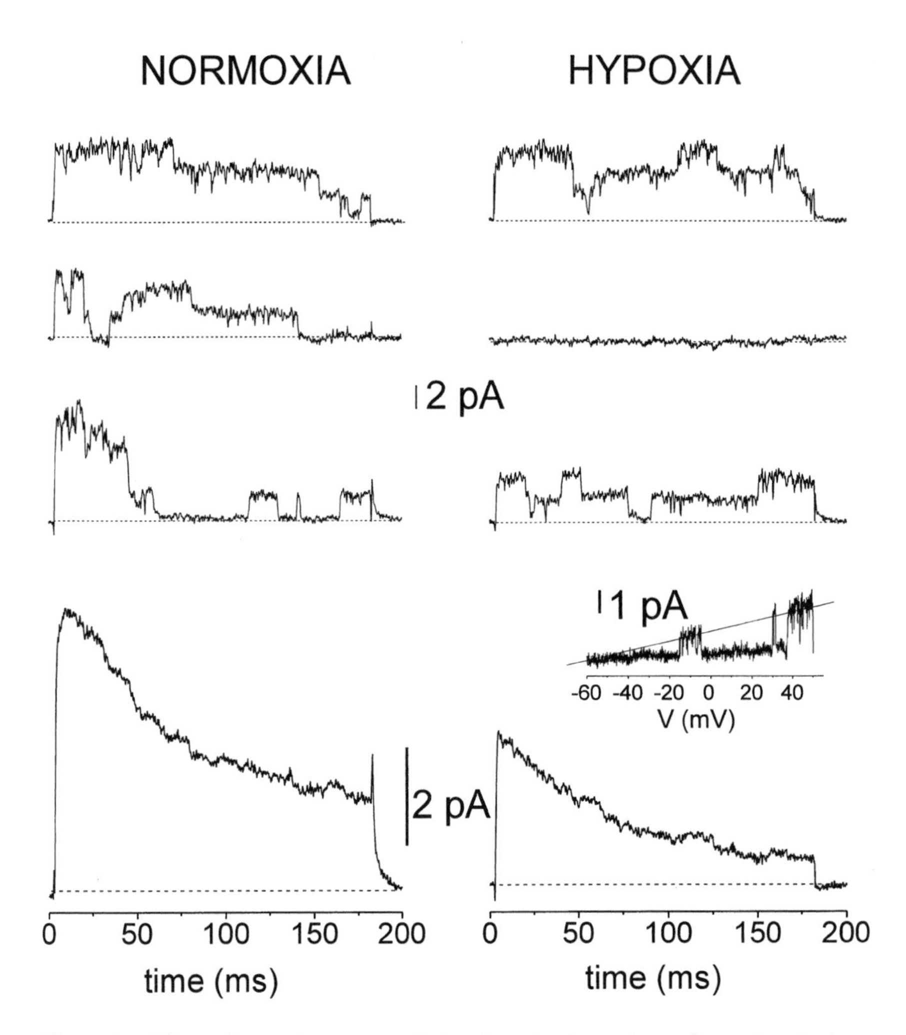

Figure 2. Effect of hypoxia on a 20 pS slow-inactivating voltage-dependent K channel. Hypoxia inhibits a 20 pS slow-inactivating outward K channel. **A. Top panels** show representative traces recorded during step depolarizing pulses (from −60 mV HP to +50 mV, 180 ms duration) in normoxia and 2 minutes after exposure to hypoxia (10% oxygen). The experiments were performed in cell-attached patch-clamp configuration. Upward current deflections from the zero current (**dotted line**) correspond to the opening of the channel. The corresponding ensemble averaged currents (from 100 consecutive traces) are shown in the **bottom panels**. This channel had a conductance of 20 pS, measured with ramp pulse depolarization (from −60 mV HP to +50 mV, 800 ms duration, 2.8 mM [K^+] in the pipette) and shown as an **inset**.

Exposure to Low Po_2 Selectively Enhances the Expression of the Kv1.2 K^+ Channel Type

We hypothesized that gene expression for Ko_2 channel would also be regulated during exposure to prolonged hypoxia. We, therefore, studied the expression of genes that code for delayed rectifier type of K channels in PC12 cells and the effect of hypoxia on regulation of these genes. Total RNA was obtained from PC12 cells in culture exposed for 18 hours to 10% oxygen and then compared to that of cells exposed to normoxia. Figure 3 shows the comparison between control and hypoxic mRNA (mea-

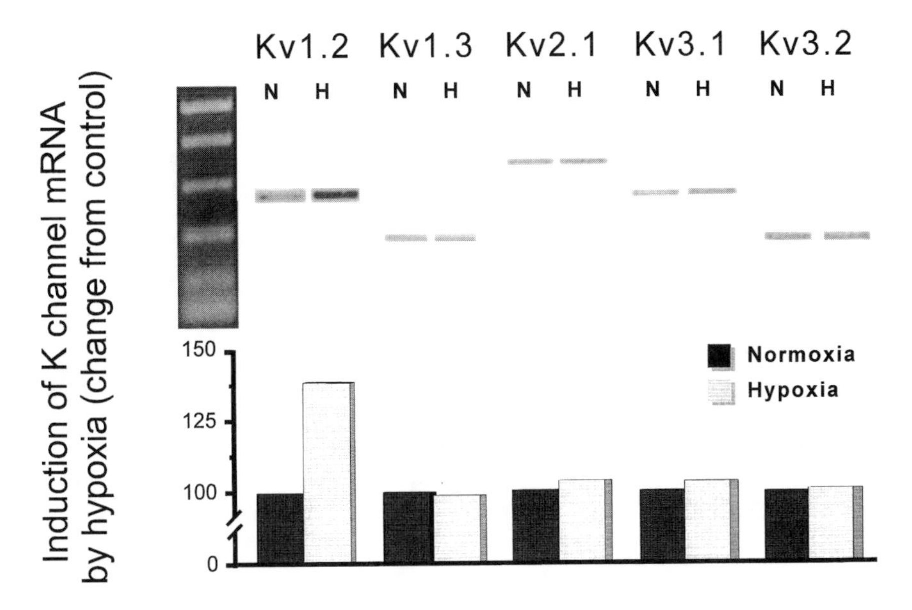

Figure 3. Regulation of expression of genes encoding the α subunit of delayed rectifier type of K channels in PC12 cells during prolonged exposure to hypoxia. **Top**: Ethidium bromide visualization of PCR products obtained by RT-PCR of total RNA of PC12 cells. The **left lane** corresponds to the PCR marker which contains six DNA fragments of 1000, 700, 500, 300, 150, and 50 bp size. PC12 cells express *Shaker* K channels genes: Kv1.2 (PCR product predicted size of 407 bp) and Kv1.3 (235 bp); *Shab* Kv2.1 (557 bp); *Shaw* Kv3.1 (414 bp), and Kv3.2 (251 bp). Agarose gel of PCR products from experiments in normoxia (N) and after prolonged exposure to hypoxia (H, 10% oxygen for 18 hours) are shown in the **top panel**. The relative intensity of the ethidium bromide fluorescence of each band is reported in arbitrary units with respect to that of the control (set as 100) and shown in the **bottom panel**. The data are the average of seven experiments for Kv1.2 and four experiments for the other genes.

sured with RT-PCR) for different K genes. The expression of Kv1.2, but not other K channel genes, increased in hypoxic conditions.

PC12 Cells as a Model System to Study the Oxygen-Dependent Cellular Functions

The current study is important in establishing the suitability of PC12 cells as an oxygen-sensitive model cell line. The model cell shown in Figure 4 summarizes the different steps involved in the oxygen sensitivity

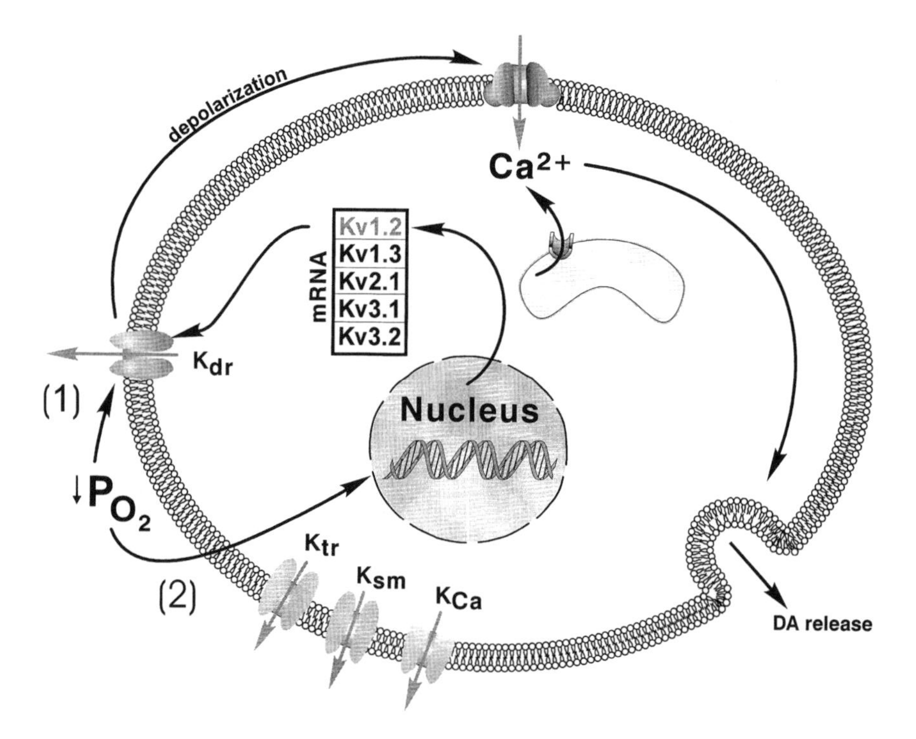

Figure 4. Cell model outlining the effect of hypoxia in PC12 cells. PC12 cells express at least four types of voltage-dependent K channels: delayed rectifier (K_{dr}), transient (K_{tr}), small conductance (K_{sm}), and Ca^{2+}-activated (K_{Ca}) channels. A decrease in partial pressure of oxygen (Po_2) selectively inhibits the K_{dr}. Inhibition of this channel induces membrane depolarization, activation of voltage-dependent Ca channels, increase in cytosolic Ca^{2+}, and release of neurotransmitter. Different genes encoding delayed rectifier type of K channels are expressed in PC12 cells. Prolonged hypoxia increased expression of the *Shaker* Kv 1.2 only.

in the PC12 clonal cell line: 1) A sudden decrease in P_{O_2} in the extracellular environment selectively inhibits an oxygen-sensitive delayed rectifier type K channel in PC12 cells. The K channel inhibition leads to membrane depolarization, activation of the voltage-dependent Ca^{2+} channels, and increase of intracellular Ca^{2+}.[11] The increase in intracellular Ca^{2+} leads to an increased release of DA and altered gene expression via Ca^{2+}-activated signal transduction pathways.[18] Thus, it appears that a critical step in oxygen sensing is membrane depolarization by inhibition of the oxygen-sensitive K channel. Different types of K^+ channels have been reported in PC12 cells[19] and in rabbit carotid body type I cells.[8] Their conductances and gating properties are very similar to those of the different K channels we recorded in PC12 cells. We found that hypoxia inhibited a 20 pS delayed rectifier K channel, but not other K channels. A similar response to hypoxia has been observed for a K channel of similar conductance in the rabbit carotid body type I cells[8] and in pulmonary artery smooth muscle cells[9]; and 2) Exposure to hypoxia over a long period of time increases expression in *Shaker* Kv1.2 gene. Kv1.2 is known to encode for slow-inactivating outward K channels of similar conductance to the oxygen-sensitive K channel which we recorded in PC12 cells.[20] These data, therefore, suggest that the *Shaker* Kv1.2 channel subunit may belong to the oxygen-sensitive K channel.

Findings from this model cell line should have significant impact on understanding how a reduction in oxygen tension is detected and transduced into the appropriate physiologic response, as well as how oxygen-sensitive cells adapt to chronic exposure to hypoxia via regulation of gene expression.

Acknowledgments

This research was supported by NIH grant R37-HL33831 to David R.E. Millhorn.

References

1. Czyzyk-Krzeska MF, Bayliss DA, Lawson EE, et al: Regulation of tyrosine hydroxylase gene expression in carotid body by hypoxia. *J Neurochem* 58:1538–1546, 1992.
2. Norris ML, Millhorn D: Hypoxia induced protein binding to O_2-responsive sequences on the tyrosine hydroxylase gene. *J Biol Chem* 270:23774–23779, 1995.
3. Yuan XJ, Goldman WF, Tod ML, et al: Hypoxia reduces potassium currents in

cultured rat pulmonary but not mesenteric arterial myocytes. *Am J Physiol* 264(8): L116-L123, 1993.

4. Zhu WH, Conforti L, Millhorn DE: Excitation-secretion in PC12 cells during hypoxia. *J Neurosci* 21(1):65a, 1995.
5. Fidone SJ, Gonzalez C: Initiation and control of chemoreceptor activity in the carotid body. In: *Handbook of Physiology, Section 3, The Respiratory System.* Vol. II, Part I. Bethesda, MD: American Physiological Society; 247, 1986.
6. Green LA, Tischler AS: PC12 pheochromocytoma cultures in neurobiological research. *Adv Cell Neurobiol* 3:373–414, 1987.
7. Lopez-Barneo J: Oxygen-sensing by ion channels and the regulation of cellular functions. *Trends Neurosci* 19:435–440, 1996.
8. Ganfornina MD, Lopez-Barneo J: Potassium channel types in arterial chemoreceptor cells and their selective modulation by oxygen. *J Gen Physiol* 100: 401–426, 1992.
9. Archer SL, Huang JMC, Reeve HL, et al: Differential distribution of electrophysiologically distinct myocytes in conduit and resistance arteries determines their response to nitric oxide and hypoxia. *Circ Res* 78:431–442, 1996.
10. Hamill OP, Marty A, Neher E, et al: Improved patch-clamp techniques for high-resolution current recordings from cells and cell-free membrane patches. *Pflügers Arch* 391:85–100, 1981.
11. Zhu WH, Conforti L, Czyzyk-Krzeska MF, et al: Membrane depolarization in PC-12 cells during hypoxia is regulated by an O_2-sensitive K^+ current. *Am J Physiol* 271:C658-C665, 1996.
12. Stühmer W, Ruppersberg JP, Schröter KH, et al: Molecular basis of functional diversity of voltage-gated potassium channels in mammalian brain. *EMBO J* 8: 3235–3244, 1989.
13. Frech GC, VanDongen AM, Schuster G, et al: A novel potassium channel with delayed rectifier properties isolated from rat brain by expression cloning. *Nature* 340:642–645, 1989.
14. Yokoyama S, Imoto K, Kawamura T, et al: Potassium channels from NG108–15 neuroblastoma-glioma hybrid cells: primary structure and functional expression from cDNAs. *FEBS Lett* 259:37–42, 1989.
15. Wiedmann R, Smith J, Williams J, et al: Shaw-like rat brain potassium channel cDNAs with divergent 3′-ends. *FEBS Lett* 288:163–167, 1991.
16. Nakayama H, Yokoi H, Fujita J: Quantification of mRNA by non-radioactive RT-PCR and CCD imaging system. *Nucleic Acids Res* 20:4939, 1992.
17. Buckler KJ, Vaughan-Jones RD: Effects of hypoxia on membrane potential and intracellular calcium in rat neonatal carotid body type I cells. *J Physiol* 476: 423–428, 1994.
18. Raymond R, Millhorn DE: Regulation of tyrosine hydroxylase gene expression during hypoxia: the role of calcium and PKC. *Kidney Int* 51:536–541, 1997.
19. Hoshi T, Aldrich RW: Voltage-dependent K^+ currents and underlying single K^+ channels in pheochromocytoma cells. *J Gen Physiol* 91:73–106, 1988.
20. Grissmer S, Nguyen AN, Aiyar J, et al: Pharmacological characterization of five cloned voltage-gated K^+ channels, type Kv1.1, 1.1, 1.3, 1.5, and 3.1, stably expressed in mammalian cell lines. *Mol Pharmacol* 45:1227–1234, 1994.

Section 4

ION CHANNELS AND FUNCTIONAL RESPONSES TO HYPOXIA

Part 2

VASCULAR SMOOTH MUSCLE

Chapter 16

Oxygen Sensing in the Pulmonary Vasculature

E. Kenneth Weir
Helen L. Reeve
Simona Tolarova
David N. Cornfield
Daniel P. Nelson
Stephen L. Archer

Introduction

The ambient oxygen tension plays a major role in determining the tone of the pulmonary vasculature and the ductus arteriosus in the fetus. The resistance of the pulmonary circulation is high because the lungs are not expanded and because the tissue is hypoxic. The pulmonary arterial oxygen tension in the fetus is about 17 to 20 mm Hg. The ductus arteriosus is open, allowing oxygenated blood, returning to the right heart from the placenta, to bypass the lungs and be shunted to the aorta. At birth, pulmonary vascular resistance drops rapidly both as a result of the mechanical expansion of the lungs associated with ventilation, and also because of the rise in alveolar oxygen tension. The flow of blood through the ductus arteriosus decreases in the minutes after birth, in part because of the drop in pulmonary vascular resistance and in part because of active

---

From: López-Barneo, J and Weir, EK: *Oxygen Regulation of Ion Channels and Gene Expression*. Armonk, NY: Futura Publishing Company, Inc., ©1998.

constriction of the smooth muscle in the wall of the ductus that is stimulated by the rise in oxygen tension. The mechanisms by which oxygen causes constriction in the ductus arterious and vasodilation in the pulmonary vasculature are only partially understood and will be discussed in this chapter.

In the adult, the pulmonary vasculature is almost fully dilated under normoxic conditions. When there is localized atelectasis or consolidation of the lung, vasoconstriction occurs in the small pulmonary arteries which are hypoxic as a result of the decrease in ventilation. Teleologically speaking, this localized hypoxic vasoconstriction is beneficial, in that it reduces the volume of desaturated blood which flows past under-ventilated alveoli and which could decrease systemic arterial oxygen tension. However, when there is generalized hypoxia in both lungs, widespread constriction and proliferation of pulmonary artery smooth muscle cells can cause pulmonary hypertension.

Hypoxic Pulmonary Vasoconstriction

The fact that pulmonary arterial pressure rises during lung hypoxia has been known for over 100 years[1]; that hypoxic pulmonary vasoconstriction (HPV) involves the entry of extracellular calcium into the smooth muscle cells of the pulmonary arteries has seemed likely for 20 years,[2] and that depolarization of the smooth muscle occurs with hypoxia has been evident for more than 10 years.[3] How is the membrane potential of the pulmonary vascular smooth muscle cell controlled and how does hypoxia cause depolarization? Ten years ago, by analogy with the control of insulin secretion in the β cell of the pancreas, it was proposed that hypoxia might change the redox status of the smooth muscle cell membrane and, thus, decrease outward potassium current, which in turn would lead to membrane depolarization.[4] The hypothesis that hypoxia can inhibit potassium current and cause membrane depolarization in pulmonary vascular smooth muscle cells appears to be correct.[5–7] Figure 1 shows single-channel data to illustrate hypoxic inhibition of a delayed rectifier potassium channel (K_{DR}). (Further details are given in Chapter 17 and 18.) While potassium channels in these cells can be opened by oxidizing agents and closed by reducing agents,[8–12] it is not yet proven that this is the mechanism involved in HPV. Some aspects of redox gating of the channels are discussed below.

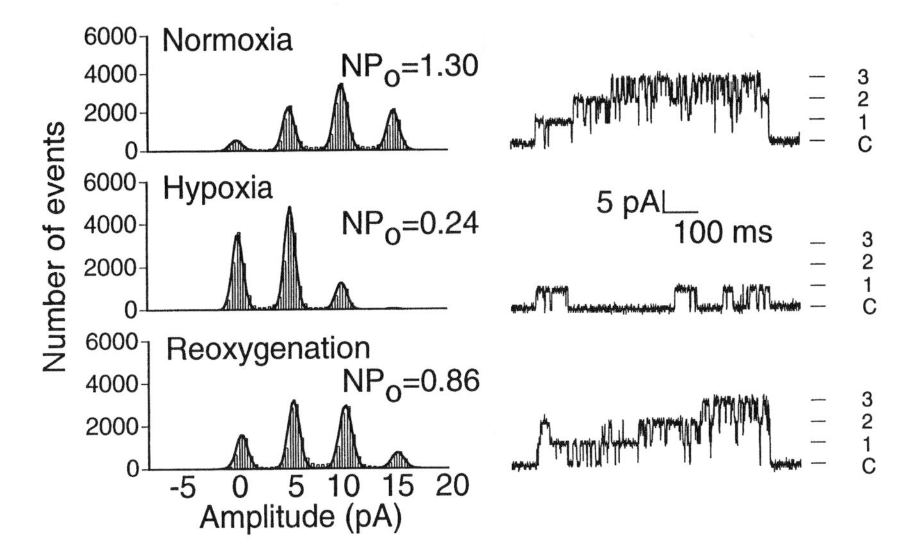

Figure 1. Hypoxia causes reversible K^+ channel inhibition. Frequency histograms and examples of actual single-channel recordings in an amphotericin-perforated vesicle obtained from a rat resistance pulmonary artery smooth muscle cell. **C** indicates channel closed; **1**, **2**, and **3** indicates number of channels open (Reproduced with permission from Reference 7.)

Oxygen-Induced Fetal Pulmonary Vasodilation

In the adult rat, the oxygen-sensitive channels appear to be in the K_{DR} group. However, in the fetal lamb, the calcium-dependent potassium (K_{Ca}) channel seems more likely to be oxygen sensitive. In the lamb in utero, ventilation of the maternal ewe with 100% oxygen causes a reduction in fetal pulmonary vascular resistance.[13] If blockers of K_{Ca} channels, tetraethylammonium (TEA) or iberiotoxin, are administered into the pulmonary artery, this oxygen-induced pulmonary vasodilatation is diminished (Figure 2). Further evidence involving K_{Ca} channels has been obtained from whole-cell patch-clamp studies of potassium current (I_K) in smooth muscle cells dispersed from small pulmonary arteries of fetal lambs.[13] The transition from hypoxia to normoxia of these cells dramatically increases I_K and this increase can be reversed by charybdotoxin (100 nM), a relatively specific blocker of K_{Ca} channels (Figure 3). The I_K measured in these cells during normoxia can be significantly increased by nitric oxide,[13] which is known to activate K_{Ca} channels.[14] Hypoxia caused

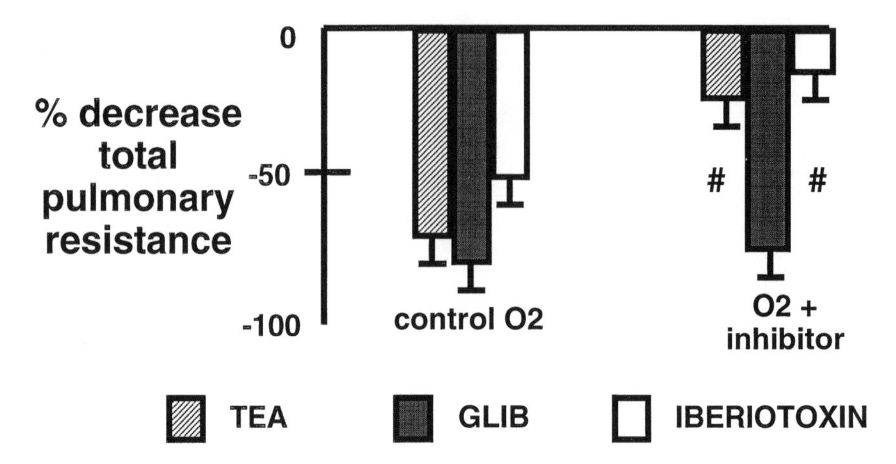

Figure 2. Effect of K^+ channel inhibition on oxygen-induced ovine fetal pulmonary vasodilation. In each of the control periods, 100% oxygen given to the maternal ewe causes a decrease in total pulmonary resistance in the fetus. Tetraethylammonium (▨; N = 5) and Iberiotoxin (□; N = 5), which are K_{Ca} channel blockers, reduce the oxygen-induced pulmonary vasodilation ($P<0.05$). Glibenclamide (■), a K_{ATP} channel blocker, has no effect. (Drawn from data in Reference 13.)

membrane depolarization in these fetal cells, which can be mimicked by charybdotoxin. This observation suggests that the K_{Ca} current may be present at the resting membrane potential and, thus, is physiologically relevant. It appears likely that there is a developmental change in the oxygen sensitivity of potassium channels in the pulmonary vascular smooth muscle, such that K_{Ca} channels are sensitive to changes in oxygen tension in the fetus and K_{DR} channels are sensitive later in life. An incidental finding in the fetal ovine smooth muscle cells was the presence of spontaneous transient outward currents (STOCs), which were not observed in cells from 2-week-old sheep.[13] STOCs are carried by the K_{Ca} channels, but their relationship to hypoxia has not yet been established.

A switch in the oxygen-sensitive potassium channel seems also to occur in the carotid body, or in different species. In the neonatal rat, K_{Ca} channels (190 pS) in the type I cell are reported to be inhibited by hypoxia, when studied in perforated vesicles.[15] In the adult rabbit, the oxygen-sensitive potassium channel is not affected by calcium and has a conductance of about 20 pS.[16] These observations suggest that the oxygen sensor, whether it is a β subunit or a membrane-associated electron transport chain such as nicotinamide adenine dinucleotide phosphate [NAD(P)H] oxidase, can be expressed with different potassium channels, in different cell types, and at different stages of development.

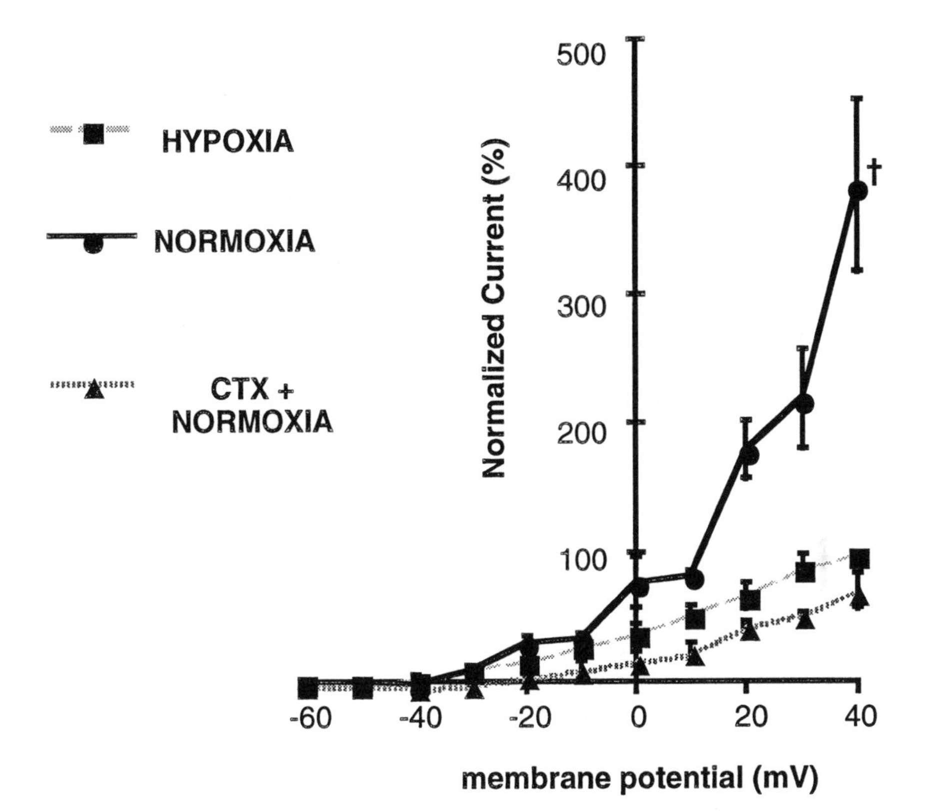

Figure 3. Effect of normoxia on K^+ currents in smooth muscle cells freshly dispersed from distal pulmonary arteries of the ovine fetus. Whole-cell current increases on changing from hypoxia (Po_2 25 mm Hg) to normoxia (Po_2 120 mm Hg). Charybdotoxin (Ctx, 100 nM) decreases the current during continued normoxia. ■ = hypoxia; ● = normoxia; ▲ = Ctx + normoxia. Current-voltage relationship different from hypoxic control ($P<0.01$). (Reproduced with permission from Reference 13.)

Oxygen-Induced Constriction of the Ductus Arteriosus

As the pulmonary vasculature dilates at birth, the ductus arteriosus constricts. Twenty-five years ago, it was demonstrated that the constriction of the ductus is directly proportional to the rise in oxygen tension.[17] When rings from the ductus of fetal rabbits at term are transferred from hypoxia (22 mm Hg) to normoxia (133 mm Hg), constriction occurs, in the presence or absence of endothelium.[18] Similar contraction can be elicited during continued hypoxia by 4-aminopyridine, the blocker of K_{DR} channels, but not by glibenclamide (K_{ATP} blocker) or tetraethylammonium (K_{Ca} blocker). The addition of oxygen on top of 4-aminopyridine did not increase the contraction further. When single smooth muscle cells from the ductus are studied under hypoxic conditions using the whole-cell patch-clamp technique, the introduction of normoxia or 4-aminopyridine (1 mM) can be seen to inhibit I_K at test potentials near the resting membrane potential.[18] The physiologic significance of the inhibition of I_K is strengthened by the fact that normoxia and 4-aminopyridine both cause membrane depolarization, while tetraethylammonium and glibenclamide do not. These findings suggest that oxygen inhibits a K_{DR} channel, causing membrane depolarization and calcium entry through the voltage-gated calcium channels. Single-channel recordings (Figure 4) from a cell-attached patch indicate that the channel inhibited by normoxia has a conductance of 58

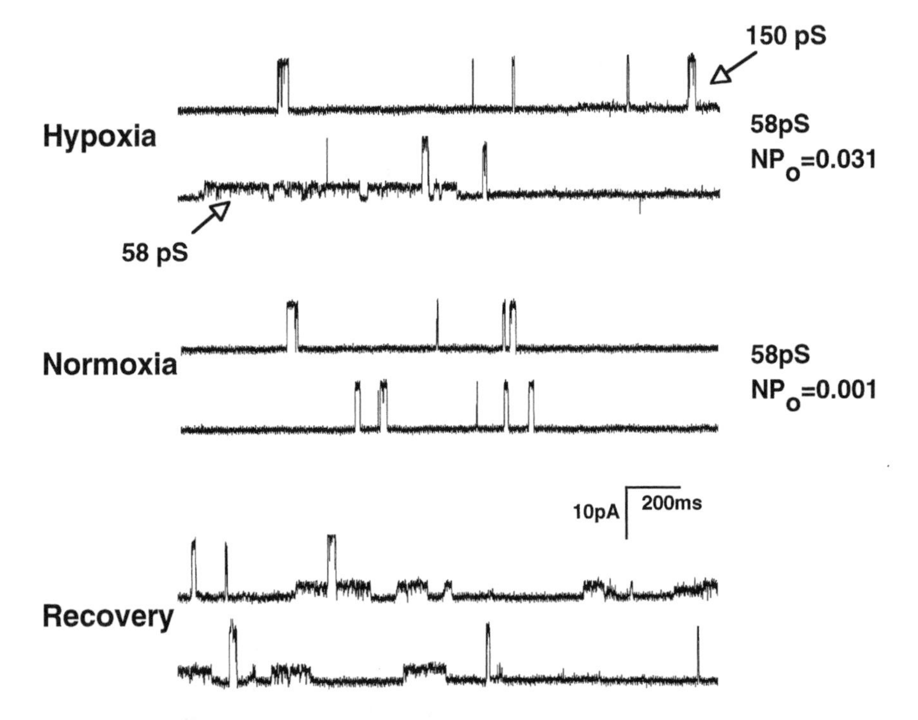

Figure 4. Cell-attached, single-channel recording from a smooth muscle cell freshly dispersed from the ductus arteriosus of a neonatal lamb (+40 mV). Two distinct channels are shown: a 150 pS channel, sensitive to tetraethyl ammonium (TEA) (5 mM), and a 58 pS channel, sensitive to 4-AP (1 mM). Normoxia inhibits the smaller conductance channel, while leaving the larger conductance channel unchanged.

pS and is sensitive to 4-aminopyridine. The 150 pS channel, sensitive to tetraethylammonium, is not inhibited by normoxia.

Entry of extracellular calcium is necessary for normoxic constriction of the ductus. Normoxia will more than double cytosolic calcium in ductal rings,[18] while simultaneously increasing tension. The use of nisoldipine (0.5 μM) or lanthanum (5 mM) will completely inhibit normoxic contraction of the rings, while RO 40–5967, a blocker of T-type calcium channels has no effect. These observations point directly at the riddle of oxygen sensing. In both the pulmonary artery and the ductus arteriosus, a change in oxygen tension leads to inhibition of one or more, 4-aminopyridine-sensitive, potassium channels in the smooth muscle cell, to membrane depolarization, and to calcium entry through the L-type voltage-gated calcium channel. The difference is that, in the pulmonary artery, it is hypoxia that inhibits the potassium channel, while in the ductus, it is normoxia. This consideration raises the question of the mechanism by which changes in oxygen tension alter the gating of the potassium channel.

Potassium Channel Gating and Oxygen

In the type I cell of the rabbit carotid body, reversible inhibition of potassium channels by hypoxia has been demonstrated in excised membrane patches.[16] The same has been shown in membrane patches excised from rat temporal cortex neurons.[19] These observations suggest that the oxygen sensor is in, or closely associated with, the membrane. The disparity between the effects of oxygen in the pulmonary artery and the ductus arteriosus makes the mitochondria less likely as the site of the oxygen sensor and again points toward the cell membrane.

There has been considerable interest in the concept that the production of oxygen radicals in proportion to the oxygen tension might determine vascular tone. Certainly, oxygen radical production, measured as luminol enhanced chemiluminescence from the surface of the rat lung, decreases immediately prior to the rise in pulmonary artery pressure.[20] Similar inhibition of chemiluminescence by anoxia has been described by others.[21] In the case of the pulmonary vasculature, the carotid body and the neuroepithelial body, it has been suggested that the production of oxygen radicals by NAD(P)H oxidase may be the mechanism by which oxygen is sensed.[22–25] It might be that the production of radicals by NADPH oxidase would produce a more oxidized environment in the vicinity of the potassium channels, favoring the open state of the channel and hyperpolarization of the membrane. Certainly, I_K in pulmonary vascular smooth muscle cells can be increased by oxidized glutathione and decreased by reduced glutathione, indicating that some of the potassium channels are redox sensitive (Figure 5).[11]

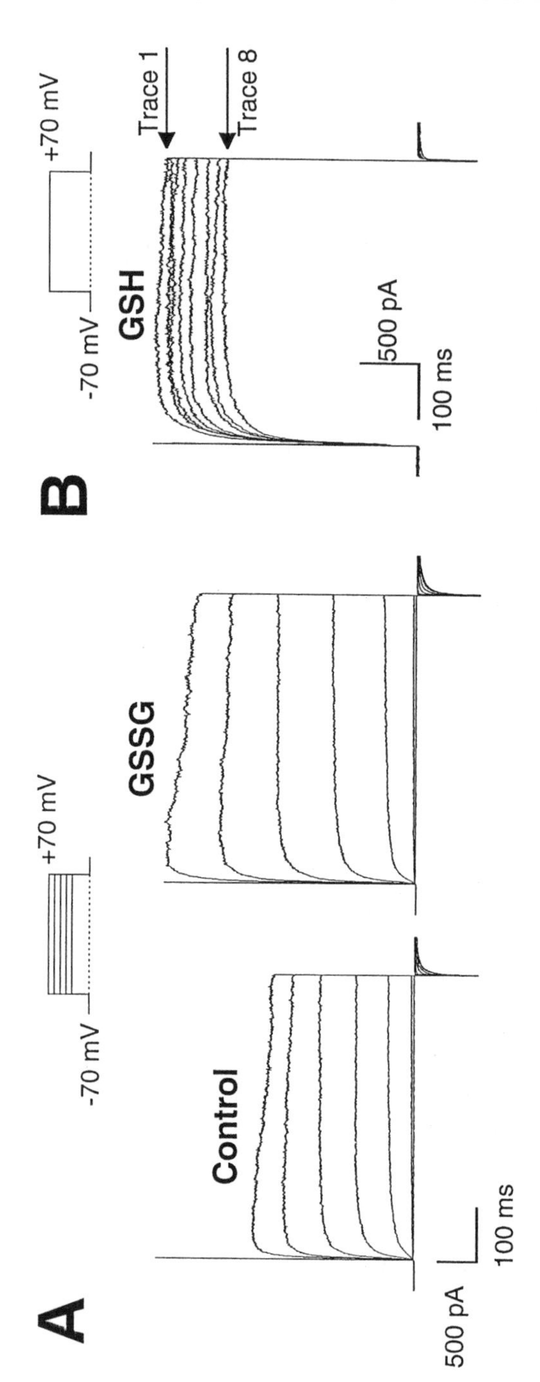
A
-70 mV
+70 mV
Control
GSSG
500 pA
100 ms
B
-70 mV
+70 mV
GSH
Trace 1
Trace 8
500 pA
100 ms

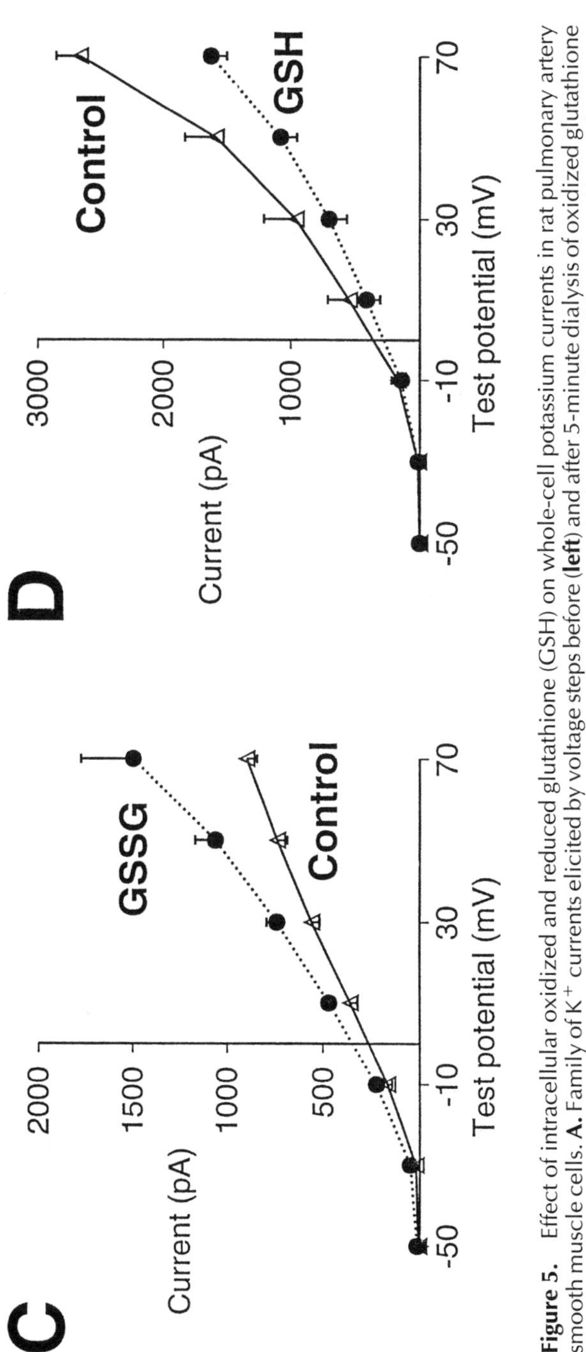

Figure 5. Effect of intracellular oxidized and reduced glutathione (GSH) on whole-cell potassium currents in rat pulmonary artery smooth muscle cells. **A.** Family of K^+ currents elicited by voltage steps before (**left**) and after 5-minute dialysis of oxidized glutathione (GSSG:2 mM) into the cell, showing an increase in outward current. **B.** Series of K^+ currents elicited by a repetitive voltage step from −70 to +70 mV, every 20 seconds after start of dialysis of reduced glutathione (GSH: 2 mM) into the cell, showing a decrease in outward current. **C.** Current-voltage relationship for mean (± SEM potassium current in the presence and absence of GSSG (2 mM). **D.** Current-voltage relationship in presence and absence of GSH (2 mM) (Reproduced with permission from Reference 11.)

Part of the evidence for implicating NADPH oxidase comes from the use of the NADPH oxidase inhibitor, diphenyleneiodonium (DPI). While DPI does inhibit potassium channels in both pulmonary vascular smooth muscle and type I cells, it also inhibits the voltage-gated calcium channels in these tissues.[26,27] Consequently, DPI has limited use in defining the

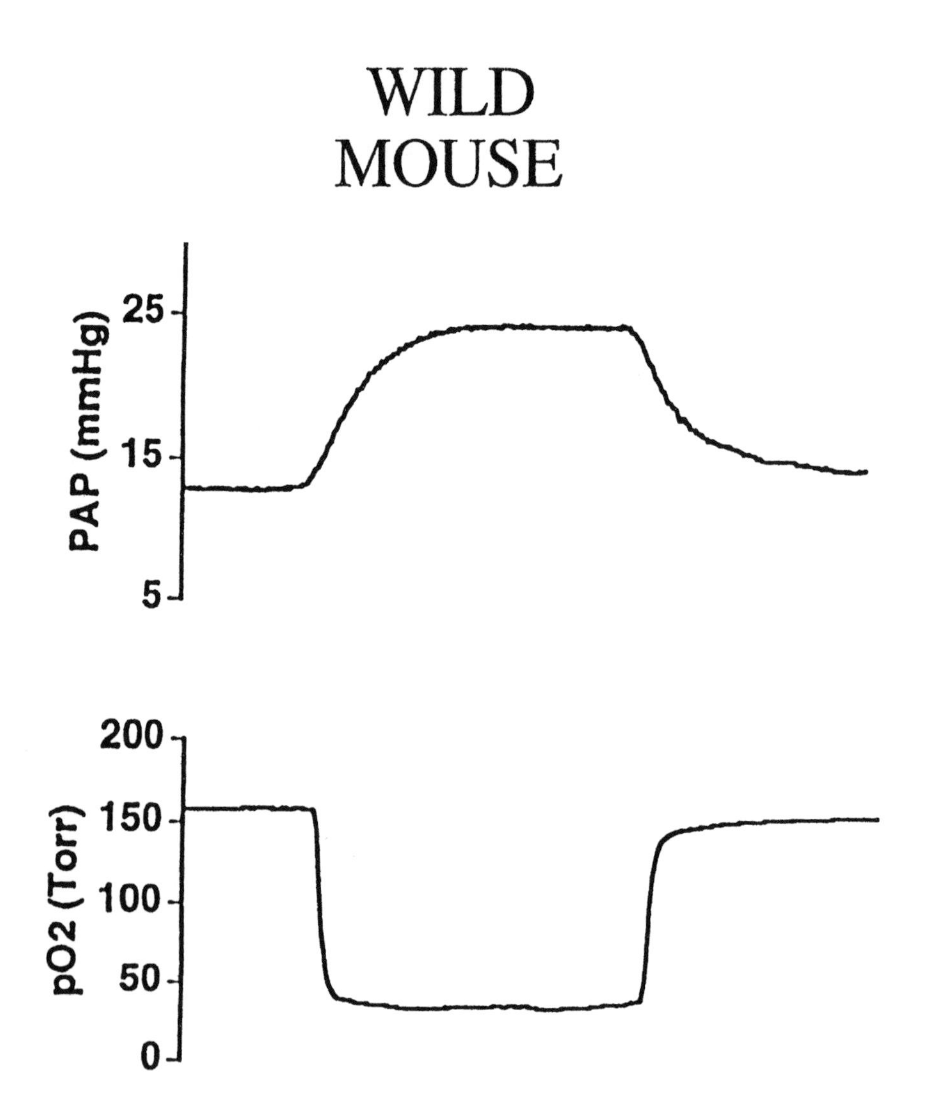

role of NADPH oxidase. A transgenic mouse has been developed which lacks the 91 kD subunit of NADPH oxidase.[28] These mice are a model of chronic granulomatous disease. We have found that the trangenic mice have a perfectly normal pulmonary pressor response, no different from that of the wild-type mice (Figure 6). Consequently, it appears, at a mini-

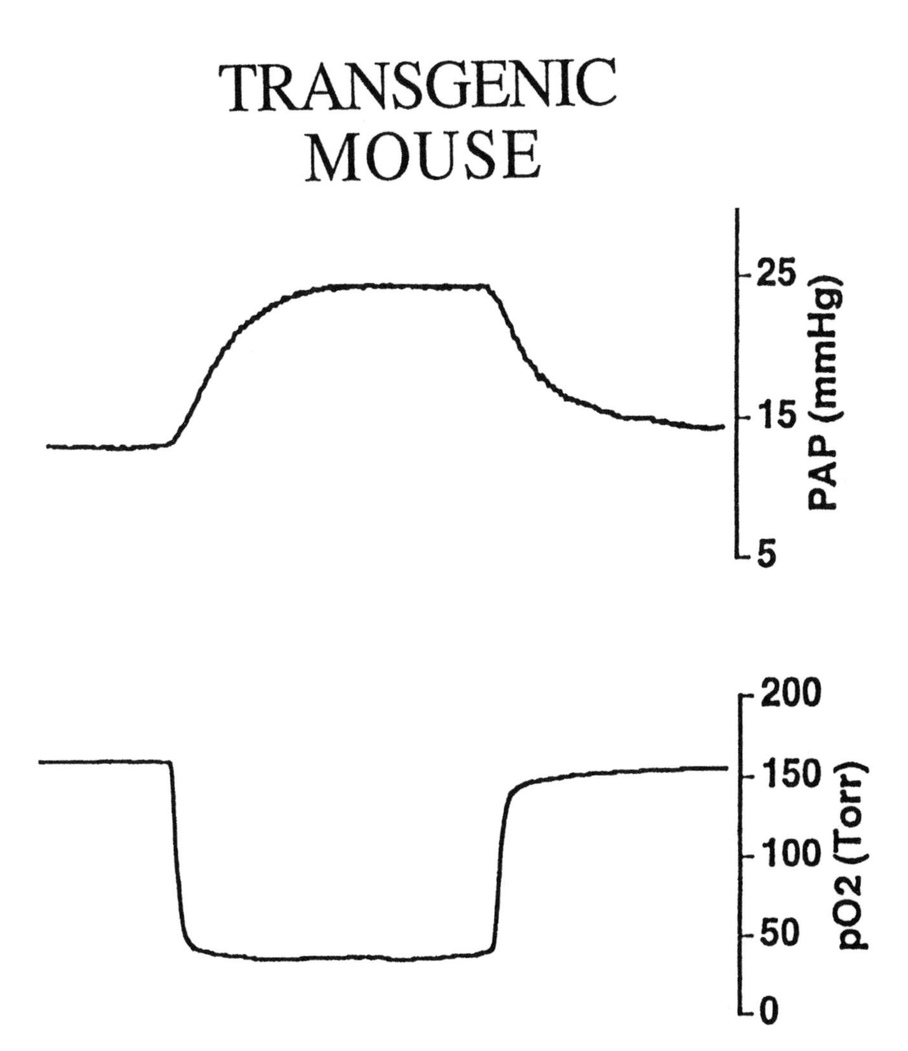

Figure 6. Pulmonary pressor response to hypoxia is the same in transgenic mice which lack nicotinamide adenine dinucleotide phosphate (NADPH) oxidase and in the wild-type mice. A representative pulmonary artery pressure trace is shown to illustrate the hypoxic pressor response in both mice.

mum, that the oxygen sensor for the pulmonary vasculature does not require all the subunits of NADPH oxidase. The redox hypothesis could still provide the sensing mechanism, either through a version of NADPH oxidase which does not require the 91 kD subunit, through NADH oxidase, or through some other oxygen-sensitive redox shift.

Redox control of potassium channels has been demonstrated in life forms as disparate as bacteria and tumor cells. In *Escherichia coli,* two potassium channels have been identified that are gated by the redox state of glutathione. Anoxia and the reducing agent dithionite inhibit potassium efflux in E. coli, whereas oxidants such as hydrogen peroxide, t-butyl hydroperoxide, and diamide increase potassium efflux. Similarly, hydrogen peroxide, and superoxide (produced by xanthine/xanthine oxidase) increase potassium current in human lung adenocarcinoma cells. Another experiment provides more information about the importance of sulfhydryl groups in the gating mechanism. Hydrogen peroxide applied to three cloned, voltage-gated potassium channels, expressed in Xenopus oocytes, increased the outward current. Two other potassium channels were unaffected. The three that were sensitive to hydrogen peroxide all have the cysteine residue in a similar amino acid sequence at the N-terminal region of the channel protein. Again, this observation is compatible with the concept that the redox status of the potassium channel can determine its gating. The question which still remains to be resolved is whether changes in oxygen tension alter potassium channel gating through a redox mechanism.

References

1. Bradford J, Dean H: The pulmonary circulation. *J Physiol* 16:34–96, 1894.
2. McMurtry I, Davidson B, Reeves J, Grover R: Inhibition of hypoxic pulmonary vasconstriction by calcium antagonists in isolated rat lungs. *Circ Res* 38:99–104, 1976.
3. Madden J, Dawson C, Harder D: Hypoxia-induced activation in small isolated pulmonary arteries from the cat. *J Appl Physiol* 59:113–118, 1985.
4. Archer S, Will J, Weir E: Redox status in the control of pulmonary vascular tone. *Herz* 11:127–141, 1986.
5. Post J, Hume J, Archer S, Weir E: Direct role for potassium channel inhibition in hypoxic pulmonary vasconstriction. *Am J Physiol* 262:C882-C890, 1992.
6. Yuan X-J, Goldman W, Tod M, Rubin L, Blaustein M: Hypoxia reduces potassium currents in cultured rat pulmonary but not mesenteric arterial myocytes. *Am J Physiol* 264:L116-L123, 1993.
7. Archer S, Huang J, Reeve H, et al: Differential distribution of electrophysiologically distinct myocytes in conduit and resistance arteries determines their response to nitric oxide and hypoxia. *Circ Res* 78:431–442, 1996.
8. Post J, Weir E, Archer S, Hume J: Redox regulation of K^+ channels and hypoxic

pulmonary vasoconstriction. In: Weir E (ed). *Ion Flux in Pulmonary Vascular Control.* New York: Plenum Press; 189–204, 1993.
9. Yuan X-J, Tod M, Rubin L: Deoxyglucose and reduced glutathione mimic effects of hypoxia on K^+ and Ca^{2+} conductances in pulmonary artery cells. *Lung Cell Mol Physiol* 11:52-L63, 1994.
10. Park M, Lee S, Ho W-K, Earm Y: Redox agents as a link between hypoxia and the responses of ionic channels in rabbit pulmonary vascular smooth muscle. *Exp Physiol* 80:835–842, 1995.
11. Weir E, Archer S: The mechanism of acute hypoxic pulmonary vasconstriction: the tale of two channels. *FASEB J* 9:183–189, 1995.
12. Reeve H, Weir E, Nelson D, Peterson D, Archer S: Opposing effects of oxidants and antioxidants on K^+ channel activity and tone in rate vascular tissue. *Exp Physiol* 80:825–834, 1995.
13. Cornfield D, Reeve H, Tolarova S, Weir E, Archer S: Oxygen causes fetal pulmonary vasodilation through activation of a calcium-dependent potassium channel. *Proc Natl Acad Sci USA* 93:8089–8094, 1996.
14. Archer S, Huang J, Hampl V, Nelson D, Shultz P, Weir E: Nitric oxide and cGMP cause vasorelaxation by activation of a charybdotoxin-sensitive K channel by cGMP-dependent protein kinase. *Proc Natl Acad Sci USA* 91:7583–7587, 1994.
15. Wyatt C, Peers C: Ca^{2+}-activated K^+ channels in isolated type I cells of the neonatal rat carotid body. *J Physiol* 483:559–565, 1995.
16. Ganfornina M, Lopez-Barneo J: Potassium channel types in arterial chemoreceptor cells and their selective modulation by oxygen. *J Gen Physiol* 100:401–426, 1992.
17. Fay F: Guinea pig ductus arteriosus. I. Cellular and metabolic basis for oxygen sensitivity. *Am J Physiol* 221:470–479, 1971.
18. Tristani-Firouzi M, Reeve H, Tolarova S, Weir E, Archer S: Oxygen-induced constriction of rabbit ductus arteriosus occurs via inhibition of a 4-aminopyridine-, voltage sensitive potassium channel. *J Clin Invest* 98:1959–1965, 1996.
19. Jiang C, Haddad G: A direct mechanism for sensing low oxygen levels by central neurons. *Proc Natl Acad Sci USA* 91:7198–7201, 1994.
20. Archer S, Nelson D, Weir E: Simultaneous measurement of O_2 radicals and pulmonary vascular reactivity in rat lung. *J Appl Physiol* 67:1903–1911, 1989.
21. Paky A, Michael J, Burke-Wolin T, Wolin M, Gurtner G: Endogenous production of superoxide by rabbit lungs: effects of hypoxia or metabolic inhibitors. *J Appl Physiol* 74:2868–2874, 1993.
22. Thomas H, Carson R, Fried E, Novitch R: Inhibition of hypoxic pulmonary vasconstriction by diphenyleneiodonium. *Biochem* Pharmacol 42:R9-R12, 1991.
23. Grimminger F, Weissmann N, Spriestersbach R, Becker E, Rosseau S, Seeger W: Effects of NADPH oxidase inhibitors on hypoxic vasconstriction in buffer-perfused rabbit lungs. *Am J Physiol* 268:L747–L752, 1995.
24. Mohazzab-H K, Wolin M: Sites of superoxide anion production detected by lucigenin in calf pulmonary artery smooth muscle. *Am J Physiol* 27:L815-L822, 1994.
25. Youngson C, Nurse C, Yeger H, Cutz E: Oxygen sensing in airway chemoreceptors. *Nature* 365:153–155, 1993.
26. Weir E, Wyatt C, Reeve H, Huang J, Archer S, Peers C: Diphenyleneiodonium inhibits both potassium and calcium currents in isolated pulmonary artery smooth muscle cells. *J Appl Physiol* 76:2611–2615, 1994.

27. Wyatt C, Weir E, Peers C: Diphenyleneiodonium blocks K^+ and Ca^{2+} currents in type I cells isolated from neonatal rat carotid body. *Neurosci Lett* 172:63–66, 1994.
28. Pollock J, Williams D, Gifford M, et al: Mouse model of x-linked chronic granulomatous disease, an inherited defect in phagocyte superoxide production. *Nature* 9:202–209, 1995.

Chapter 17

Mechanisms of Hypoxic Pulmonary Vasoconstriction:

The Role of Oxygen-Sensitive Voltage-Gated Potassium Channels

Xiao-Jian Yuan

Introduction

Hypoxic pulmonary vasoconstriction (HPV) serves a regulatory function by matching perfusion to ventilation and shunting blood flow away from the poorly oxygenated regions of the lung. It is a critical regulatory mechanism of the lung to ensure maximal oxygenation under normal physiologic conditions. Persistent alveolar hypoxia, however, causes pulmonary hypertension which is characterized pathologically by vasoconstriction, vascular remodeling, and endothelial dysfunction. The hypoxia-mediated pulmonary hypertension causes right heart failure in patients with a variety of cardiopulmonary diseases, including chronic obstructive pulmonary disease, the fourth leading cause of death in the United States. Although extensively studied since 1876 when HPV was first observed, the precise mechanism by which hypoxia causes pulmonary vasoconstriction is still unclear. Hypoxia causes pulmonary vasoconstriction in isolated pulmonary arteries (PA) with or without endothelium,[1–4] and

From: López-Barneo, J and Weir, EK: *Oxygen Regulation of Ion Channels and Gene Expression.* Armonk, NY: Futura Publishing Company, Inc., ©1998.

induces contraction in single PA smooth muscle cells.[5,6] These results support the hypothesis that HPV is an intrinsic property of PA smooth muscle: the mechanism of HPV involves direct oxygen sensing by PA smooth muscle, and intact endothelial function plays a prominent role in modulating pulmonary vasomotor tone.[2]

Elevation of cytoplasmic free calcium concentration ($[Ca^{2+}]_i$) is a major trigger for both vasoconstriction and cell proliferation in vascular smooth muscle, including PA smooth muscle. $[Ca^{2+}]_i$ is primarily regulated by Ca^{2+} influx through sarcolemmal Ca^{2+} channels and Ca^{2+} release from intracellular stores (mainly sarcoplasmic reticulum [SR], but also including mitochondria). By governing Ca^{2+} influx through voltage-gated Ca^{2+} channels, membrane potential (E_m) is an important regulator of vascular tone.[7,8] Similar to neurons and cardiac myocytes, in vascular smooth muscle, E_m is predominantly controlled by potassium (K^+) permeability, which is determined by sarcolemmal K^+ channel conductance and transmembrane K^+ gradient. In PA smooth muscle cells, at least three types of K^+ currents have been described: 1) voltage-gated K^+ (K_V) currents ($I_{K(V)}$), composed of A-type, delayed-rectifier and noninactivating currents[9–11]; 2) Ca^{2+}-activated K^+ (K_{Ca}) currents ($I_{K(Ca)}$)[12]; and 3) adenosine triphosphate (ATP)-sensitive K^+ (K_{ATP}) currents ($I_{K(ATP)}$).[13] Although all of these K^+ currents, as well as Cl^- currents and Na^+ pump activity, participate in the regulation of E_m, $I_{K(V)}$ has been shown to be the major determinant of resting E_m in vascular smooth muscle cells.[11,14–16] This chapter emphasizes the role of $I_{K(V)}$ in the regulation of E_m and $[Ca^{2+}]_i$ in PA smooth muscle cells and its relationship to HPV.

Characteristics of $I_{K(V)}$ and $I_{K(Ca)}$ and Their Roles in Regulating Membrane Potential and $[Ca^{2+}]_i$

Electrophysiologic Differentiation of A-Type and Steady-State $I_{K(V)}$

Whole-cell $I_{K(V)}$ (Figure 1A, left panel) can be isolated when $I_{K(Ca)}$ and $I_{K(ATP)}$ are minimized by using 10 mM ethylenegylcoltetracetic acid (EGTA) and 5 mM ATP in Ca^{2+}-free pipette (intracellular) solution in PA smooth muscle cells superfused with Ca^{2+}-free, 1 mM EGTA-containing solution.[15] Two exponentials are required for best fit of the decay of the $I_{K(V)}$ (Figure 1A, middle panels), a fast component with a time constant of 30 ms (τ_1) and a slow component with a time constant of 434 ms (τ_2) at +80 mV in this cell (these values are based on two-component exponential fit). Apparently, the currents also include a noninactivating component.[11] The equation used for the two-component fit is: $I_K = A_0 + A_1e^{(-t/\tau 1)} + A_2e^{(-t/\tau 2)}$, where A_1 (1063 pA in this experiment) and A_2 (555 pA) represent current amplitudes for two inactivation components at time (t) = 0, τ_1 and τ_2 represent respective inactivation time constants, and A_0 (1218 pA) corresponds to the amplitude of the steady-state current.

Upon depolarization to +80 mV, the $I_{K(V)}$ is rapidly activated and has a transient component ($I_{K(tr)}$) (Figure 1B, inset) that resembles A-type $I_{K(V)}$,[15,17,18] and a steady-state component ($I_{K(ss)}$) (Figure 1B) that corresponds to the delayed rectifier and noninactivating $I_{K(V)}$.[9,11,16] Both components of $I_{K(V)}$, $I_{K(tr)}$ and $I_{K(ss)}$, are activated by very negative potentials (−40 to −60 mV) (Figure 1A, right panel), and are reversibly inhibited by the K_V channel blocker, 4-aminopyridine (4-AP, 5 mM) (Figure 1C, upper panels). The K_{Ca} channel blocker, charybdotoxin (ChTX, 20 nM), negligibly affects the currents (Figure 1B, lower panels).[15]

Inhibition of $I_{K(V)}$ Causes Membrane Depolarization and Increases $[Ca^{2+}]_i$ at Rest

By blocking the K_V channels that are active under resting conditions, 4-AP significantly and reversibly depolarizes PA smooth muscle cells and elicits Ca^{2+}-dependent action potentials (Figure 1D, left panel). Removal of extracellular Ca^{2+} abolishes the transient action potentials (that apparently result from enhanced Ca^{2+} influx), but does not affect the steady-state depolarization (that results from reduced $I_{K(V)}$).[15] In intact PA smooth muscle cells that are devoid of dialysis with the pipette (intracellular) solution, 4-AP reversibly increases $[Ca^{2+}]_i$ (Figure 1E), while in isolated perfused lungs, 4-AP significantly increases pulmonary arterial pressure.[19] Both responses are apparently caused by the evoked membrane depolarization and Ca^{2+}-dependent action potentials. Consistent with its lack of effect on resting E_m (Figure 1D, right panel), ChTX (20–100 nM) has no effect on $[Ca^{2+}]_i$ as well (Figure 1E, right panel). These data indicate that $I_{K(V)}$ is the major determinant of E_m and $[Ca^{2+}]_i$ at rest in PA smooth muscle cells. K_{Ca} channels, which are relatively closed under resting conditions, contribute to the regulation of E_m and vascular tone when $[Ca^{2+}]_i$ is increased.

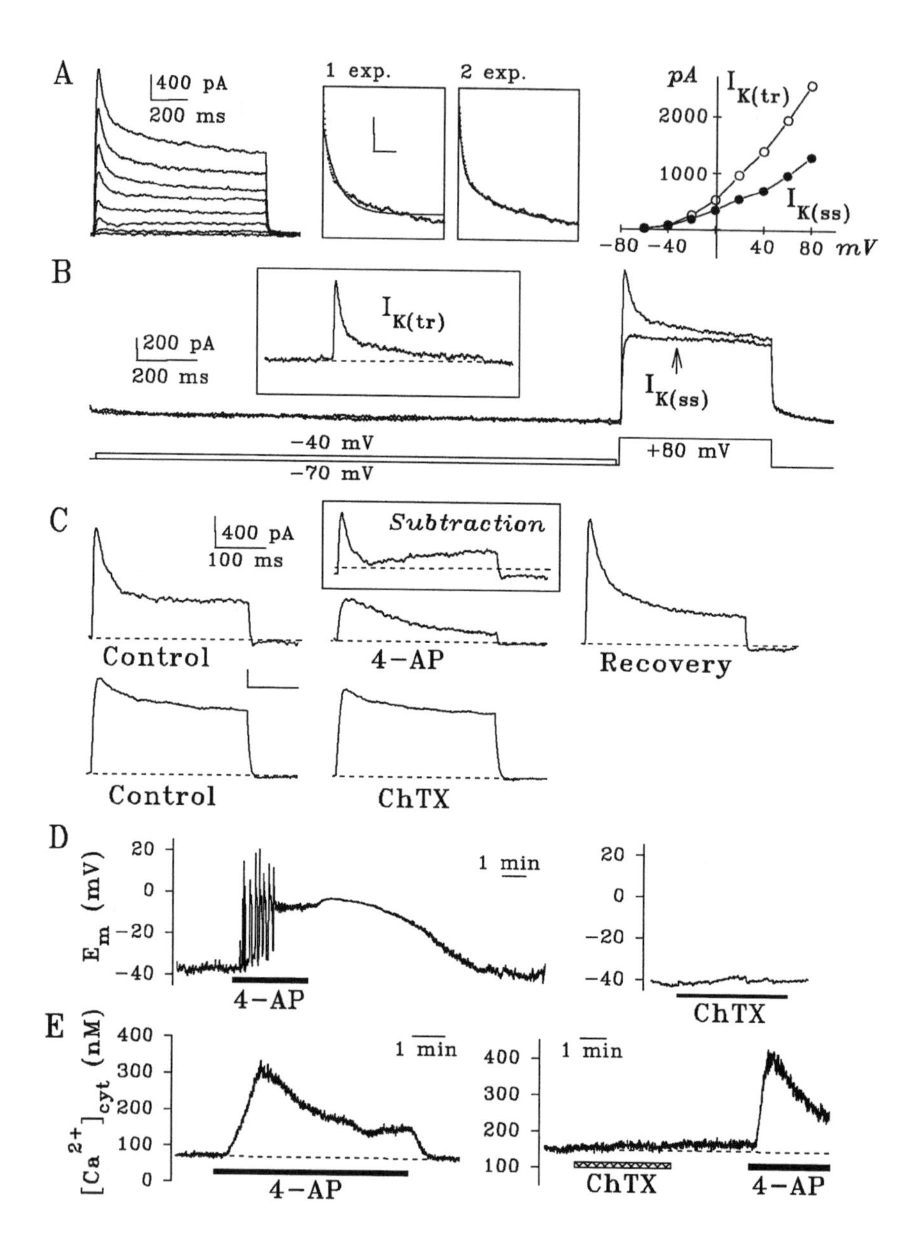
A
400 pA
200 ms
1 exp.
2 exp.
pA
$I_{K(tr)}$
2000
1000
$I_{K(ss)}$
−80 −40
40 80 mV
B
200 pA
200 ms
$I_{K(tr)}$
$I_{K(ss)}$
−40 mV
+80 mV
−70 mV
C
400 pA
100 ms
Subtraction
Control
4−AP
Recovery
Control
ChTX
D
E_m (mV)
20
0
−20
−40
1 min
4−AP
ChTX
E
$[Ca^{2+}]_{cyt}$ (nM)
400
300
200
100
0
1 min
4−AP
ChTX
4−AP

Figure 1. $I_{K(V)}$ and regulation of E_m and $[Ca^{2+}]_i$. **A.** A family of currents (**left panels**) and the corresponding I-V curve (**right panel**) obtained by depolarizing the cell to test potentials between −60 and +80 mV (holding potential, −70 mV). The cell was superfused and dialyzed with Ca^{2+}-free and EGTA-containing solutions. One-component (1 exp., **left inset**) and two-component (2 exp., **right inset**) exponential fits (**smooth lines** superimposed on the current records) of inactivation of $I_{K(V)}$, elicited by a 900-ms voltage step to +80 mV, are shown in **middle panels**. $I_{K(tr)}$ (**open circle**) and $I_{K(ss)}$ (**closed circle**) denote the transient and steady-state currents measured at the beginning (10–50 ms) and end (850–890 ms) of the test pulse (900 ms), respectively. **B**. Predepolarization to −40 mV inactivates $I_{K(tr)}$. **Inset** shows the current component that was inactivated by predepolarizing the cell from −70 mV to −40 mV before the +80 mV test pulse was applied. **C**. Representative current traces, elicited by a +80-mV test pulse, were recorded before, during, and after application of 5 mM 4-AP (**upper panels**) and 20 nM charybdotoxin (ChTX) (**lower panels**). **Inset** shows the 4-AP-sensitive component of $I_{K(V)}$ (*Subtraction*), obtained by subtracting the currents recorded before and during application of 4-AP. **Broken lines** represent zero-current levels. **D**. E_m was measured before, during, and after applications of 5 mM 4-AP (**left panel**) and 20 nM ChTX (**right panel**) in the presence of 1.8 mM Ca^{2+}. **E.** $[Ca^{2+}]_i$, measured in the peripheral area of a cell, was recorded in cells superfused with solutions containing 10 mM 4-AP (**left panel**) or 10 nM ChTX (**right panel**). **Broken lines** represent $[Ca^{2+}]_i$ values measured before application of 4-AP or ChTX. (Modified with permission from Reference 15).

Activation of $I_{K(Ca)}$ When $[Ca^{2+}]_i$ is Increased

When $[Ca^{2+}]_i$ is increased to ~500 nM by adding $CaCl_2$ in the pipette (intracellular) solution, both $I_{K(V)}$ and $I_{K(Ca)}$ can be elicited by depolarization (−40 to +80 mV) (Figure 2A). The activation kinetics of the currents is slower than that of $I_{K(V)}$ alone, but the amplitude of the currents is much greater (compare Figure 1A with Figure 2A). ChTX, a selective K_{Ca} channel blocker, significantly decreases the currents by 55% at +80 mV (Figure 2A). This reduction is clearly caused by the inhibitory effect of ChTX on $I_{K(Ca)}$, since ChTX has no effect on $I_{K(V)}$. The ChTX-sensitive $I_{K(Ca)}$ (Figure 2A, inset), obtained by subtracting the currents recorded before and during introduction of ChTX, exhibits relatively slow activation kinetics similar to the $I_{K(Ca)}$ generated by the cloned K_{Ca} channels (*hSlo*).[20] The large, long-lasting inward tail currents elicited under these conditions may be due to the Ca^{2+}-activated Cl^- currents which have been described in these cells.[21] Although having minimal effect on E_m at resting $[Ca^{2+}]_i$ (50–100 nM) (Figure 1D, right panel), ChTX significantly and reversibly depolarizes PA smooth muscle cells (Figure 2B) when $[Ca^{2+}]_i$ is raised to ~500

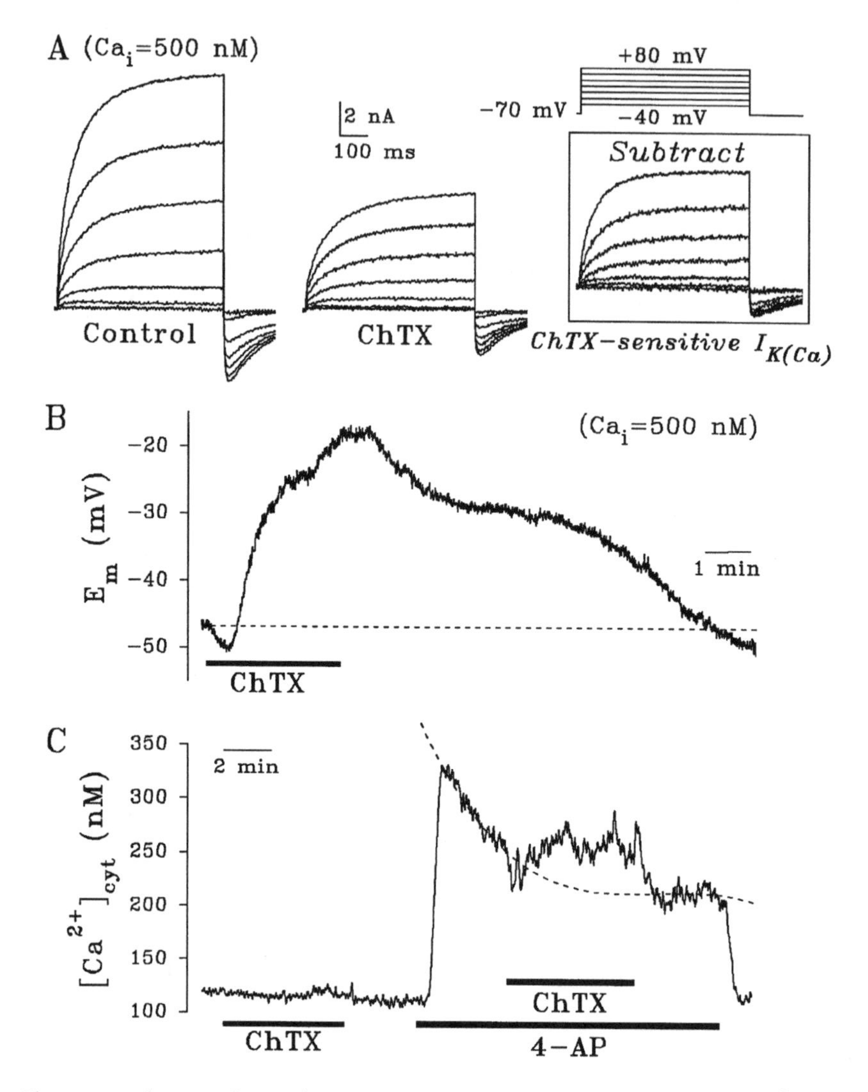

Figure 2. Pharmacologic characteristics of $I_{K(Ca)}$ and effects on E_m and $[Ca^{2+}]_i$. **A.** A family of $I_{K(Ca)}$, elicited by depolarizing the cell to test potentials from −40 to +80 mV, was recorded before and during application of 10 nM charybdotoxin (ChTX). The cells were superfused with 1.8 mM Ca^{2+}-containing bath solution and dialyzed with 500 nM Ca^{2+}-containing pipette (intracellular) solution. **Inset** shows the current component that was inhibited by ChTX (Subtract). **B.** E_m was measured before, during, and after application of 10 nM ChTX in a cell dialyzed with 500 nM Ca^{2+}-containing intracellular solution. **C.** $[Ca^{2+}]_i$ is measured in the peripheral area of a cell super-

nM. Consistently, inhibition of K_{Ca} channels by ChTX, which is without effect on resting $[Ca^{2+}]_i$ (Figure 1E, right panel, and Figure 2C), significantly enhances the 4-AP-induced increase in $[Ca^{2+}]_i$ (Figure 2C).

Thus, the 4-AP-sensitive K_V channels, which are active at rest while resting $[Ca^{2+}]_i$ is very low ($\leq$100 nM), are the major contributors to the regulation of resting E_m. Inhibition of the K_V channels depolarizes PA smooth muscle cells, increases $[Ca^{2+}]_i$, and triggers pulmonary vasoconstriction. The ChTX-sensitive K_{Ca} channels are the major negative feedback regulators of E_m (by eliciting membrane repolarization) when $[Ca^{2+}]_i$ is increased or the vessel is stimulated. Inhibition of K_{Ca} channels, thus, helps to maintain the membrane depolarization and evoked pulmonary vascular tone.

Molecular Basis for $I_{K(V)}$ and $I_{K(Ca)}$

At the molecular level, K^+ channels are composed of two structurally distinct subunits, the large pore-forming α-subunits and the smaller cytoplasmic β-subunits ($\alpha_4\beta_4$).[18,22,23] Biophysical properties of K^+ channels encoded by certain α-subunits can be dramatically altered by the association with β-subunits.[18] By using reverse transcription polymerase chain reaction (RT-PCR), at least five K_V channel α-subunit gene transcripts from the *Shaker* family, $K_V1.1$, $K_V1.2$, $K_V1.4$, $K_V1.5$, and $K_V1.6$, as well as a K_{Ca} channel α-subunit gene transcript, *rSlo*, are identified in rat PA smooth muscle cells.[24] In addition, the transcripts of three K_V channel β-subunits, $K_V\beta1$, $K_V\beta2$, and $K_V\beta3$, are also identified in these cells.[24] These data suggest that the native K^+ channels in PA smooth muscle cells are encoded by multiple α- and β-subunit genes. The homo- and/or heteromultimeric assembly of α-subunits, as well as the association of α- and β-subunits, contributes to the remarkable diversity of K^+ channels and the numerous electrophysiologic and pharmacologic properties of K^+ channels in vivo.[18, 22–25]

Accordingly, the 4-AP-sensitive steady-state $I_{K(V)}$ ($I_{K(ss)}$, including delayed rectifier and noninactivating currents) may be attributed to, at least,

Figure 2. *(continued)* fused with solutions containing 10 mM 4-AP and/or 20 nM ChTX. **Broken line** depicts the monoexponential fitting of the $[Ca^{2+}]_i$ decay curve in the absence of ChTX. Although ChTX alone had no effect on $[Ca^{2+}]_i$, application of 20 nM ChTX in the presence of 10 mM 4-AP enhanced the elevated $[Ca^{2+}]_i$.(Modified with permission from Reference 15).

the $K_V1.1$, $K_V1.2$, $K_V1.5$, and $K_V1.6$ gene products. The A-type $I_{K(V)}$ ($I_{K(tr)}$) is probably conferred by $K_V1.4$ and/or $K_V1.5$ associated with K_V β-subunits. The ChTX-sensitive $I_{K(Ca)}$ is likely endowed by the *rSlo* gene product. The recent finding that the K_V channel β-subunits belong to an NAD(P)H oxidoreductase superfamily[26] suggests that the β-subunits may serve as an intermediate in sensing changes in oxygen tension and redox status to govern the native K_V (or other K^+) channel functions. Whether genes of the K^+ channels, such as other K_V (K_V2, K_V3, K_V4, K_V5, K_V6, K_V8, K_V9, IsK, etc.) channels, inward rectifier K^+ channels (K_{ir}), and other K_{Ca} channels, are expressed in PA smooth muscle cells is unknown and requires further study.

Effects of Acute Hypoxia on $I_{K(V)}$, Membrane Potential, and $[Ca^{2+}]_i$

Potassium channel activity mediated alteration of E_m and $[Ca^{2+}]_i$ in PA smooth muscle cells is pivotal in regulating pulmonary vasomotor tone.[7,15] HPV is dependent on extracellular Ca^{2+} and can be inhibited by Ca^{2+} channel blockers or hyperpolarizing agents.[3,27] Hypoxia induces depolarization and elicits action potentials in isolated PA,[28] suggesting that membrane depolarization and activation of voltage-gated Ca^{2+} channels are early steps in HPV.

Hypoxia-Induced Inhibition of K_V Channels Initiates Depolarization and Increases $[Ca^{2+}]_i$

Post et al[29] first reported that hypoxia decreased K^+ currents in canine PA smooth muscle cells. This effect was abolished either by buffering intracellular Ca^{2+} with [1,2-bis(2)aminophenoxy]ethane *N,N,N',N'*-tetraacetic acid (BAPTA, 10 mM) or by blocking Ca^{2+} influx with nisoldipine, suggesting that a Ca^{2+}-dependent mechanism was involved in the response. A further study[30] indicated that the hypoxia-induced decrease of K^+ currents resulted from inhibition of K_V channels that was mediated by Ca^{2+} release from intracellular Ca^{2+} stores (the caffeine-sensitive SR). In rat PA smooth muscle cells, our early observations showed that hypoxia inhibited K^+ currents[31] in the absence of extracellular and intracellular Ca^{2+} (Figure 3A), suggesting that the Ca^{2+}-independent K_V channels were involved in this response.[31–33] Similar observations have recently been reported in rabbit PA smooth muscle cells[34] and in PA smooth muscle cells isolated from chronically hypoxic rats.[35] Hypoxia, however, does not affect $I_{K(V)}$ in smooth muscle cells isolated from systemic arteries, including mesenteric artery,[31] renal artery,[29] and ear artery.[36]

In single-channel recording mode, at least two K^+ currents can be elicited in cell-attached membrane patches: the large conductance $I_{K(Ca)}$ (200–250 pS) and the small conductance $I_{K(V)}$ (45–55 pS).[16,30,37] Consistent with the whole-cell studies, hypoxia decreases the single-channel $I_{K(V)}$ in cell-attached patches of PA smooth muscle cells.[30,38] In neurons[39] and chemoreceptor cells,[40] hypoxia inhibits $I_{K(V)}$ recorded from both on-cell and excised membrane patches, suggesting a direct regulation of channel activity by acute hypoxia.

The sequence of events involved in the early steps of HPV appears to be initiated with membrane depolarization (Figure 3B) triggered by blockade of the K_V channels in PA smooth muscle cells. The resultant increase of voltage-gated Ca^{2+} conductance (Ca^{2+}-dependent action potentials, Figure 3B, inset) raises $[Ca^{2+}]_i$ (Figure 3C)[33, 41] and, thus, causes pulmonary vasoconstriction.[3,29,42] In this process, as reported by several laboratories using PA smooth muscle cells obtained from different species, K_V channels have been recognized as the target for acute hypoxia to initiate membrane depolarization.[30–35] K_V channel inhibition is also associated with the membrane depolarization and pulmonary vasoconstriction mediated by chronic hypoxia.[35,43]

Hypoxia-Induced Inhibition of K_{Ca} Channels Helps to Maintain Depolarized Membrane Potential and Elevated $[Ca^{2+}]_i$

Elevation of $[Ca^{2+}]_i$, induced by enhanced Ca^{2+} influx and release, activates K_{Ca} channels. The resultant increase in $I_{K(Ca)}$ elicits membrane repolarization to limit vasoconstriction and also induces hyperpolarization to cause vasodilation.[44,45] K_{Ca} channels in PA smooth muscle cells are synergistically regulated by E_m and $[Ca^{2+}]_i$ and possess a large conductance (200–250 pS).[12,30] The huge $I_{K(Ca)}$, elicited by the increased $[Ca^{2+}]_i$ (Figure 2A) and depolarized E_m, would limit the hypoxia-induced membrane depolarization to a transient process if normal function of K_{Ca} channels were preserved during hypoxia. However, the observed response of E_m to hypoxia (e.g., Figure 3B) is a sustained depolarization, which can be explained by the results that hypoxia, in addition to blocking

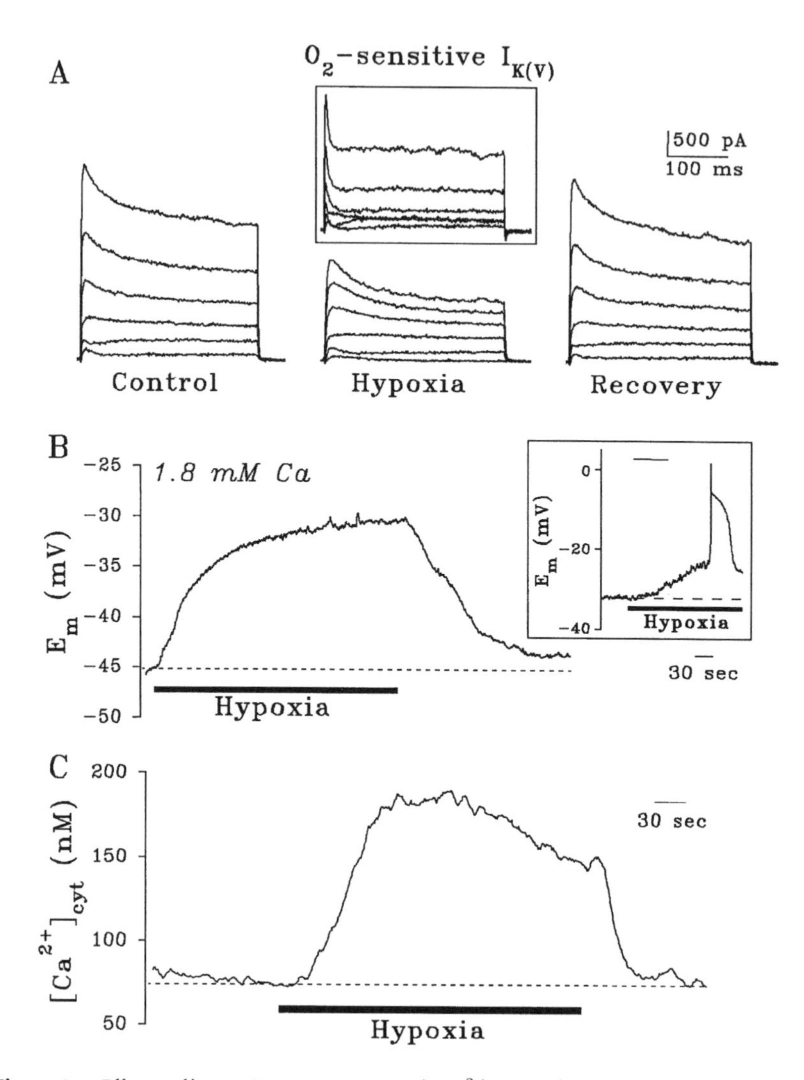

Figure 3. Effects of hypoxia on $I_{K(V)}$, E_m, and $[Ca^{2+}]_i$ in pulmonary artery (PA) smooth muscle cells. **A.** A family of currents, elicited by depolarizing the cell to test potentials between −60 and +80 mV (holding potential, −70 mV), was recorded before, during, and after reduction of Po_2 from 155 to 15 Torr in the extracellular solution. **Inset** shows the current components that were inhibited by hypoxia. **B.** E_m was measured in a cell superfused with 1.8 mM Ca^{2+}-containing solution under normoxic and hypoxic conditions. **Inset** shows the hypoxia-induced Ca^{2+} action potential recorded in some of the cells. **C.** $[Ca^{2+}]_i$ was measured in the peripheral area of a cell superfused with normoxic or hypoxic solutions. **Broken lines** represent $[Ca^{2+}]_i$ values measured before Po_2 was reduced. (Modified with permission from Reference 31).

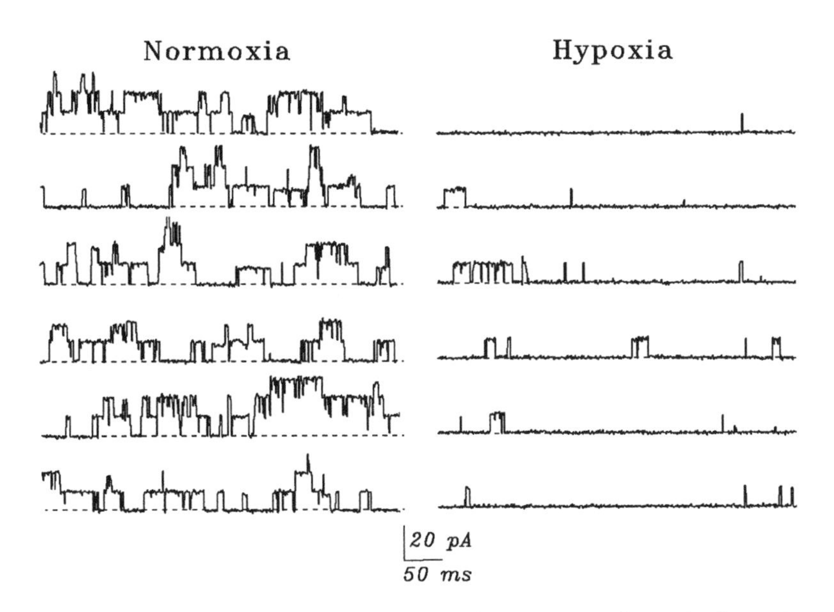

Figure 4. Effect of hypoxia on single-channel $I_{K(Ca)}$ in a cell-attached membrane patch from a pulmonary artery (PA) smooth muscle cell exposed to a symmetrical K^+ gradient. Single-channel $I_{K(Ca)}$ recorded in a patch before and after the cell was exposed to hypoxia (Po_2 = 32 Torr). The membrane patch was held at +70 mV. Current levels when channels were closed are indicated by horizontal **broken lines**. Upward deflection represents outward currents. Hypoxia reduces the steady-state open probability, NxP_{open}, from 1.10708 to 0.2532.

K_V channels for initiating E_m depolarization, also inhibits $I_{K(Ca)}$ in cell-attached membrane patches of PA smooth muscle cells (Figure 4). Similar observations have been reported in rabbit PA smooth muscle cells[36] and carotid body cells.[46] Hypoxia-induced inhibition of $I_{K(Ca)}$ appears to depend on cell integrity, since the effect disappears in excised (inside-out) membrane patches.[30, 36] Thus, hypoxia-induced inhibition of K_{Ca} channels, although not involved in triggering membrane depolarization, certainly plays an important role in maintaining membrane depolarization.

Roles of Ca^{2+} Channels, Cl^- Channels and K_{ATP} Channels in Hypoxic Pulmonary Vasoconstriction

Franco-Obregon and Lopez-Barneo[47] recently demonstrated that hypoxia directly augments the activity of voltage-gated Ca^{2+} channels in smooth muscle cells isolated from small PA. Hypoxia increases the amplitude of the L-type Ca^{2+} currents and shifts the current-voltage relationship in the direction of more negative potentials. These results provide an additional explanation for the hypoxia-induced rise in $[Ca^{2+}]_i$.

In addition to augmented Ca^{2+} influx with membrane depolarization[29–35] and/or enhanced Ca^{2+} channel activity,[47] hypoxia also releases Ca^{2+} from intracellular Ca^{2+} stores (sarcoplasmic reticulum and mitochondria).[41,48] Although the concentration of Ca^{2+} provided by the transient $[Ca^{2+}]_i$ increase from intracellular Ca^{2+} stores is sufficient to trigger contraction, sustained Ca^{2+} influx through opened voltage-gated Ca^{2+} channels is necessary for both initiating and maintaining contraction. Increased $[Ca^{2+}]_i$, in addition to activating calmodulin and causing contraction, also activates other Ca^{2+}-dependent membrane proteins, e.g., Ca^{2+}-activated Cl^- channels. Since the equilibrium potential for Cl^-, the most predominant anion in cytoplasmic and intercellular fluids, is more positive (-27 to 0 mV) than resting E_m (-55 to -40 mV) in PA smooth muscle cells, activation of Cl^- channels would result in inward currents by enhancing Cl^- efflux.[21] Whether Cl^- channels are directly affected by hypoxia is unknown, but the inward Cl^- currents, resulting from opened Ca^{2+}-activated Cl^- channels when $[Ca^{2+}]_i$ is raised, would contribute considerably to the maintenance of membrane depolarization during hypoxia. Therefore, Ca^{2+}-activated Cl^- channels act as a positive feedback mechanism in hypoxia-induced membrane depolarization in PA smooth muscle cells.

Intracellular ATP content is a major regulator of K_{ATP} channel activity in vascular smooth muscle cells.[25] Inhibition of cellular metabolism decreases ATP production[49] and activates K_{ATP} channels.[25,50] This appears to be a very important mechanism involved in hypoxia- (or ischemia-) mediated hyperpolarization and vasodilation in coronary[50] and cerebral[25] arteries. In the pulmonary vasculature, activation of K_{ATP} channels has been suggested to cause membrane hyperpolarization and vasodilation during anoxia, which decreases ATP production.[51] Whether K_{ATP} channels are involved in an early stage of initiating membrane depolarization during hypoxia is unknown.

Hence, acute hypoxia inhibits K_V channels and decreases $I_{K(V)}$ (both $I_{K(tr)}$ and $I_{K(ss)}$) in PA smooth muscle cells. The resultant membrane depolarization promotes Ca^{2+} influx through voltage-gated Ca^{2+} channels, increases $[Ca^{2+}]_i$, and initiates hypoxic pulmonary vasoconstriction. Acute hypoxia also inhibits K_{Ca} channels and reduces $I_{K(Ca)}$, which helps to maintain membrane depolarization, increased $[Ca^{2+}]_i$, and evoked pulmonary vascular tone. Activation of Ca^{2+}-activated Cl^- channels promotes

Cl^- efflux because of the substantially less negative equilibrium potential (−27 to 0 mV). The resultant inward Cl^- current causes further membrane depolarization and plays a positive feedback role in maintaining elevated $[Ca^{2+}]_i$ and pulmonary vasoconstriction. Since Ca^{2+} is a stimulator for smooth muscle cell proliferation, increased $[Ca^{2+}]_i$ in PA smooth muscle cells may also be related to pulmonary vascular remodeling.

Effect of Chronic Hypoxia on K_V Channels

An early work by McMurtry et al[52] reported that the pressor response to acute hypoxia was impaired in lungs from chronically hypoxic rats, whereas the pressor response to vasoconstrictor agonists (angiotensin II, prostaglandin $F_{2\alpha}$, and norepinephrine) was enhanced. They suggested that this reduced pressor response to acute hypoxia might result from abnormalities in the mechanism that couples acute hypoxia to contraction of the pulmonary vascular smooth muscle. As mentioned above, inhibition of K_V channels in PA smooth muscle cells is a critical mechanism by which acute hypoxia initiates membrane depolarization, increases $[Ca^{2+}]_i$, and elicits pulmonary vasoconstriction. Therefore, an alteration in the activity and function of K_V channels may also be involved in the development of chronic hypoxia-mediated pulmonary vasoconstriction and hypertension. Indeed, reduced $I_{K(V)}$ and more depolarized E_m have been observed in PA smooth muscle cells isolated from chronically hypoxic rats (4 weeks in normobaric chamber containing 10% oxygen in nitrogen).[35,43] Thus, chronic and acute hypoxia may share the same cellular mechanisms in mediating pulmonary vasoconstriction, i.e., chronic hypoxia-mediated HPV may also be related to inhibition of K_V channels.

A change in the number of functional K_V channels occurs within hours because of the rapid turnover rate of the channel mRNAs and proteins (e.g., the half-life of $K_V1.5$ mRNA and protein is only 0.5 and 4 hours, respectively).[53] In pituitary cells, membrane depolarization downregulates $K_V1.5$ gene expression.[54] Hypoxia is known to affect gene expression of several oxygen-sensitive proteins (e.g., erythropoietin, vascular endothelial growth factor, inducible nitric oxide synthase, and various glycolytic enzymes). The cellular and molecular mechanisms responsible for the chronic hypoxia-mediated pulmonary vasoconstriction may involve transcriptional regulation of K_V channel genes.

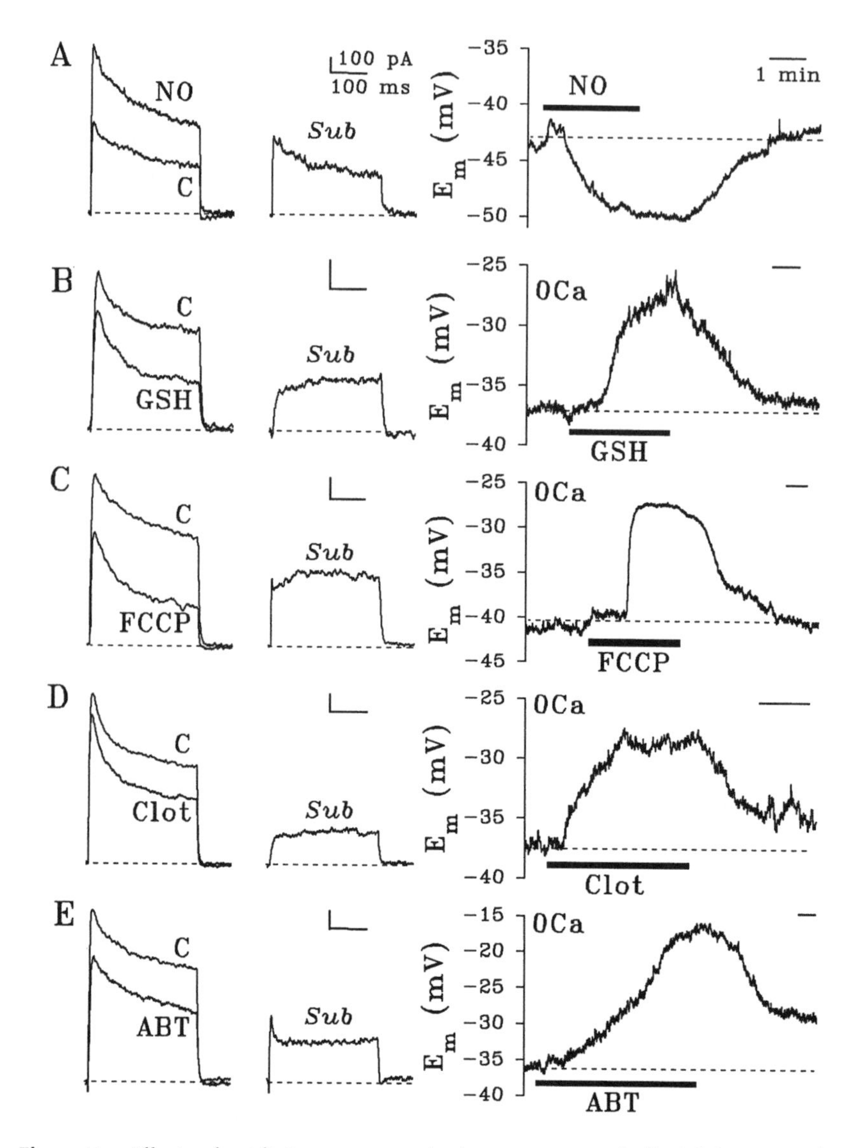

Figure 5. Effects of oxidizing agents, reducing agents, metabolic inhibitors, and P-450 inhibitors on $I_{K(V)}$ and E_m in pulmonary artery (PA) smooth muscle cells. Currents were elicited by depolarizing the cells from a holding potential of −70 mV to a test potential of +80 mV before (**C**) and during applications of 0.3 μM nitric oxide (NO, **A**), 5 mM reduced glutathione (GSH, **B**), 5 μM carbonyl cyanide-*p*-trifluoromethoxy-phenyl-hydrazone (FCCP, **C**), 1 μM clotrimazole (Clot, **D**), and 1 mM 1-amino-benzotriazole (ABT, **E**), respectively (**left panels**). Subtractions between the currents recorded before and during treatments are shown in **middle panels**. E_m (**right panels**)

Mechanisms Involved in Acute Hypoxia-Induced Inhibition of K_V Channels

Acute reduction of oxygen tension (Po_2) inhibits K_V channels not only in PA smooth muscle cells, but also in carotid body type I cells,[40,55,56] neurons,[39] and neuroepithelial bodies.[57] This implies that an oxygen-sensing system exists in a variety of cell types and plays an important role in various specific cell functions, ranging from ventilation-perfusion matching to chemotransduction (see Chapter 11). The precise mechanism involved in the acute hypoxia-induced inhibition of K_V channels remains unclear, but it may be related to: 1) change of cellular redox status[32,42,58–60]; 2) inhibition of cellular metabolism[32,61]; 3) release of intracellularly stored Ca^{2+}[30]; 4) inhibition of NADPH oxidase[56,57]; and/or 5) inhibition of cytochrome P-450[62] or nonheme iron-containing moieties that are associated with or adjacent to the channel proteins (see Chapters 11, 16, and 21).[39]

Redox Regulation

Changes of cellular redox status regulate pulmonary vascular reactivity and may be involved in the development of HPV.[63,58] Hypoxia increases the ratios of the reduced to the oxidized forms of glutathione (GSH/GSSG) and/or nicotinamide adenine dinucleotide phosphate ($NADPH/NADP^+$) in isolated perfused lungs[42] and, thus, shifts the cells to a more reduced state. Oxidants (e.g., diamide, NO [nitric oxide], hydrogen peroxide) increase $I_{K(V)}$ (Figure 5A, left panel),[37,42,60] cause membrane hyperpolarization (Figure 5A, right panel) and pulmonary vasodilation,[64] and inhibit HPV,[63,59] while reducing agents (e.g., GSH, dithiothreitol, N-acetyl-L-cysteine) decrease $I_{K(V)}$ (Figure 5B, left panel),[17,18,32,42,60] cause membrane depolarization (Figure 5B, right panel)[32] and pulmonary vasoconstriction, and mimic HPV.[58]

Cysteine residues in K_V channel α- and β-subunits are sensitive to redox change (see Chapter 3). In cloned K_V channels (α-subunits),

Figure 5. *(continued)* was measured using current-clamp mode in the cells superfused with solutions containing NO (**A**), GSH (**B**), FCCP (**C**), Clot (**D**) and ABT (**E**), respectively. (Modified with permission from References 32, 37, 61, and 62).

cysteine is present in all portions (external, internal, and transmembrane segments). Cysteine-based disulfide bridges in channel protein molecules may contribute to the gating behavior and permeation properties of K_V channels.[17,18,65] Oxidizing and reducing agents influence the integrity of disulfide bonds within the channel proteins, thereby altering either the kinetic or the conductive properties of the channels. Cysteine residues in K_V channel protein molecules might be cycled between the reduced form, cysteine (Cys-SH), and the oxidized form, cystine (Cys-S-S-Cys), based on the redox status of cytosol and/or membrane. During normoxia, cysteine residues tend to be oxidized, forming sulfide bonds with other cysteine residues or combining with other sulfur-containing residues. During hypoxia, the cellular redox status shifts to a more reduced state because of the increased ratios of GSH/GSSG and $NADPH/NADP^+$,[42,58] and the sulfide bonds (Cys-S-S-Cys) tend to be reduced to sulfhydryl groups (Cys-SH), which confers inactivation on the slowly- or noninactivating K_V channels[17,18] and facilitates blocking of K_V channel conduction by β-subunits.[66]

The extracellular surface of the cell membrane is normally more oxidized, while the cytoplasmic side of the membrane is more reduced because of ample GSH in the cytosol. Thus, alveolar hypoxia may readily create a reduced environment at the extracellular surface of PA smooth muscle cells. The imbalance between extracellular and intracellular sites of the *local* redox potential results in the change of K_V channel activity.

Figure 6. Schematic diagram depicting the proposed cellular mechanisms involved in acute hypoxic pulmonary vasoconstriction (**A**) and in acute hypoxia-induced inhibition of K_V channels (**B**). **A.** Hypoxic pulmonary vasoconstriction (HPV) appears to be initiated by blockade of K_V channels and the attendant depolarization and rise in $[Ca^{2+}]_i$. The response is maintained by hypoxia-induced blockade of K_{Ca} channels, which inhibits repolarization, by activation of Ca^{2+}-activated Cl^- channels, which elicits further depolarization, and by hypoxia-induced release of Ca^{2+} from sarcoplasmic reticulum and mitochondria. $I_{Cl(Ca)}$ denotes Ca^{2+}-activated Cl^- currents. **B.** K_V channels may be blocked during hypoxia by an extracellular gating domain that is attached to both the NADPH-P-450 oxidoreductase and the channel α-subunits (**a**), an intracellular inactivation domain that can be inlaid to the channel pore (**a** and **b**), a decreased production of the intermediate, oxygen-sensitive channel regulator (ODCR), which keeps the channel open during normoxia (**a** and **b**), and/or a conformational change of a nicotinamide adenine dinucleotide phosphate (NADPH)-P-450 oxidoreductase that is attached to the channel α-subunits and functions as a β-subunit (**c**).

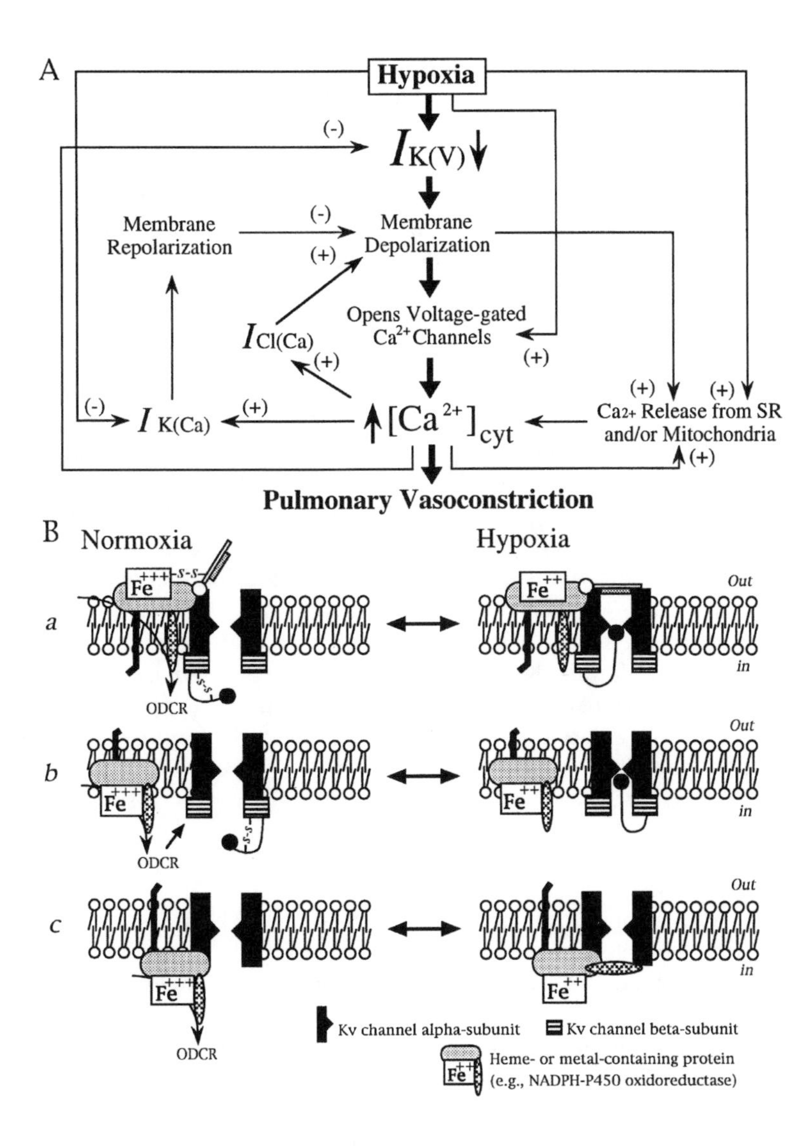
A
Hypoxia
(-)
$I_{K(V)}$
Membrane Repolarization
(-)
Membrane Depolarization
(+)
Opens Voltage-gated Ca^{2+} Channels
$I_{Cl(Ca)}$
(+)
(+)
(+)
(+)
Ca2+ Release from SR and/or Mitochondria
(-)
$I_{K(Ca)}$
(+)
$[Ca^{2+}]_{cyt}$
(+)
Pulmonary Vasoconstriction
B
Normoxia
Hypoxia
a
b
c
Out
in
ODCR
Kv channel alpha-subunit
Kv channel beta-subunit
Heme- or metal-containing protein (e.g., NADPH-P450 oxidoreductase)

Metabolic Regulation

McMurtry and associates demonstrated in their early works that inhibition of oxidative phosphorylation and the citric acid cycle induced pulmonary vasoconstriction during normoxia,[67] while inhibition of glycolysis potentiated HPV.[68] They proposed that alveolar hypoxia reduced the phosphate potential [ATP/(ADP + Pi)], an indicator of the energy status of PA smooth muscle cells, by decreasing oxidative phosphorylation. This hypoxia-induced change in energy status might subsequently decrease K^+ conductance, increase Ca^{2+} influx, and cause pulmonary vasoconstriction.[69] Indeed, the metabolic inhibitors, 2-deoxy-D-glucose,[32] carbonyl cyanide-*p*-trifluoromethoxyphenyl-hydrazone (FCCP) (Figure 5C),[61] rotenone,[42] and antimycin A[42] all mimic the inhibitory effect of hypoxia on $I_{K(V)}$ in PA smooth muscle cells. On the contrary, intracellular application of ATP enhances $I_{K(V)}$,[70] suggesting that K_V channels are regulated by changes in ATP production. Although a global decrease of intracellular ATP content occurs slowly,[49] hypoxia and metabolic inhibition may produce a rapid depletion of local or compartmentalized ATP contents.[71] Most ion channels are regulated by phosphorylation.[72] The K_V channels in PA smooth muscle cells may be modulated by a phosphorylation-dephosphorylation mechanism controlled by the local ATP level produced by a membrane-associated metabolic pathway. In fact, a tyrosine kinase site and a protein kinase C site are present in the intracellular domains of the *Shaker* subfamily K_V channels that are expressed in PA smooth muscle cells. This provides molecular evidence that K_V channel activity can be rapidly regulated by protein kinase-dependent phosphorylation and dephosphorylation.

Ca^{2+}-Mediated Regulation

Divalent cations (Mg^{2+} and Ca^{2+}) have recently been shown to block native K^+ channels in vascular smooth muscle cells[30,73] and cloned K_V channels expressed in *Xenopus* oocytes.[74] Post et al[30] provided compelling evidence that Ca^{2+}, ~1 μM, applied to the cytoplasmic surface of inside-out membrane patches from canine PA smooth muscle cells, directly blocked the 4-AP-sensitive K_V channels. They proposed that hypoxia elicits an early increase in $[Ca^{2+}]_i$, which subsequently induces membrane depolarization by blocking the Ca^{2+}-sensitive K_V channels. The resultant activation of voltage-gated Ca^{2+} channels augments Ca^{2+} influx, raises $[Ca^{2+}]_i$ in PA smooth muscle cells, and finally causes pulmonary vasoconstriction.

Oxygen atoms are required for Ca^{2+} binding to Ca^{2+}-dependent proteins. Proteins often bind Ca^{2+} through ~6 oxygen atoms provided by the charged glutamate and aspartate residues.[75] The Ca^{2+}-binding sites in a variety of Ca^{2+}-dependent proteins (e.g., calmodulin and inositol phospholipid-specific phospholipase C) include an important motif, namely the EF hand. This helix-loop-helix Ca^{2+}-binding motif is characterized by two α helices separated by a Ca^{2+}-binding loop. The Ca^{2+}-binding loop is composed of residues containing side-chain oxygen groups.[75] Oxygen atoms are also involved in forming an oxygen cage that may determine K^+ selectivity in K^+ channel proteins.[76] Whether hypoxia can affect Ca^{2+} binding to the contractile apparatus and alter K^+ selectivity in K^+ channel proteins is unknown and needs further study.

Cytochrome P-450 and NADPH-Dependent Oxidoreductase

The cytochrome P-450 monooxygenase system (P-450) is a family of heme-thiolate enzymes that catalyze oxidative reactions. The activity of P-450 requires a reducing agent, NADPH, as an electron donor and molecular (atmospheric) oxygen in a 1:1 stoichiometry. P-450 is prevalent in lungs and in various vascular beds.[77] Various P-450 metabolites of arachidonic acid have been shown to play an important role in regulating vascular tone, primarily by affecting K^+ channel activity.[77,78] Activation of P-450 is oxygen dependent, and half-saturation of P-450 with oxygen occurs at a P_{O_2} of 20 to 100 Torr,[79] which is similar to the range of P_{O_2} that affects K_V channels, E_m, $[Ca^{2+}]_i$, and pulmonary vascular tone.[3,29–31,41,42] Indeed, P-450 has been suggested to function as a pulmonary oxygen sensor in the triggering of HPV.[79,80]

In PA smooth muscle cells, inhibition of P-450 by the structurally distinct inhibitors of P-450, the imidazole antimycotics (clotrimazole and miconazole) and the suicide substrate inhibitor (1-aminobenzotriazole), significantly decreases $I_{K(V)}$ and causes membrane depolarization (Figure 5D and E).[62] Induction of P-450 enzyme significantly increases membrane hyperpolarization, while depletion of the enzyme significantly reduces membrane hyperpolarization.[81] Taken together with the observations that carbon monoxide inhibits HPV[82] and hypoxia inhibits P-450 (4A family),[77] these data suggest that P-450 or a heme-protein may be involved in hypoxia-mediated regulation of K_V channel activity and in initiating HPV.

P-450 is always attached to an NADPH-reductase which is required to reduce $NAD(P)^+$ to NAD(P)H. It is possible that the cytochrome P-450-NADPH oxidoreductase complex is localized either very closely with or attached to K_V channel α-subunits and functions as a regulatory molecule (similar to K_V channel β-subunit). The complex requires oxygen to produce an intermediate, namely an oxygen-dependent channel regulator (ODCR), which can be rapidly and efficiently delivered to the binding sites of the channel protein. The ODCR, constantly produced by the complex, links enzyme activity to channel activity and, under normoxic conditions, keeps the channels open. During hypoxia, the production of ODCR is reduced because of inhibited enzyme activity, and the channels are, therefore, closed. In this scenario, the oxygen sensor is the oxidoreductase and the effector (receptor) is the K_V channel protein (Figure 6B). The coupler is the ODCR which can be oxygen radicals and/or epoxides. The observations supporting this hypothesis include: 1) carbon monoxide inhibits HPV,[82] while P-450 inhibitors decrease $I_{K(V)}$ and depolarize PA smooth muscle cells[62]; 2) NADPH-oxidase is activated in HPV,[83] while the enzyme inhibitor, diphenyleneiodonium, decreases $I_{K(V)}$[84] and blocks HPV[85]; and 3) the NADPH-P-450 oxidoreductase system is oxygen sensitive.[77–82]

The recent discovery that NO synthase (NOS) is a P-450 type hemoprotein[86,87] raises the possibility that hypoxia (acute and/or chronic) may regulate K_V channel function by affecting either P-450- or NOS-dependent metabolites (in this case, ODCR may be either epoxyeicosatrienoic acid or NO). This possibility is supported by observations that: 1) NO reversibly activates K_V channels in PA smooth muscle cells[37] and causes membrane hyperpolarization and pulmonary vasodilation[64]; and 2) the P-450-derived epoxides (e.g., epoxyeicosatrienoic acid) activate K^+ channels[77,88] and cause membrane hyperpolarization and pulmonary vasodilation.[78,81]

The localized change of redox potential may also be determined by localized distribution of NADPH-P-450 oxidoreductase (or NOS) that produces oxidants and reductants to regulate local redox potential. Consumption of NADPH also contributes to the regulation of local redox potentials. Thus, it is plausible that K_V channel activity is regulated by local redox potential that is controlled by local production of oxidants or reductants from attached or adjacent NADPH-P-450 oxidoreductase complexes.

Role of β-Subunits and Hypoxia-Induced Inhibition of $I_{K(V)}$

Recent identification of K_V channel β-subunits[22,89,90] and their molecular similarity to an NADPH-dependent oxidoreductase[26,91] suggested that hypoxia may alter the function of K_V channels (the pore-forming α-subunit) via the associated β-subunits.[18] A cysteine residue is identified in K_V β-subunits, which is sensitive to oxidation and is critical in binding the inactivating domains (either K_V α- or β-subunit inactivating domain) to the inner mouth of the channel pore (see Chapters 2 and 3). The K_V channels rapidly inactivate when the cysteine residue is in a reduced state, whereas the K_V channels do not rapidly inactivate (either slowly-inactivating or noninactivating) when the cysteine residue is in an oxidized state.[18] In addition, coexpression of K_V β-subunits ($hK_V\beta1.2$ or $hK_V\beta1.3$) with K_V α-subunits ($hK_V1.2$) significantly reduces the current amplitude, suggesting that K_V β-subunits also act as open-channel blockers.[66] The sensitivity of the cysteine residues in K_V β-subunits and the ability of hypoxia to alter redox status raise the possibility that hypoxia may regulate $I_{K(V)}$ through β-subunits. Molecularly, the *Shaker* K_V channel β-subunits, which are also expressed in PA smooth muscle cells, have 45% to 60% homologies to several members of an NADPH-dependent oxidoreductase superfamily.[26] It is, thus, plausible that: 1) β-subunits have oxidoreductase function, which produces ODCR during normoxia to keep channels open; and 2) an NADPH-P-450 oxidoreductase may be attached to the K_V channel α-subunits and function as a β-subunit; the conformational change of the enzyme during hypoxia blocks the K_V channels.

Conclusion

In conclusion, a pivotal procedure in HPV is the increase in $[Ca^{2+}]_i$ in PA smooth muscle cells. $[Ca^{2+}]_i$ is controlled by Ca^{2+} influx through sarcolemmal Ca^{2+} channels and Ca^{2+} release from intracellular stores. E_m regulates $[Ca^{2+}]_i$ in large part through the voltage-dependence of Ca^{2+} channels. The activity of K_V channels is a major determinant of resting E_m, and hypoxia selectively inhibits K_V channels in PA smooth muscle cells. Thus, the reduced $I_{K(V)}$ depolarizes the cells, opens voltage-gated Ca^{2+} channels, increases $[Ca^{2+}]_i$, and *initiates* pulmonary vasoconstriction. The rise in $[Ca^{2+}]_i$ also activates Ca^{2+}-activated Cl^- channels to further depolarize the cells and activates K_{Ca} channels to repolarize the cells. Hypoxia-induced inhibition of K_{Ca} channels and activation of Ca^{2+}-activated Cl^- channels by elevated $[Ca^{2+}]_i$ help to *maintain* the depolarization and, thus, the pulmonary vascular tone (Figure 6A).

Hypoxia decreases ATP generation (via decreased citric acid cycle metabolism and oxidative phosphorylation), alters cellular redox potential, reduces cytochrome P-450 activity and diminishes oxidant production. Interestingly, $I_{K(V)}$ is decreased by metabolic inhibitors (2-deoxy-D-glucose and FCCP), reducing agents (GSH), and cytochrome P-450 inhibitors (clotrimazole and 1-aminobenzotriazole), but increased by ATP and oxidants (diamide and NO). Molecularly, K_V channels are comprised of pore-forming α-subunits and auxiliary β-subunits. At least five K_V channel α-subunit genes ($K_V1.1$, $K_V1.2$, $K_V1.4$, $K_V1.5$, and $K_V1.6$) and three β-subunit genes ($K_V\beta1$, $K_V\beta2$, and $K_V\beta3$) are expressed in pulmonary arterial smooth muscle cells. A K_{Ca} channel gene, r*Slo,* is also expressed in these cells. The recent findings that the K_V channel β-subunits belong to an NAD(P)H-oxidoreductase superfamily and that an NADPH-oxidase is activated during HPV suggests that the β-subunits may serve as an intermediate in sensing changes in oxygen tension and redox status to govern the native K_V channel functions.

Therefore, the mechanisms by which acute hypoxia decreases $I_{K(V)}$ may include: 1) localized inhibition of cellular metabolism; 2) change in redox potential; 3) alteration of the activity of cytochrome P-450 or NADPH-oxidoreductase (or a membrane-delimited, heme- and metal-containing protein); and/or 4) conformational change of the channel protein (Figure 6B). The mechanisms by which chronic hypoxia inhibits K_V channels also include the transcriptional and/or translational inhibition of K_V channel genes.[92]

Acknowledgments

Supported by the National Institutes of Health (HL-54043), the American Heart Association (Established Investigator Grant), the Francis Families Foundation, and the American Physiological Society. The author thanks A.M. Aldinger, BS, and J. Wang, MD for the technical assistance, and M.L. Tod, PhD for the critical comments on the review.

References

1. Madden JA, Dawson CA, Harder DR: Hypoxia-induced activation in small isolated pulmonary arteries from the cat. *J Appl Physiol* 59:113–119, 1985.
2. Rodman DM, Yamaguchi T, O'Brien F, et al: Hypoxic contraction of isolated rat pulmonary artery. *J Pharmacol Exp Ther* 248:952–959, 1989.
3. Yuan X-J, Tod ML, Rubin LJ, et al: Contrasting effects of hypoxia on tension in rat pulmonary and mesenteric arteries. *Am J Physiol* 259:H281-H289, 1990.
4. Marshall C, Marshall BE: Hypoxic pulmonary vasoconstriction is not dependent on the endothelium. *Proc Soc Exp Bioi Med* 201:267–270, 1992.
5. Murray TR, Chen L, Marshall BE, et al: Hypoxic contraction of cultured pulmonary vascular smooth muscle cells. *Am J Respir Cell Mol Biol* 3:457–465, 1990.
6. Madden JA, Vadula MS, Kurup VP: Effects of hypoxia and other vasoactive agents on pulmonary and cerebral artery smooth muscle cells. *Am J Physiol* 263:L384-L393, 1992.
7. Nelson MT, Patlak JB, Worley JF, et al: Calcium channels, potassium channels,

and voltage dependence of arterial smooth muscle tone. *Am J Physiol* 259:C03-C18, 1990.
8. Fleischmann BK, Murray RK, Kotlikoff MI: Voltage window for sustained elevation of cytosolic calcium in smooth muscle cells. *Proc Natl Acad Sci USA* 91: 11914–11918, 1994.
9. Smirnov SV, Aaronson PI: Alteration of the transmembrane K^+ gradient during development of delayed rectifier in isolated rat pulmonary arterial cells. *J Gen Physiol* 104:241–264, 1994.
10. Yuan X-J, Goldman WF, Tod ML, et al: Ionic currents in rat pulmonary and mesenteric arterial myocytes in primary culture and subculture. *Am J Physiol* 264:L107-L115, 1993.
11. Evans AM, Osipenko ON, Gurney AM: Properties of a novel K^+ current that is active at resting potential in rabbit pulmonary artery smooth muscle cells. *J Physiol* 496(2):407–420, 1996.
12. Albarwani S, Robertson BE, Nye PCG, et al: Biophysical properties of Ca^{2+}- and Mg^{2+}-ATP-activated K^+ channels in pulmonary arterial smooth muscle cells isolated from the rat. *Pflugers Arch* 428:446–454, 1994.
13. Clapp LH, Gurney AM: ATP-sensitive K^+ channels regulate resting potential of pulmonary arterial smooth muscle cells. *Am J Physiol* 262:H916-H920, 1992.
14. Fleischmann BK, Washabau RJ, Kotlikoff MI: Control of resting membrane potential by delayed rectifier potassium currents in ferret airway smooth muscle cells. *J Physiol* 469:625–638, 1993.
15. Yuan X-J: Voltage-gated K^+ currents regulate resting membrane potential and $[Ca^{2+}]_i$ in pulmonary arterial myocytes. *Circ Res* 77:370–378, 1995.
16. Gelband CH, Hume JR: Ionic currents in single smooth muscle cells of the canine renal artery. *Circ Res* 71:745–758, 1992.
17. Ruppersberg J, Stocker M, Pongs O, et al: Regulation of fast inactivation of cloned mammalian $I_K(A)$ channels by cysteine oxidation. *Nature* 352:711–714, 1991.
18. Rettig J, Heinemann SH, Wunder F, et al: Inactivation properties of voltage-gated K^+ channels altered by presence of β-subunit. *Nature* 369:289–294, 1994.
19. Hasunuma K, Rodman DM, McMurtry IF: Effects of K^+ channel blockers on vascular tone in the perfused rat lung. *Am Rev Respir Dis* 144:884–887, 1991.
20. McCobb DP, Fowler NL, Featherstone T, et al: A human calcium-activated potassium channel gene expressed in vascular smooth muscle. *Am J Physiol* 269: H767-H777, 1995.
21. Yuan X-J: Role of calcium-activated chloride current in regulating pulmonary vasomotor tone. *Am J Physiol* 272:L959–L968, 1997.
22. Isom LL, De Jongh KS, Catteral WA: Auxiliary subunits of voltage-gated ion channels. *Neuron* 12:1183–1194, 1994.
23. Pongs O: Molecular biology of voltage-dependent potassium channels. *Physiol Rev* 72(suppl):S69-S88, 1992.
24. Yuan X-J, Wang J, Juhaszova M, et al: Functional expression of voltage-gated K^+ channels in pulmonary artery myocytes (abstr). *Am J Resp Crit Care Med* 155(4):A792, 1997.
25. Nelson MT, Quayle JM: Physiological roles and properties of potassium channels in arterial smooth muscle. *Am J Physiol* 268:C799-C822, 1995.
26. McCormack T, McCormack K: *Shaker* K^+ channel β subunits belong to an NAD(P)H-dependent oxidoreductase superfamily. *Cell* 79:1133–1135, 1994.
27. McMurtry IF, Davidson B, Reeves JT, et al: Inhibition of hypoxic pulmonary

vasoconstriction by calcium antagonists in isolated rat lungs. *Circ Res* 38: 99–104, 1976.
28. Harder DR, Madden JA, Dawson C: Hypoxic induction of Ca^{2+}-dependent action potentials in small pulmonary arteries of the cat. *J Appl Physiol* 59: 1389–1393, 1985.
29. Post JM, Hume JM, Archer SL, et al: Direct role for potassium channel inhibition in hypoxic pulmonary vasoconstriction. *Am J Physiol* 262:C882-C890, 1992.
30. Post JM, Gelband CH, Hume JR: $[Ca^{2+}]_i$ inhibition of K^+ channels in canine pulmonary artery, novel mechanisms for hypoxia-induced membrane depolarization. *Circ Res* 77:131–139, 1995.
31. Yuan X-J, Goldman WF, Tod ML, et al: Hypoxia reduces potassium currents in cultured rat pulmonary but not mesenteric arterial myocytes. *Am J Physiol* 264: L116-L123, 1993.
32. Yuan X-J, Tod ML, Rubin LJ, et al: Deoxyglucose and reduced glutathione mimic the effects of hypoxia on K^+ and Ca^{2+} conductances in pulmonary artery cells. *Am J Physiol* 267:L52-L63, 1994.
33. Yuan X-J, Salvaterra CG, Tod ML, et al. The sodium gradient, potassium channels, and regulation of calcium in pulmonary and mesenteric arterial smooth muscles: effects of hypoxia. In: Weir EK, Hume JR, Reeves JT (eds): *Ion Flux in Pulmonary Vascular Control.* New York: Plenum Press; 205–222, 1993.
34. Osipenko ON, Evans AM, Gurney AM: Regulation of the resting potential of rabbit pulmonary artery myocytes by a low threshold, O_2-sensitive potassium current. *Br J Pharmacol* 120:1461–1470, 1997.
35. Smirnov SV, Robertson TP, Ward JPT, et al: Chronic hypoxia is associated with reduced delayed rectifier K^+ current in rat pulmonary artery muscle cells. *Am J Physiol* 266:H365-H370, 1994.
36. Park MK, Lee SH, Lee SJ, et al: Different modulation of Ca-activated K channels by the intracellular redox potential in pulmonary and ear arterial smooth muscle cells of the rabbit. *Pflugers Arch* 430:308–314, 1995.
37. Yuan X-J, Tod ML, Rubin LJ, et al: NO hyperpolarizes pulmonary artery smooth muscle cells and decreases the intracellular Ca^{2+} concentration by activating voltage-gated K^+ channels. *Proc Natl Acad Sci USA* 93:10489–10494, 1996.
38. Archer SL, Huang JM, Reeve HL, et al: Differential distribution of electrophysiologically distinct myocytes in conduit and resistance arteries determines their response to nitric oxide and hypoxia. *Circ Res* 78:431–442, 1996.
39. Jiang C, Haddad GG: A direct mechanism for sensing low oxygen levels by central neurons. *Proc Natl Acad Sci USA* 91:7198–7201, 1994.
40. Ganfornina MD, Lopez-Barneo J: Single K^+ channels in membrane patches of arterial chemoreceptor cells are modulated by O_2 tension. *Proc Natl Acad Sci USA* 88:2927–2930, 1991.
41. Salvaterra CG, Goldman WF: Acute hypoxia increases cytosolic calcium in cultured pulmonary arterial myocytes. *Am J Physiol* 264:L323-L328, 1993.
42. Archer SL, Huang J, Henry Y, et al: A redox-based O_2 sensor in rat pulmonary vasculature. *Circ Res* 73:1100–1112, 1993.
43. Michelakis ED, Huang J, Reeve HL, et al: Down-regulation of a redox based oxygen sensor explains the selective loss of hypoxic pulmonary vasoconstriction in chronic hypoxia (abstr). *Circulation* 94(8 suppl):I-231, 1996.
44. Nelson MT, Cheng H, Rubart M, et al: Relaxation of arterial smooth muscle by calcium sparks. *Science* 270:633–637, 1995.
45. Lee SH, Earm YE: Caffeine induces periodic oscillations of Ca^{2+}-activated K^+

current in pulmonary arterial smooth muscle cells. *Pflugers Arch* 426:189–198, 1994.
46. Wyatt CN, Peers C: Ca^{2+}-activated K^+ channels in isolated type I cells of the neonatal rat carotid body. *J Physiol* 483(3):559–565, 1995.
47. Franco-Obregon A, Lopez-Barneo J: Differential oxygen sensitivity of calcium channels in rabbit smooth muscle cells of conduit and resistance pulmonary arteries. *J Physiol* 491:511–518, 1996.
48. Duchen MR, Biscoe TJ: Relative mitochondrial membrane potential and $[Ca^{2+}]_i$ in type I cells isolated from the rabbit carotid body. *J Physiol* 450:33–61, 1992.
49. Ohe M, Mimata T, Haneda T, et al: Time course of pulmonary vasoconstriction with repeated hypoxia and glucose depletion. *Respir Physiol* 63:177–186, 1986.
50. Daut J, Maier-Rudolph W, von Beckerath N, et al: Hypoxic dilation of coronary arteries is mediated by ATP-sensitive potassium channels. *Science* 247: 1341–1344, 1990.
51. Wiener CM, Dunn A, Sylvester JT: ATP-dependent K^+ channels modulate vasoconstrictor responses to severe hypoxia in isolated ferret lungs. *J Clin Invest* 88: 500–504, 1991.
52. McMurtry IF, Petrun MD, Reeves JT: Lungs from chronically hypoxic rats have decreased pressor response to acute hypoxia. *Am J Physiol* 235(1):H104-H109, 1978.
53. Takimoto K, Fomina AF, Gealy R, et al: Dexamethasone rapidly induces Kv1.5 K^+ channel gene transcription and expression in clonal pituitary cells. *Neuron* 11:359–369, 1993.
54. Levitan ES, Gealy R, Trimmer JS, et al: Membrane depolarization inhibits Kv1.5 voltage-gated K^+ channel gene transcription and protein expression in pituitary cells. *J Biol Chem* 270(11):6036–6041, 1995.
55. Lopez-Barneo J, Lopez-Lopez JR, Urena J, et al: Chemotransduction in the carotid body: K^+ current modulated by Po_2 in type I chemoreceptor cells. *Science* 241: 580–582, 1988.
56. Cross A, Henderson L, Jones OT, et al: Involvement of an NAD(P)H oxidase as a Po_2 sensor protein in the rat carotid body. *Biochem J* 272:743–747, 1990.
57. Youngson C, Nurse C, Yeger H, et al: Oxygen sensing in airway chemoreceptors. *Nature* 365:153–155, 1993.
58. Archer SL, Will JA, Weir EK: Redox status in the control of pulmonary vascular tone. *Herz* 11(3):127–141, 1986.
59. Wolin MS, Burke-Wolin TM, Kaminski PM, et al: Reactive oxygen species and vascular oxygen sensors. In: Weir EK, Archer SL, Reeves JT (eds). Nitric Oxide and Radicals in the Pulmonary Vasculature. Armonk, NY: Futura Publishing Company, Inc.; 245–263, 1996.
60. Post JM, Weir EK, Archer SL, et al: Redox regulation of K^+ channels and hypoxic pulmonary vasoconstriction. In: Weir EK, Hume JR, Reeves JT (eds). Ion Flux in Pulmonary Vascular Control. New York: Plenum Press; 189–204, 1993.
61. Yuan X-J, Sugiyama T, Goldman WF, et al: A mitochondrial uncoupler increases K_{Ca} currents but decreases K_V currents in pulmonary artery myocytes. *Am J Physiol* 270:C321-C331, 1996.
62. Yuan X-J, Tod ML, Rubin LJ, et al: Inhibition of cytochrome *P*-450 reduces voltage-gated K^+ currents in pulmonary arterial myocytes. *Am J Physiol* 268:C259-C270, 1995.
63. Weir EK, Eaton JW, Chesler E: Redox status and pulmonary vascular reactivity. *Chest* 88:249S-252S, 1985.

64. Zhao Y, Wang J, Rubin LJ, et al: Inhibition of K_V and K_{Ca} channels antagonizes NO-induced relaxation in pulmonary artery. *Am J Physiol* 272:H904–H912, 1997.
65. Sullivan JM, Traynelis SF, Chen H-SV, et al: Identification of two cysteine residues that are required for redox modulation of the NMDA subtype of glutamate receptor. *Neuron* 13:929–936, 1994.
66. DeBiasi M, Wang Z, Accili E et al: Open channel block of human heart hKv1.5 by the β-subunit hKvβ1.2. *Am J Physiol* 272:H2932–H2941, 1997.
67. Rounds S, McMurtry IF: Inhibitors of oxidative ATP production cause transient vasoconstriction and block subsequent pressor responses in rat lungs. *Circ Res* 48:393–400, 1981.
68. Stanbrook HS, McMurtry IF: Inhibition of glycolysis potentiates hypoxic vasoconstriction in rat lungs. *J Appl Physiol* 55:1467–1473, 1983.
69. McMurtry IF, Rounds S, Stanbrook HS: Studies of the mechanism of hypoxic pulmonary vasoconstriction. *Advanc Shock Res* 8:21–33, 1981.
70. Evans AM, Clapp LH, Gurney AM: Augmentation by intracellular ATP of the delayed rectifier current independently of the glibenclamide-sensitive K-current in rabbit arterial myocytes. *Br J Pharmacol* 111:972–974, 1994.
71. Korge P, Campbell KB: Local ATP regeneration is important for sarcoplasmic reticulum Ca^{2+} pump function. *Am J Physiol* 267:C357–C366, 1994.
72. Levitan IB: Modulation of ion channels by protein phosphorylation and dephosphorylation. *Annu Rev Physiol* 56:193–212, 1994.
73. Gelband CH, Ishikawa T, Post JM, et al: Intracellular divalent cations block smooth muscle K^+ channels. *Circ Res* 73:24–34, 1993.
74. Lopatin AN, Nichols CG: Internal Na^+ and Mg^{2+} blockade of DRK1 (K_V1.2) potassium channels expressed in *Xenopus* oocytes. *J Gen Physiol* 103:203–216, 1994.
75. Clapham DE: Calcium signaling. *Cell* 80:259–268, 1995.
76. Miller C: Potassium selectivity in proteins: oxygen cage or in the F ace? *Science* 261:1692–1693, 1993.
77. Harder DR, Narayanan J, Birks EK, et al: Identification of a putative microvascular oxygen sensor. *Circ Res* 79:54–61, 1996.
78. Campbell WB, Gebremedhin D, Pratt PF, et al: Identification of epoxyeicosatrienoic acids as endothelium-derived hyperpolarizing factors. *Circ Res* 78: 415–423, 1996.
79. Sylvester JT, McGowan C: The effects of agents that bind to cytochrome *P*-450 on hypoxic pulmonary vasoconstriction. *Circ Res* 43:429–437, 1978.
80. Miller MA, Hales CA: Role of cytochrome *P*-450 in alveolar hypoxic pulmonary vasoconstriction in dogs. *J Clin Invest* 64:666–673, 1979.
81. Chen G, Cheung DW: Modulation of endothelium-dependent hyperpolarization and relaxation to acetylcholine in rat mesenteric artery by cytochrome P450 enzyme activity. *Circ Res* 79:827–833, 1996.
82. Gonzalez C, Almaraz L, Obeso A, et al: Carotid body chemoreceptors: from natural stimuli to sensory discharges. *Physiol Rev* 74(4):829–898, 1994.
83. Marshall C, Mamary AJ, Verhoeven AJ, et al: Pulmonary artery NADPH-oxidase is activated in hypoxic pulmonary vasoconstriction. *Am J Resp Cell Mol Biol* 15:633–644, 1996.
84. Weir EK, Wyatt C, Reeve H, et al: Diphenyleneiodonium inhibits both potassium and calcium currents in isolated pulmonary artery smooth muscle cells. *J Appl Physiol* 76:2611–2615, 1994.

85. Thomas H, Carson R, Fried E, et al: Inhibition of hypoxic pulmonary vasoconstriction by diphenyleneiodonium. *Biochem Pharmacol* 42:R9-R12, 1991.
86. White KA, Marletta MA: Nitric oxide synthase is a cytochrome P-450 type hemoprotein. *Biochem* 31:6627–6631, 1992.
87. Bredt DS, Hwang PM, Glatt CE, et al: Cloned and expressed nitric oxide synthase structurally resembles cytochrome P-450 reductase. *Nature* 351:714–718, 1991.
88. Hu S, Kim H: Activation of K^+ channel in vascular smooth muscles by cytochrome P450 metabolites of arachidonic acid. *Eur J Pharmol* 230:215–221, 1993.
89. Rehm H, Lazdunski M: Purification and subunit structure of a putative K^+ channel protein identified by its binding properties for dendrotoxin I. *Proc Natl Acad Sci USA* 85:4919–4923, 1988.
90. Scott VES, Rettig J, Parcej DN, et al: Primary structure of a β subunit of α-dendrotoxin-sensitive K^+ channels from bovine brain. *Proc Natl Acad Sci USA* 91:1637–1641, 1994.
91. Chouinard SW, Wilson GF, Schlimgen AK, et al: A potassium channel β subunit related to the aldo-keto reductase superfamily is encoded by the *Drosophila Hyperkinetic* locus. *Proc Natl Acad Sci USA* 92:6763–6769, 1995.
92. Wang J, Juhaszova M, Rubin LJ, et al: Hypoxia inhibits gene expression of voltage-gated K^+ channel α subunits in pulmonary artery smooth muscle cells. *J Clin Invest* 100:2347–2353, 1997.

Chapter 18

Diversity of Potassium Channel Expression in Pulmonary Vascular Smooth Muscle Cells

Stephen L. Archer
Helen L. Reeve
James Huang
Daniel P. Nelson
Simona Tolarova
Evangelos Michelakis
E. Kenneth Weir

Introduction

Several facets of the pulmonary vascular bed set it apart from other circulations. First, the pulmonary circulation is a low resistance circuit which accommodates the entire cardiac output at low pressure and resistance (approximately 20% that of the systemic vasculature). In normal individuals, the pulmonary circulation is capable of accommodating four- or fivefold increases in cardiac output without any increase in pulmonary vascular resistance (PVR).[1] While some of the properties of the pulmonary

From: López-Barneo, J and Weir, EK: *Oxygen Regulation of Ion Channels and Gene Expression.* Armonk, NY: Futura Publishing Company, Inc., ©1998.

circuit relate to anatomy of the vessels, recent studies, using patch-clamp electrophysiology, have demonstrated an important role for ion channels in the vascular smooth muscle cell (SMC). As will be discussed subsequently, the many types of potassium (K) channels in pulmonary artery (PA) SMC are important targets for vasoconstrictor (e.g., hypoxia) and vasodilator (e.g., nitric oxide [NO]) stimuli. Control of tone in the PA is substantially (but not wholly) modulated by the electrical properties of the PA SMC, both in health[2] and disease.[3]

The importance of ion channels to pulmonary vascular physiology is particularly evident in the mechanism of hypoxic pulmonary vasoconstriction (HPV) (see recent review[2]). On exposure of a lobe of lung to hypoxia, as in pneumonia or atelectasis, there is rapid, regional constriction of small, muscular PAs in the affected segment. This diverts blood flow to better ventilated regions of the lung. HPV is a means of matching ventilation and perfusion. If the entire lung is hypoxic, then PA pressure rises and blood is shifted toward the less dependent zones. In contrast, most systemic beds either dilate to hypoxia or show no response.[4]

Although HPV can be altered by neuro-humoral factors, including prostaglandins, leukotrienes, endothelins, and NO, the essence of the response is intrinsic to the PA SMC.[5–7] Recently, we have learned that HPV is dependent on the coordinated activity of voltage-gated potassium (Kv) and calcium (Ca^{2+}) channels.[2] HPV is initiated by inhibition of a Kv channel.[7,8] This K channel, yet to be precisely identified, is a rapidly activating, slow inactivating, Kv channel which is also inhibited by 4-aminopyridine (4-AP). Inhibition of this Kv channel by hypoxia or 4-AP depolarizes the plasma membrane, resulting in a rise in cytosolic Ca^{2+} and vasoconstriction. Indeed, it has been known for 20 years that Ca^{2+} influx into the SMCs, necessary for HPV, occurred via the voltage-gated Ca^{2+} channel.[9–11]

NO, a potent pulmonary vasodilator, causes relaxation in part by activating another class of K channels, the calcium-sensitive potassium (K_{Ca}) channel.[12] NO, synthesized primarily by endothelial NO synthase (NOS), contributes substantially to pulmonary vasodilatation at birth.[13] The fall in PVR with the first breath is due in large part to NO and cyclic guanine monophosphate (cGMP)-dependent activation of a cGMP-dependent protein kinase which in turn phosphorylates and activates K_{Ca} channels.[13] In the adult circulation, NO does not determine basal tone (which remains quite low, even if one uses arginine analogs to acutely[14] or chronically[15] inhibit NOS). Rather, NO production increases in response to vasoconstrictors and pulmonary hypertension, and serves a homeostatic, hemodynamic function. The rise in pressure caused by all classes of vasoconstrictors is enhanced by inhibition of NOS. Recently, we have shown that the sensitivity of the pulmonary circulation to dexfenfluramine, an anorectic agent implicated in a recent outbreak of pulmonary hypertension in Europe,[16] is greatly increased by NOS inhibition.[3]

Thus, NO and hypoxia are an electrophysiologic "ying and yang," K-channel opener, K-channel closer, respectively (although neither stimulus is exclusively mediated through its effects of K channels). This chapter reviews recent data from our laboratory which shows that the hypoxia-inhibited, delayed-rectifier (K_{DR}) and the NO-activated, K_{Ca} channels are differentially distributed along the pulmonary vascular bed, proceeding from proximal, conduit to small, resistance PAs. It is the regional diversity of K channel distribution which explains why HPV is greatest in resistance PAs and NO most potent in conduit PAs.[17] The concept of K channel diversity has recently been reviewed[18] and is relevant not only for control of vascular tone, but also for growth and remodeling in pulmonary and systemic vessels.[19–21]

Before discussing the concept of K channel diversity, it is useful to briefly review the electrophysiologic properties of PA SMCs and the various pharmacolgic probes used in their study.

Potassium Channels and Regulation of Membrane Potential in Pulmonary Artery Smooth Muscle Cell

Membrane potential (E_m) in vascular SMC is largely controlled by K channels (although the chloride channels may play a role). It is probable that the precise type of K channel controlling E_m varies within a species from bed to bed and during development from fetus to adult. There are also likely to be some interspecies differences. In the adult rat PA, for example, E_m is largely controlled by a delayed rectifier-type Kv channel; in contrast, in the fetal sheep, E_m is controlled more by K_{Ca} channels.[13] Regardless of the type of K channel controlling E_m, some common mechanisms apply.

When K channels open, positively charged K ions exit down a concentration gradient (intracellular K 145 mM, extracellular K 4–5 mM). This leaves negatively charged macromolecules trapped in the cell interior. This makes the interior of the cell more negative, relative to the exterior: "membrane hyperpolarization." E_m negative to ~ -20 mV leads to closure of the voltage-gated Ca^{2+} channel, reducing Ca^{2+} influx and inhibiting vasoconstriction. K-channel blockers and openers cause pulmonary vasoconstriction [7,22] and vasodilatation,[23] respectively, largely through their effects on the E_m and the Ca^{2+} channel. Although it has long been suspected that K conductance is important to the regulation of pulmonary vascular tone,[24–26] the application of patch-clamp techniques provided the first, direct evidence of the involvement of K channels in regulation of the pulmonary circulation. These techniques show that K channels in PA SMC are inhibited by hypoxia, leading to depolarization and pulmonary vasoconstriction[7] (Figure 1). This has subsequently been confirmed by others,[27] using dithionite as a surrogate for hypoxia.

PA SMC cells contain various types of K channels including: K_{Ca}[7], K_{DR},[17,27–30] and adenosine triphosphate-gated K channels (K_{ATP}).[31] K_{Ca} channels are voltage-gated but, at any voltage level, their activity is greatly enhanced by increases in $[Ca^{2+}]_i$. Although not normally active at resting E_m,(activation threshold ~ −20 mV), vasoconstriction brings these channels into play by increasing $[Ca^{2+}]_i$ and depolarizing the membrane. Once activated, these large conductance, "maxi-K" channels tend to restore E_m toward basal levels. K_{DR} channels are a family of Kv channels, which control the resting E_m in PA SMC.[8,29,30,32] They appear to include the hypoxia-inhibited K channel(s) involved in HPV.[17] K_{ATP} channels, although inactive in normoxia,[22] do contribute to anoxic PA relaxation.[33] The K_{Ca} channels are inhibited by tetraethylammonium (TEA) or charybdotoxin (CTX). TEA is a cationic blocker which interferes with the outer pore of the K_{Ca} channel (and competes with CTX for this aspect of the channel).[34] At low doses (1–5 mM), TEA is a preferential K_{Ca} inhibitor.[30,35,36] Synthetic CTX (<100 nM) is a relatively selective, peptide K_{Ca} inhibitor.[37] It blocks the channel externally by interaction of basic amino acids with fixed negative charges in the channel and is similarly effective in binding the channel in both open and closed conditions.[34] Although CTX is quite specific, it can block Kv channels in some neural tissue,[38] but it appears to have no effect on the 4-AP sensitive channels in SMC. Neither does CTX block K_{ATP} or small conductance, apamin-sensitive K_{Ca} channels.[34] Concerns regarding nonspecificity of CTX are minimized by use of the synthetic (vs wild) toxin, as contamination with other components of the scorpion venom is avoided.[39]

→

Figure 1. Hypoxia pulmonary vasconstriction is initiated by K channel inhibition, resulting in membrane depolarization and activation of the Ca^{2+} channel. AOS = activated oxygen species; GSH:GSSG = reduced and oxidized glutathione; NAD(P)H/NAD(P)–nicotinamide adenine dinucleotide (phosphate) reduced and oxidized; ETC = electron transport chain.

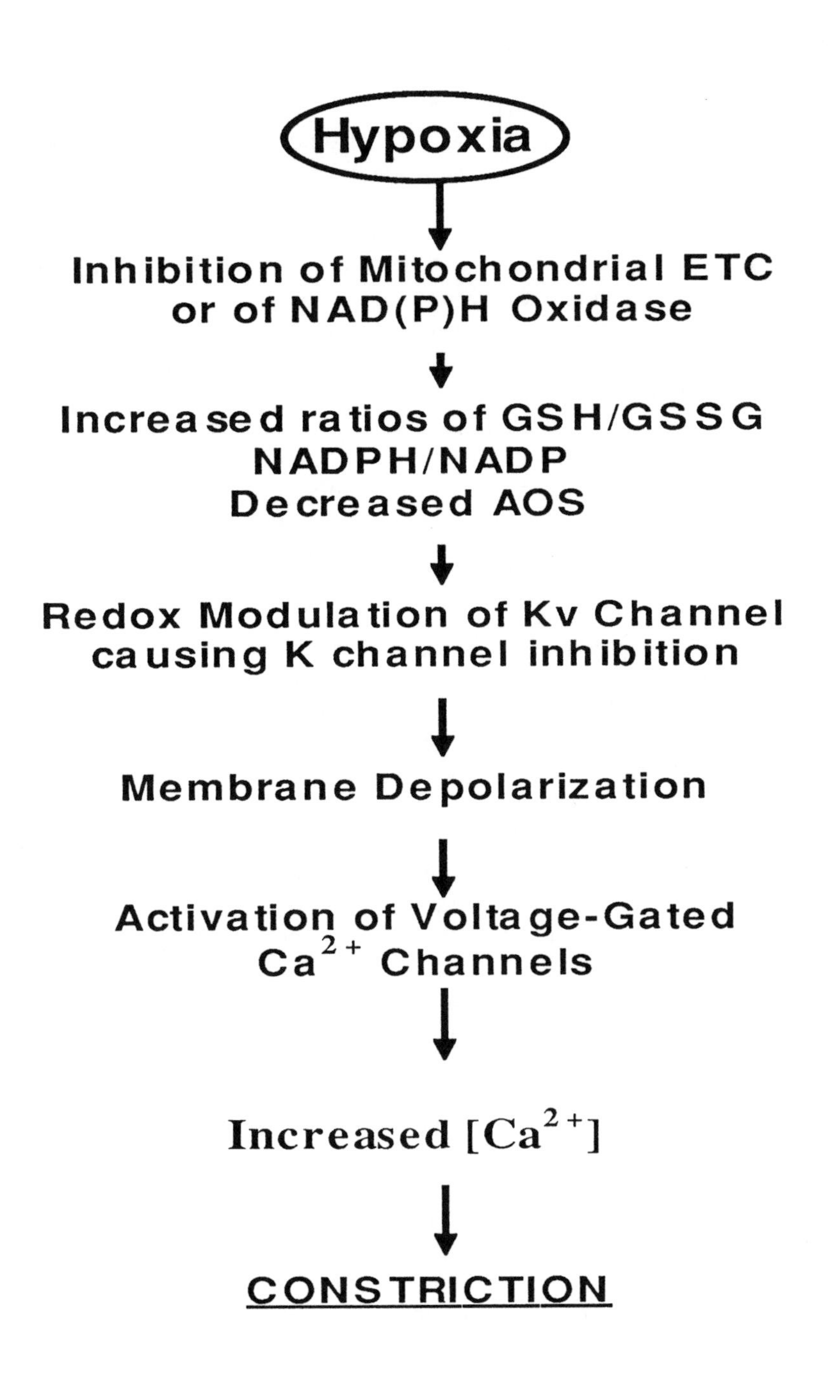
Hypoxia
Inhibition of Mitochondrial ETC
or of NAD(P)H Oxidase
Increased ratios of GSH/GSSG
NADPH/NADP
Decreased AOS
Redox Modulation of Kv Channel
causing K channel inhibition
Membrane Depolarization
Activation of Voltage-Gated
Ca^{2+} Channels
Increased $[Ca^{2+}]$
CONSTRICTION

K_{DR} channels, originally described in neural tissue, were so named because they displayed a voltage-activation delay. However, these channels have now been cloned and can be better identified using a molecular classification. In this scheme, the channel types are grouped in relation to the *Drosophila* K channel they resemble, as Kv 1, Kv 2, Kv 3, Kv 4 (related to *Drosophila* K channel families *Shaker*, *Shab*, *Shaw*, and *Shal*, respectively). The Kv1 group is divided into individual, homomultimeric channel types, i.e., Kv1.1,1.2, . . . 1.5.[40,41] The channel proteins from different genes within a single Kv family can combine, increasing the diversity of the channel protein finally expressed. K channel function is regulated through the assembly of channel subunit isoforms into either homo-or heterotetrameric structures, each characterized by distinct pharmacologic and kinetic properties.[42] Deletion of a small segment in the amino-terminal domain of the Kv1.4 gene prevents the formation of hybrid channels within the subfamily, but has no effect on homomultimerization or voltage-dependent gating, demonstrating that the amino-terminal region of mammalian K channels provides a recognition site necessary for hetero-, but not homomultimeric channel assembly within a subfamily and prevents coassembly between subfamilies.[42] Similarly, it appears that the Kv 1.5 channel in PA SMC is slightly different than the same channel in heart.[43] While a high level of identity to other K channels of the Kv1.5 class is preserved in the core region between transmembrane segments S1 to S6; homology decreases to between 74% and 82% in the amino and carboxyl (NH2 and COOH) terminal segments.[43]

Many K_{DR} channels are preferentially inhibited by low dose 4-AP (1–5 mM).[44,30,35,36] Although the K_i for 4-AP's effects on the K_{DR} channel (in isolated cells) is <1 mM,[35] it appears that higher doses are needed to block the K_{DR} in tissues. Doses of 4-AP less than 1 mM have no effect on pulmonary artery pressure (PAP) in isolated lungs, while doses of 5 to 10 mM cause much more constriction than TEA.[22] Although high doses of TEA and 4-AP are not "specific" for K_{Ca} and K_{DR} channels, low doses do inhibit different components of the potassium current (I_K) in PA SMC.[32]

There are, nonetheless, concerns about the specificity of 4-AP for the K_{DR} and so other toxins can be used (although ultimately molecular or immunological techniques offer the optimal precision in assessing the particular Kv channel involved in a given response). β Dendrotoxin, a component of the venom of elapid snakes, such as the Green Mamba, is a specific K_{DR} blocker in some vascular SMCs (45% inhibition of K_{DR} at 1 μM).[45] α Dendrotoxin blocks K_{DR} in neurons, but not in SMC.[45] Tityustoxin, a venom component from the Brazilian scorpion, Tityus serrulatus, blocks noninactivating Kv channels; whereas alpha-dendrotoxin and CTX block inactivating Kv channels.[46]

Nitric Oxide and Cyclic Guanine Monophosphate as Hyperpolarizing Factors

Endogenous NO is an important regulator of pulmonary vascular tone[14, 47–51] and inhaled, exogenous NO is an effective treatment for several forms of pulmonary hypertension (PHT).[52–56] NO causes vasodilatation by activating guanylate cyclase and increasing cGMP levels in vascular SMC[47,57–59] cGMP-mediated relaxation has traditionally been attributed to increased Ca^{2+} extrusion from the cell by Ca^{2+}-ATPase,[60] desensitization of actin and myosin to $[Ca^{2+}]_i$, or enhanced Ca^{2+} sequestration by the sarcoplasmic reticulum (SR).[61,62]

There is substantial evidence that E_m is an important determinant of the ability of vessels to synthesize or respond to endothelium-derived relaxing factor (EDRF) or NO. Potassium chloride (KCl), which depolarizes the membrane by decreasing the gradient for K efflux, inhibits EDRF activity in bioassay[63] and impairs bradykinin-evoked elevations of $[Ca^{2+}]_i$ in endothelial cells.[64,65] Even relaxation to authentic NO is attenuated by KCl,[12] suggesting it is membrane hyperpolarization, not NO synthesis, which is prevented by KCl. There has been controversy whether NO does[66–68] or does not[69,70] cause membrane hyperpolarization. Some of this variability is explained by our observation of electrophysiologic diversity among PA SMC (i.e., not all cells are the same). There is almost certainly true variability among vascular beds and between species as to whether cyclic nucleotides (cyclic adenosine monophosphate [cAMP] or cGMP) cause relaxation through effects on K channels and if so, which of the nucleotides is most important. In some vascular beds, prostacyclin is the predominant hyperpolarizing factor, in others cAMP, in others cGMP, in others, perhaps epoxyeicosatrienoic acids. The class of K channel activated by NO and cyclic nucleotides also varies among species and vascular beds. There is evidence, that the K_{ATP} channel is activated by cGMP[71] and that glyburide, a K_{ATP} blocker, inhibits NO-induced hyperpolarization in mesenteric arteries.[72] In the PA SMC, the K_{Ca} channel appears to be an important target for cGMP-protein phosphokinase (PK), but the possibility that the K_{ATP} channel is also important has not been excluded. The evidence supporting cGMP and NO as hyperpolarizing factors is persuasive, including studies of intact vessels[66,68–70,73,74] and patch-clamp documentation of the ability of cGMP and NO to activate K channels.[12,75–77] Figure 2 illustrates the proposed basis for that part of NO-induced relaxation which depends on K channels. It must be stated that the contribution of K channel activation to the net effect of NO varies substantially among species, vascular beds, and with maturation.

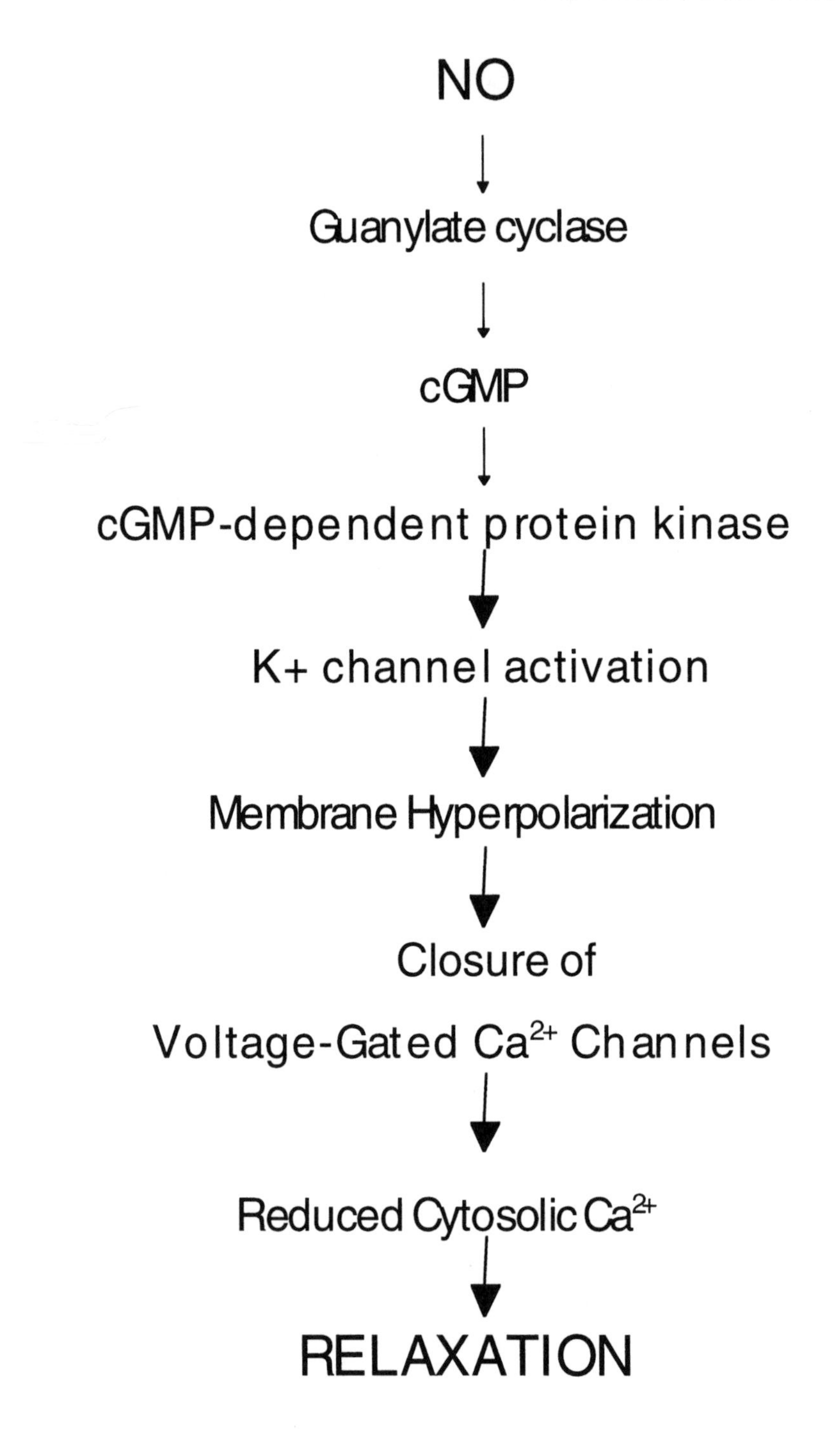
NO
Guanylate cyclase
cGMP
cGMP-dependent protein kinase
K+ channel activation
Membrane Hyperpolarization
Closure of
Voltage-Gated Ca2+ Channels
Reduced Cytosolic Ca2+
RELAXATION

Does Nitric Oxide Affect the Ion Channel Directly or Through Cyclic Guanine Monophosphate?

Cyclic nucleotides alter the activity of ion channels either by direct interaction with the channel protein, as in the cation channels of the retinal rod cells,[78] or indirectly, via cGMP-PK. These kinases control ion channel function by phosphorylating the channel or its regulatory factors. cGMP-PK is a serine/threonine kinase, abundant in SMC, which is activated by low levels of cGMP (<1 mM).[79,80] It phosphorylates a specific site on ion channels and other intracellular proteins (e.g. arg-arg-X-serine).[79,80] Activation of K_{Ca} channels in response to cGMP-PK, has been described in colonic cells,[81] as well as carotid[76] and pulmonary[12] SMC. The independent reports in diverse types of SMC suggest this mechanism is widely conserved and, thus, likely to be important. Furthermore, studies by Khan et al and by our laboratory suggest that interrupting this K_{Ca} activation pathway impairs cGMP-induced relaxation.[12,13,77] In all reports, save one,[82] cGMP appears to be essential for NO-induced activation of K channels-and this occurs by stimulating cGMP-PK.[12,75,76] We also found that a cGMP phosphodiesterase inhibitor (zaprinast), authentic cGMP, or a cGMP-PK activator all mimicked the effects of NO on K channels, indicating NO itself was not essential to the K channel activation. The observation that inhibitors of guanylate cyclase diminish the effects of EDRF-NO[83–85] suggests that much of NO's effects are channeled through the cGMP pathway. Consistent with our hypothesis, inhibiting guanylate cyclase with methylene blue reduces the effects of NO on K channel activity[12] and LY83583 (another inhibitor of guanylate cyclase) also attenuates NO-induced relaxation, in PA rings. The involvement of cGMP-PK in channel activation suggests the mechanism of channel activation involves phosphorylation, the hallmark of kinase activation. In support of this, we have found that inhibition of phosphatases (by okadaic acid, an inhibitor of protein phosphatases 1 and 2A[86]) increases basal I_K in NO-sensitive K_{Ca} cells (but not in K_{DR} cells).[12] This is strong evidence for the importance of phosphorylation in cGMP-induced channel activation.

Interfering with K channel activation (i.e., by giving TEA) impairs NO and cGMP-induced relaxation in mesenteric arteries,[77] conduit PA rings,[12] and isolated lungs. TEA's effects are somewhat specific for cGMP-

Figure 2. Proposed mechanism of NO effects on K^+ and Ca^{2+} channels.

dependent vasodilators, as TEA reduced relaxation caused by zaprinast, a cGMP-dependent dilator, but not relaxation to papaverine, a vasodilator which does not act through cGMP.[12] In addition, TEA does not interfere with the ability of NO to increase levels of cGMP.

Nitric Oxide and Clues to the Existence of Diversity

In the course of pursuing the mechanism of NO's effects on K channels, it became apparent that there are different types of PA SMC cells. We initially noted that not all cells in the PA (even cells from the same digestion) responded to NO with K channel activation. This finding was initially perplexing until the explanation emerged from studies of the pharmacology of K currents in "responder" and "nonresponder" cells. In cells with I_K predominated by K_{Ca} channel activity (current inhibited by CTX or TEA), NO consistently increased I_K. However, I_K was not increased by NO in cells in which I_K was predominated by K_{DR} channels (as determined by the fact the current was readily inhibited by 4-AP, but not TEA).[12] It has emerged that in some cells, I_K in the resting condition is carried mainly by K_{DR} channels, in others by K_{Ca} channels and in others by both channel types (Figure 3). This lead us to name these cell "types" K_{DR}, K_{Ca}, and mixed.[17] Simple electrophysiologic criteria (current density, capacitance, Figure 3) and morphology differentiate K_{DR}, K_{Ca}, and mixed cells.[17]

Elongate cells with low current density, have I_Ks which are sensitive

Figure 3. Whole cell electrophysiology demonstrates three cell types in the conduit pulmonary artery (PA). Three distinct cell types exist in the conduit PA. The names of the cells reflect the type of K channel conducting the majority of the whole cell current: K_{Ca}; K_{DR}; and mixed. Cells are characterized by (from **left to right**): **Column A.** Morphology of the macroscopic currents (example shown was obtained by stepped depolarization from −70 to +70 mV). Note the small, noisy, **spiky current** in K_{Ca} cells is inhibited by TEA, but not 4-AP. In contrast, the large, **smooth-profile current** in K_{DR} cells is much more sensitive to 4-AP than TEA. In mixed cells, 4-AP inhibits approximately half the total current, leaving the noisy, TEA-inhibitable portion intact. **Column B.** Current-voltage curves (mean ± SEM; n = 7 K_{Ca}, 5 mixed, and 20 K_{DR} cells) elicited by stepped depolarization from −70 to +0 mV. *$P<0.05$ curve differs from control. Note the current is much greater in the K_{DR} cells, even though they are smaller than the K_{Ca} cells. **Column C.** Cell capacitance and current density. $P<0.01$ value differs from all other groups. Note the K_{Ca} cells are large but have low current density. (Reproduced with permission from Reference 17.)

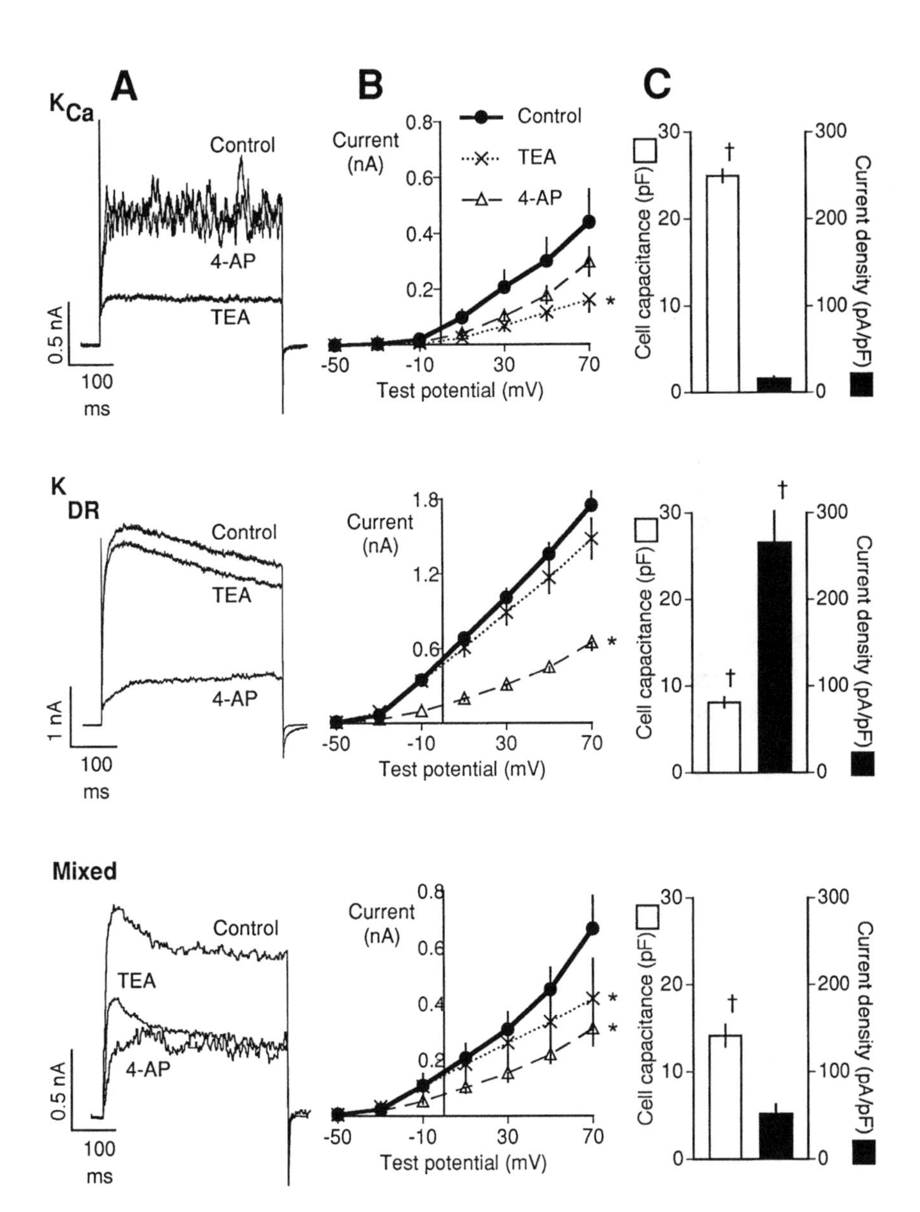

A
B
C
K_{Ca}
Control
4-AP
TEA
0.5 nA
100 ms
Current (nA)
Test potential (mV)
Cell capacitance (pF)
Current density (pA/pF)
K_{DR}
1 nA
Mixed

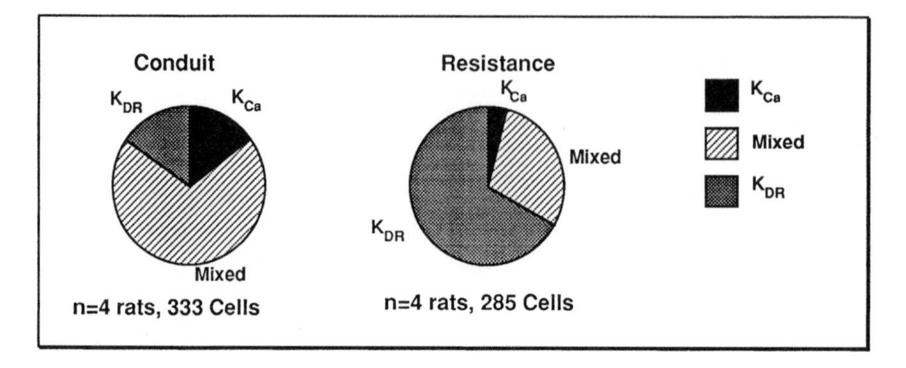

Figure 4. There are more K_{DR} cells in resistance than conduit pulmonary arteries (PAs). The results of a survey performed by light microscopy on enzymatically-dispersed PA smooth muscle cells (SMC), harvested from conduit and resistance rat PAs. Cells were classified by morphology into three groups, using criteria of length and shape. The names were ascribed based on previous patch-clamp studies which indicated that a certain morphology corresponded to a particular current phamacology (Figure 3). (Reproduced with permission from Reference 17.)

to CTX and low doses of TEA, consistent with a major role for the K_{Ca} channel. These cells are located in the proximal PA and respond to NO with increased I_K (Figure 4). In contrast, cells in resistance arteries have a characteristic perinuclear bulge, larger I_Ks and greater sensitivity to low doses of 4-AP, consistent with a major contribution from K_{DR} channels. The use of whole-cell current density provides an objective measure of net current, corrected for cell size. Current density objectively separates cells into 3 groups: K_{Ca} 15.6 $\pm$ 2.2; K_{DR} 265.3 $\pm$ 36.6; and mixed 51.7 $\pm$ 10.8 pA/pF (Figure 3). Differences in morphology do not reflect variations in digestion, as all three cell types can be seen in a single dispersion from a single ring, in which all cells are treated identically. Furthermore, cells from conduit and resistance arteries have marked structural differences, despite identical harvesting and dispersion protocols. Overdigested cells, identified by their round appearance, were not included in the electrophysiologic or morphological survey. Furthermore, scanning electron microscopy shows differences among cell types which cannot be explained as "artifacts."

The prevalence of K_{Ca} and K_{DR} cells varies between conduit (main or first division PAs) and resistance (4th-5th division, $<$400 mm, intraparenchymal PAs) arteries (Figure 4). K_{Ca} cells are more common in the conduit and K_{DR} cells are more common in resistance PAs. Although a cell's I_K may be predominated by one channel type, each cell contains several K channel types and the I_K is a mosaic, derived from all active K channels. Thus, although K_{Ca} *cells* are most common in conduit arteries and K_{DR} cells in resistance PAs, $-K_{Ca}$ *channels* occur in cells in all segments of the PA. The occurrence of diverse electrophysiologic cell types within and between vascular segments may contribute to regional differences in vascular reactivity to stimuli which modulate tone through effects on the K channels, such as NO-cGMP[12] and hypoxia.[7,8,29,32]

What Are the Functional Consequences of K Channel Diversity in the Pulmonary Circulation?

If regional differences in K channel distribution are of functional importance, one might expect segmental differences in the response of the pulmonary vasculature to stimuli which alter tone at least in part due to their effects on K channels,[7,8,12,29] i.e., hypoxia and NO. Certainly, this is true for HPV. Hypoxia inhibits K_{DR} channels while activating K_{Ca} channels.[17] As predicted by our hypothesis, hypoxia constricts resistance PA rings (rich in K_{DR} cells), while primarily relaxing conduit rings (rich in K_{Ca} cells).[17] NO, while effective in both conduit and resistance segments, is more potent in K_{Ca}-enriched conduit PAs.[17]

Evidence of Vascular Cell Diversity from Other Laboratories

Although the existence of cell diversity in arteries is a recent concept, much work has already been done. Frid et al found at least three populations of PA SMC, based on immunological and morphological criteria, within the media of the calf conduit PA.[19] They noted diversity in cells based on the distribution of contractile and cytoskeletal proteins (alpha actin, myosin, calponin, desmin, and metavinculin), as they surveyed from lumen toward adventitia. They also showed that exposure of calves to hypoxia (a stimulus for pulmonary hypertension and cell proliferation) caused proliferation in only one of the populations of SMC in the vessel wall.[20] Unlike our experiments, cells were studied in section (rather than following isolation), and no data relating to cell function were acquired. Thus, we do not know if the three cell types we reported in conduit PA correlate with those of Frid et al.

Neylon et al found two cell types in cultures of adult rat aortic SMC. In observing cells over many passages, they found two different cell populations. There were elongate cells which depolarized in response to vasoactive agonists (endothelin 1 and alpha-thrombin) due to influx of sodium and Ca^{2+} and epithelial-like cells which hyperpolarized (in response to the same stimuli), probably due to activation of K_{Ca} channels.[21] They speculated that the "hyperpolarization-prone" cells could be important in healing vascular injuries, as they tended to grow rapidly and might resist vasoconstriction. The cell morphology they described in nondispersed, cultured cells is not comparable to the morphology in our dispersed, isolated cells.

Neither our studies, nor those of Frid or Neylon, provide a clear explanation for the diversity of cell types within the vessel wall. We speculate that the disparity in the proportion of SMC cell subtypes between conduit and resistance PAs could be related to the different embryologic origin of the conduit PA (6th aortic arch) and resistance PA (lung bud).[87] Consequently, the conduit PA may have reactivity closer to that of systemic vessels (both dilate in response to hypoxia, while the resistance PAs constrict).

There is also strong evidence for diversity of K channel expression in nonvascular tissues, particularly neurons (see recent review[88]). In certain neurons, there is differential distribution of certain Kv channels between the soma and the dendrites.[89] Thus, it appears that it is a common strategy to have great variability in K channel expression within and between tissue types.

In conclusion, the pulmonary vasculature is a mosaic of electrophysiogically diverse SMCs. Differences in the localization of K_{Ca} and K_{DR}-enriched cells appears to contribute to the observed localization of HPV to resistance arteries. SMC cell diversity also exists in systemic arteries and in species other than the rat. K channel diversity is a common and important means for regional control of vascular tone, response to changes in oxygen tension, and possibly vascular remodeling.

References

1. Reeves J, Dempsey J, Grover RL: Pulmonary circulation during exercise. In: Weir EK, Reeves JT (eds). *Pulmonary Vascular Physiology and Pathophysiology.* Mount Kisco, NY: Futura Publishing Co.; 107–120, 1989.
2. Weir EK, Archer SL: The mechanism of acute hypoxic pulmonary vasoconstriction: the tale of two channels. *FASEB J* 9:183–189, 1995.
3. Weir EK, Reeve HL, Huang JMC, et al: The anorexic agents, aminorex, fenfluramine, and dexfenfluramine inhibit potassium current in rat pulmonary vascular smooth muscle and cause pulmonary vasoconstriction. *Circulation* 94: 2216–2220, 1996.
4. Hampl V, Weir EK, Archer SL: Endothelium-derived nitric oxide is less important

for basal tone regulation in the pulmonary than the renal circulation of the adult rat. *J Vasc Med Biol* 5:22–30, 1994.
5. Madden JA, Vadula MS, V Kurup: Effects of hypoxia and other vasoactive agents on pulmonary and cerebral artery smooth muscle cells. *Am J Physiol* 263:L384-L393, 1992.
6. Vadula M, Kleinman SJ, Madden J: Effect of hypoxia and norepinephrine on cytoplasmic free Ca^{2+} in pulmonary and cerebral arterial myocytes. *Am J Physiol* 265:L591–L597, 1993.
7. Post J, Hume J, Archer S, et al: Direct role for potassium channel inhibition in hypoxic pulmonary vasoconstriction. *Am J Physiol* 1992; 262:C882–C890.
8. Archer SL, Huang J, Henry T, et al: A redox-based oxygen sensor in rat pulmonary vasculature. *Circ Res* 73:1100–1112, 19993.
9. McMurtry I, Davidson A, Reeves J, et al: Inhibition of hypoxic pulmonary vasoconstriction by calcium channel antagonists in isolated rat lungs. *Circ Res* 38: 99–104, 1976.
10. McMurtry IF, Bay K: 8644 potentiates and A23187 inhibits hypoxic vasoconstriction in rat lungs. *Am J Physiol* 249:H741–H746, 1985.
11. Tolins M, Weir EK, Chesler E, et al: Pulmonary vascular tone is increased by a voltage-dependent calcium channel potentiator. *J Appl Physiol* 60:942–948, 1986.
12. Archer SL, Huang JMC, Hampl V, et al: Nitric oxide and cGMP cause vasorelaxation by activation of a charybdotoxin-sensitive K channel by cGMP-dependent protein kinase. *Proc Natl Acad Sci USA* 91:7583–7587, 1994.
13. Cornfield DN, Reeve HL, Tolarova S, et al: Oxygen causes fetal pulmonary vasodilation through activation of a calcium-dependent potassium channel. *Proc Natl Acad Sci USA* 93:8089–8094, 1996.
14. Archer SL, Tolins JP, Reye L, et al: Hypoxic pulmonary vasoconstriction is enhanced by inhibition of the synthesis of an endothelium derived relaxing factor. *Biochem Biophys Res Comm* 164:1198–1205, 1989.
15. Hampl V, Archer SL, Nelson DP, et al: Chronic EDRF inhibition and hypoxia: effects on the pulmonary circulation and systemic blood pressure. *J Appl Physiol* 75:1748–1757, 1993.
16. Abenhaim L, Moride Y, Brenot F, et al: Appetite-suppressant drugs and the risk of primary pulmonary hypertension. *N Engl J Med* 335:609–616, 1996.
17. Archer SL, Huang JMC, Reeve HL, et al: Differential distribution of electrophysiologically distinct myocytes in conduit and resistance arteries determines their response to nitric oxide and hypoxia. *Circ Res* 78(3):431–442, 1996.
18. Archer SL: Diversity of phenotype and function of vascular smooth muscle cells. *J Lab Clin Med* 6:524–529, 1996.
19. Frid MG, Moiseeva EP, Stenmark KR: Multiple phenotypically distinct smooth muscle cell populations exist in the adult and developing bovine pulmonary arterial media in vivo. *Circ Res* 75:669–681, 1994.
20. Whorley JD, Frid MG, Orton EC, et al: Hypoxia selectively induces proliferation in a specific subpopulation of smooth muscle cells in the bovine neonatal pulmonary arterial media. *J Clin Invest* 96:273–281, 1995.
21. Neylon CB, Avdonin PV, Dilley RJ, et al: Different electrical responses to vasoactive agonists in morphologically distinct smooth muscle cell types. Circ Res 75: 733–741, 1994.
22. Hasunuma K, Rodman D, McMurtry IF: Effects of K channel blockers on vascular tone in the perfused rat lung. *Am Rev Resp Dis* 144:884–887, 1991.

23. Chang JK, Moore P, Fineman JR, et al: K channel pulmonary vasodilation in fetal lambs: role of endothelium-derived nitric oxide. *J Appl Physiol* 73(1):188–94, 1992.
24. Lloyd TC: P_{O_2}-dependent pulmonary vasoconstriction caused by procaine. *J Appl Physiol* 21:1439–1442, 1966.
25. Hottenstein O, Mitzner W, Bierkamper G: Hypoxia alters membrane potential in the rat main pulmonary artery smooth muscle: a possible calcium mechanism (abstr). *Physiologist* 24:276, 1982.
26. Archer SL, Will J, Weir EK: Redox status in the control of pulmonary vascular tone. *Herz* 11:127–141, 1986.
27. Yuan X-J, Goldman W, Tod ML, et al: Ionic currents in rat pulmonary and mesenteric arterial myocytes in primary culture and subculture. *Am J Physiol* 264: L107–L115, 1993.
28. Yuan X-J, Goldman W, Tod ML, et al: Hypoxia reduces potassium currents in cultured rat pulmonary but not mesenteric arterial myocytes. *Am J Physiol* 264: L116–L123, 1993.
29. Reeve HL, Weir EK, Nelson DP, et al: Opposing effects of oxidants and antioxidants on K+ channel activity and tone in vascular tissue. *J Exp Physiol* 80: 825–834, 1995.
30. Yuan X-J: Voltage-gated K currents regulate resting membrane potential and $[Ca^{2+}]i$ in pulmonary artery myocytes. *Circ Res* 77:370–378, 1995.
31. Clapp L, Gurney A: Outward currents in rabbit pulmonary artery cells disassociated with a new technique. *Exp Physiol* 76:667–693, 1991.
32. Smirnov S, Robertson T, Ward J, et al: Chronic hypoxia is associated with reduced delayed rectifier K current in rat pulmonary artery muscle cells. *Am J Physiol* 266:H365–H370, 1994.
33. Wiener CM, Dunn A, Sylvester JT: ATP-dependent K channels modulate vasoconstrictor responses to severe hypoxia in isolated ferret lungs. *J Clin Invest* 88: 500–504, 1991.
34. Sugg EE, Garcia ML, Reuben JP, et al: Synthesis and structural characterization of charybdotoxin, a potent peptidyl inhibitor of the high conductance Ca^{2+}-activated K channel. *J Biol Chem* 265:18745–18748, 1990.
35. Gelband CH, Hume JR: Ionic currents in single smooth muscle cells of the canine renal artery. *Circ Res* 71:745–758, 1992.
36. Post JM, Gelband CH, Hume JR: $[Ca^{2+}]i$ inhibition of K channels in canine pulmonary artery: Novel mechanism for hypoxia-induced membrane depolarization. *Circ Res* 77:131–139, 1995.
37. Garcia ML, Galvez A, Garcia-Calvo M, et al: Use of toxins to study potassium channels. *J Bioenerg Biomembr* 23:615–646, 1991.
38. Vazquez J, Feigenbaum P, King G, et al: Characterization of the high affinity binding sites for charybdotoxin in synaptic plasma membranes from rat brain. *J Biol Chem* 265:15564–15571, 1990.
39. Garcia ML, Knaus H-G, Munujos P, et al: Charybdotoxin and its effects on potassium channels. *Am J Physiol* 269:C1–C10, 1995.
40. Chandy KG, Gutman GA: Nomenclature for mammalian potassium channel genes. *Trends Pharmacol* 14:434–440, 1993.
41. Grissmer S, Nguyen AN, Aiyar J, et al: Pharmacological characterization of five cloned voltage-gated K channels, types Kv 1.1, 1.2, 1.3, 1.5, and 3.1, stably expressed in mammalian cell lines. *J Pharm Exp Ther* 45:1227–1234, 1994.

42. Lee TE, Philipson LH, Kuznetsov A, et al: Structural determinant for assembly of mammalian K channels. *Biophys J* 66(3 Pt 1):667–673, 1994.
43. Overturf KE, Russell SN, Carl A, et al: Cloning and characterization of a Kv1.5 delayed rectifier K channel from vascular and visceral smooth muscles. *Am J Physiol* 267(5 Pt 1):C1231–C1238, 1994.
44. Hille B: *Ionic Channels of Excitable Membranes.* Sunderland, MA: Sinauer Associates, Inc.; 1–607, 1992.
45. Ren J, Karpinski E, Benishin CG: Inhibition of a K current by b-dendrotoxin in primary and subcultured vascular smooth muscle cells. *J Phar Exp Ther* 269: 209–221, 1993.
46. Rogowski RS, Krueger BK, Collins JH, et al: Tityustoxin K alpha blocks voltage-gated noninactivating K channels and unblocks inactivating K channels blocked by alpha-dendrotoxin in synaptosomes. *Proc Natl Acad Sci USA* 91(4): 1475–1479, 1994.
47. Ignarro LJ, Burke TM, Wood KS, et al: Association between cyclic GMP accumulation and acetylcholine-elicited relaxation of bovine intrapulmonary artery. *J Pharmacol Exp Ther* 228:682–690, 1984.
48. Ignarro LJ, Byrns RE, Wood KS: Endothelium-dependent modulation of cGMP levels and intrinsic smooth muscle tone in isolated bovine intrapulmonary artery and vein. *Circ Res* 60:82–92, 1987.
49. Adnot S, Raffestin B, Eddahibi S, et al: Loss of endothelium-dependent relaxant activity in the pulmonary circulation of rats exposed to chronic hypoxia. *J Clin Invest* 87:155–162, 1991.
50. Russ RD, Walker BR: Maintained endothelium-dependent pulmonary vasodilation following chronic hypoxia in the rat. *J Appl Physiol* 74(1):339–344, 1993.
51. Hampl V, Cornfield D, Cowan N, et al: Hypoxia potentiates nitric oxide synthesis and transiently increases cytosolic calcium levels in pulmonary artery endothelial cells. *Eur Resp J* 8:515–522, 1995.
52. Higenbottam T, Pepke-Zaba J, Scott J, et al: Inhaled "endothelium-derived relaxing factor" in primary hypertension (PPH). *Am Rev Respir Dis* 137(suppl): 107–120, 1988.
53. Kinsella J, Neish S, Shaffer E, et al: Low dose inhalational nitric oxide in persistent pulmonary hypertension of the newborn. *Lancet* 340:819–820, 1992.
54. Roberts J, Polaner D, Lang P, et al: Inhaled nitric oxide in persistent pulmonary hypertension of the newborn. *Lancet* 340:818–819, 1992.
55. Rossaint R, Falke K, Lopez F, et al: Inhaled nitric oxide for the adult respiratory distress syndrome. *N Engl J Med* 328:399–405, 1993.
56. Wessel DL, Adatia I, Thompson JE, et al: Delivery and monitoring of inhaled nitric oxide in patients with pulmonary hypertension. *Crit Care Med* 22(6): 930–938, 1994.
57. Murad F, Arnold W, Mittal CK, et al: Properties and regulation of guanylate cyclase and some proposed functions for cyclic GMP. *Adv Cyclic Nucleotide Res* 11:175–204, 1979.
58. Murad F: Cyclic guanosine monophosphate as a mediator of vasodilatation. *J Clin Invest* 78:1–5, 1986.
59. Ignarro LJ, Buga GM, Byrns RE, et al: Endothelium-derived relaxing factor and nitric oxide possess identical pharmacologic properties as relaxants of bovine arterial and venous smooth muscle. *J Pharm Exp Ther* 246:218–226, 1988.
60. Suematsu E, Hirata M, Kuriyama H: Effects of cAMP- and c-GMP-dependent protein kinases, and calmodulin on Ca^{2+} uptake by highly purified sarcolemmal

vesicles of vascular smooth muscle. *Biochimica et Biophysica Acta* 773:83–90, 1984.

61. Raeymaekers L, Hofmann F, Casteels R: Cyclic GMP-dependent protein kinase phosphorylates phospholamban in isolated cardioplasmic reticulum from cardiac and smooth muscle. *Biochem J* 252:269–273, 1988.
62. Twort CHC, van Breemen C: Cyclic guanosine monophosphate-enhanced sequestration of Ca^{2+} by sarcoplasmic reticulum in vascular smooth muscle. *Circ Res* 62:961–964, 1988.
63. Furchgott RF: Role of the endothelium in the response of vascular smooth muscle to drugs. *Ann Rev Pharmacol* 24:175–197, 1984.
64. Johns A, Lategan TW, Lodge NJ, et al: Calcium entry through receptor operated channels in bovine pulmonary artery endothelial cells. *Tissue Cell* 19:733–745, 1987.
65. Adams DJ, Barakeh J, Laskey R, et al: Ion channels and regulation of intracellular calcium in vascular endothelial cells. *FASEB J* 3:2389–2400, 1989.
66. Tare M, Parkington H, Coleman H, et al: Hyperpolarization and relaxation of arterial smooth muscle caused by nitric oxide derived from the endothelium. *Nature* 346:69–71, 1990.
67. Garland JG, McPherson GA: Evidence that nitric oxide does not mediate the hyperpolarization and relaxation to acetylcholine in the rat small mesenteric artery. *Br J Pharmacol* 105:429–435, 1992.
68. Krippeit-Drews P, Morel N, Godfraind T: Effects of nitric oxide on membrane potential and contraction of rat aorta. *J Cardiovasc Pharmacol* 20(suppl): S72–S75, 1992.
69. Komori K, Lorenz RR, Vanhoutte PM: Nitric oxide, ACh, and electrical and mechanical properties of canine arterial smooth muscle. *Am J Physiol* 255: H207–H212, 1988.
70. Brayden JE: Membrane hyperpolarization is a mechanism of endothelium-dependent cerebral vasodilatation. *Am J Physiol* 259:H668–H673, 1990.
71. Kubo M, Nakaya Y, Matsuoka S, et al: Atrial natriuretic factor and isosorbide dinitrate modulate the gating of ATP-sensitive K channels in cultured vascular smooth muscle cells. *Circ Res* 74(3):471–476, 1994.
72. Murphy ME, Brayden JE: Nitric oxide hyperpolarizes rabbit mesenteric arteries via ATP-sensitive potassium channels. *J Physiol* 486:47–58, 1995.
73. Kauser K, Stekiel WJ, Rubanyi G, et al: Mechanism of action of EDRF on pressurized arteries: effect on K conductance. *Circ Res* 65(1):199–204, 1989.
74. Chen G, Yamamoto Y, Miwa K, et al: Hyperpolarization of arterial smooth muscle induced by endothelial humoral substances. *Am J Physiol* 260: H1888–H1892, 1991.
75. Tanaguchi J, Furukawa K-I, Shigekawa M: Maxi K channels are stimulated by cyclic guanosine monophosphate-dependent protein kinase in canine coronary artery smooth muscle cells. *Pflugers Arch* 423:167–172, 1993.
76. Robertson BE, Schubert R, Hescheler J, et al: cGMP-dependent protein kinase activates Ca-activated K channels in cerebral artery smooth muscle cells. *Am J Physiol* 265:C299-C303, 1993.
77. Khan SA, Mathews WR, Meisheri KD: Role of calcium-activated K channels in vasodilation induced by nitroglycerine, acetylcholine, and nitric oxide. *J Pharmacol Exp Ther* 267(3):1327–1335, 1993.
78. Miller WH: Physiological effects of cyclic GMP in the vertebrate retinal rod outer segment. *Adv Cyclic Nucleotide Res* 15:495–511, 1983.

79. Cornwell TL, Lincoln TM: Regulation of intracellular Ca^{2+} levels in cultured vascular smooth muscle cells: Reduction of Ca^{2+} by atriopeptin and 8-bromo-cyclic GMP is mediated by cyclic GMP-dependent protein kinase. *J Biol Chem* 264:1146–1155, 1989.
80. Lincoln TM, Cornwell TL: Intracellular cyclic GMP receptor proteins. *FASEB 7:* 328–338, 1993.
81. Thornbury K, Ward S, Dalziel H, et al: Nitric oxide and nitrosocysteine mimic nonadrenergic, noncholinergic hyperpolarization in canine proximal colon. *Am J Physiol* 261:G553–G557, 1991.
82. Bolotina VM, Najibi S, Pagano PJ, et al: Nitric oxide directly activates calcium-dependent potassium channels in vascular smooth muscle. *Nature* 368: 850–853, 1994.
83. Gruetter CA, Barry BK, McNamara DB, et al: Relaxation of bovine coronary artery and activation of coronary arterial guanylate cyclase by nitric oxide, nitro-prusside, and a carcinogenic nitrosoamine. *J Cycl Nucleo Res* 5:211–224, 1979.
84. Ignarro LJ, Harbison RG, Wood KS, et al: Activation of purified soluble guanylate cyclase by endothelium-derived relaxing factor from intrapulmonary artery and vein: Stimulation by acetycholine, bradykinin, and arachidonic acid. *J Pharmacol Exp Ther* 237:893–899, 1986.
85. Hyman AL, Kadowitz PJ, Lippton HL: Methylene blue selectively inhibits pulmonary vasodilator responses in cats. *J Appl Physiol* 66:1513–1517, 1989.
86. Ashizawa N: Relaxing action of okidaic acid, a black sponge toxin on arterial smooth muscle. *Biochem Biophys Res Comm* 162:971–976, 1989.
87. Hislop A, Reid LM: Formation of the pulmonary vasculature. In: Hodson WA (ed). *Development of the Lung*. New York: Marcel Dekker; 37–86, 1977.
88. Michelakis E, Reeves HL, Weir EK, et al: Diversity of potassium channels in vascular smooth muscle cells. *Can Physiol J* 75(7):889–897, 1997.
89. Sheng M, Tsaur ML, Jan YN, et al: Contrasting subcellular localization of the Kv1.2 K channel subunit in different neurons of rat brain. *J Neurosci* 14(4): 2408–2417, 1994.

Chapter 19

Calcium Channels, Cytosolic Calcium, and the Vasomotor Responses to Hypoxia

Alfredo Franco-Obregón
Juan Ureña
Tarik Smani
Satoru Iwabuchi
José López-Barneo

Introduction

The regional distribution of circulation in the body is determined in part by local variations in blood oxygen tension.[1] As is characteristic of most systemic vascular beds, the main trunk and larger branches of the pulmonary artery vasodilate in response to hypoxia. By contrast, the more distal resistance branches of the pulmonary artery vasoconstrict in response to low alveolar oxygen tension (Po_2) (Figure 1). The differential responses of the systemic and pulmonary vasculatures to low Po_2 subserve distinct physiologic roles. In the systemic vasculature, regional hypoxia acts to increase the perfusion of blood to oxygen-deprived tissues of the body. However, the combined pulmonary responses favor the diversion of blood toward the better ventilated alveolar regions. Despite

---

From: López-Barneo, J and Weir, EK: *Oxygen Regulation of Ion Channels and Gene Expression.* Armonk, NY: Futura Publishing Company, Inc., ©1998.

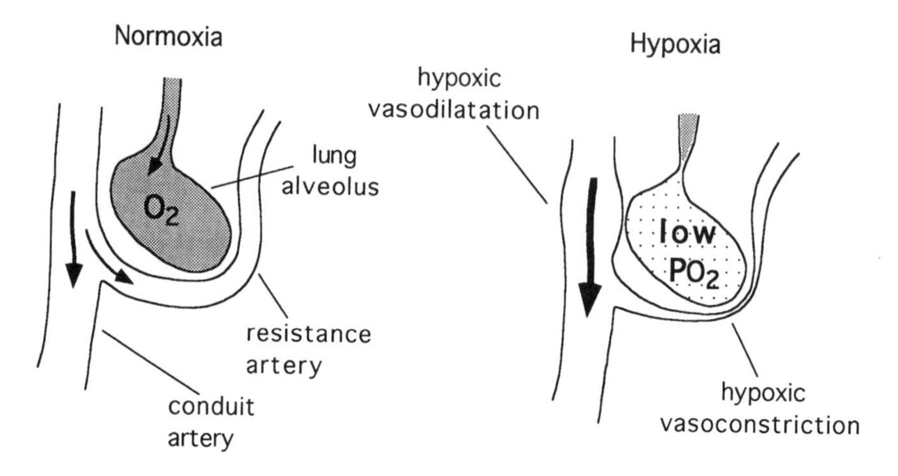

Figure 1 Schematic representation of the distinct vasomotor responses to hypoxia in the pulmonary arterial tree.

their physiologic and clinical importance, the mechanisms underlying the hypoxia-induced changes in arterial tone remain largely obscure due to complex interactions between the endothelium and the arterial smooth muscle layer in the development of these responses.

In addition to blood Po_2, local arterial resistance is also exquisitely sensitive to endothelium-derived vasoactive factors which exert their physiologic effects in the smooth muscle layer of arteries.[2,3] Both endothelium-derived relaxing (EDRFs) and constricting (EDCFs) factors have been described. The best characterized EDRF is nitric oxide (NO) which causes smooth muscle relaxation.[4] Analogously, endothelin-1, the most potent EDCF known, increases arterial smooth muscle tone.[5,6] Recently, NO has been shown to inhibit the production of endothelin-1,[2] whereas endothelin-1 positively influences the synthesis of NO. Possibly due to these complex feedback interactions, transgenic mice deficient in either endothelial NO synthase[7] or endothelin-1[8] are hypertensive at birth.

Understandably, much attention has been paid to the possible modulation of the endothelium-derived vasoactive factors by blood Po_2.[9] However, despite these efforts, there remains some uncertainty regarding the role of endothelium-derived factors in the oxygen-dependent vasomotor responses, since none of these factors have been demonstrated to be indispensable for the elaboration of the vasomotor responses to hypoxia.[3,9] Alternatively, arterial smooth muscle cells may be directly responsive to changes in blood Po_2. In support of this second hypothesis, hypoxic vasomotor responses can be partially recapitulated in arterial samples denuded of the endothelium,[10,11] as well as in isolated arterial smooth muscle cells,[12] suggesting that the endothelium plays a modulatory, rather than obligatory, role in the manifestations of the vasomotor responses to low PO_2. Moreover, any mechanism(s) responsible for setting arterial tone, regardless of whether dependent on endothelium-derived vasoactive factors or inherent to the smooth muscle cell itself, must first impinge on the modulation of cytosolic calcium Ca^{2+} concentration in vascular smooth muscle which, in turn, determines the state of smooth muscle contraction.[13] Here, we examine the evidence supporting a role for oxygen-regulated Ca^{2+} channels of the smooth muscle cell membrane in the elaboration of the vasomotor responses to hypoxia.

Ion Channels in Smooth Muscle Cells and the Regulation of Arterial Tone

The modulation of ion channel activity as a determinant step in the transduction process is a key feature of most models proposed to explain vasomotor responses.[14] In this respect, both Ca^{2+} and potassium K^+ channel classes have been implicated in the regulation of arterial tone.[15,16] Many vasoactive stimuli seem to exert their effects through modifications of transmembrane Ca^{2+} entry into arterial smooth muscle cells either directly, by modulating the activity of voltage-gated Ca^{2+} channels, or indirectly, by altering the activity of K^+ channels that regulate the smooth muscle cell resting potential.[15] For example, the relationship between membrane potential and force generation closely matches the voltage dependence of L-type Ca^{2+} channel opening.[17] In addition, the activity of L-type Ca^{2+} channels has been demonstrated near the resting membrane potential of vascular smooth muscle cells (-30 to -50 mV).[18] A role for K^+ channels in the maintenance of arterial tone is supported by pharmacologic studies demonstrating that blocking the activity of either Ca^{2+}-activated K^+ channels[19] or delayed rectifier K^+ channels[20] induces vasoconstriction. Adenosine triphosphate (ATP)-sensitive, K^+ (K_{ATP}) channels have also been implicated in the maintenance of arterial tone. Depression in cellular metabolism due to ischemia or hypoxemia can trigger K_{ATP} channel activity, which causes smooth muscle cell hyperpolarization, vasorelaxation, and the increased perfusion of metabolically active regions of the body. Agents that augment the activity of K_{ATP} channels also induce vasorelaxation.[16] Thus, the modulation of Ca^{2+} and K^+ channel classes present in the smooth muscle cell membrane is a strategy commonly used in the regulation of arterial tone.

Oxygen Sensing by Ion Channels and the Vasomotor Responses to Hypoxia.

An obvious possibility to explain the vasomotor responses to changes in blood oxygenation is that P_{O_2} regulates the activity of ion channel classes already known to be involved in the maintenance of arterial tone.[14] Initially, such studies were conducted in dispersed pulmonary arterial smooth muscle cells, away from the influence of the endothelium. In pulmonary arterial myocytes, the activity of both delayed rectifier[20–22] and Ca^{2+}-activated[23] K^+ currents is attenuated by a reduction in P_{O_2}, which is consistent with the appearance of hypoxic pulmonary vasoconstriction (HPV) (see Chapters 16–18). No effect of hypoxia has been observed in the K^+ currents of smooth muscle cells isolated from the renal[23] and mesenteric[21] systemic arteries. In regards to systemic arteries, there are several pharmacologic studies suggesting that hypoxic dilatation in the coronary circulation may be mediated by the opening of K_{ATP} channels (see Chapter 20).[24,25] Moreover, it has been recently shown in dispersed coronary myocytes that prolonged hypoxic exposures (>2 minutes) induce K_{ATP} channel activity.[26] However, it is plausible to propose that other mechanisms, apart from the regulation of K_{ATP} channel activity, must still exist to explain the effects of low P_{O_2} since the sensitivity to hypoxia in most arteries occurs rapidly without a compromise of energy metabolism (see below).

Contrasting Effects of Hypoxia on the Cytosolic Ca^{2+} Concentration of Conduit and Resistance Pulmonary Myocytes

We have studied whether cytosolic Ca^{2+} concentration is modulated by ambient oxygen tension in such a way as to account for the opposed responses of the pulmonary artery to hypoxia (see above and Figure 1). The initial observations came from microfluorimetric studies in freshly dispersed pulmonary arterial smooth muscle cells isolated from the main trunk (conduit myocytes) and the fine branches (resistance myocytes) of the pulmonary arterial tree. Measurements of cytosolic Ca^{2+} in both conduit (Figure 2A) and resistance (Figure 2B) pulmonary myocytes reveal the existence of oscillations of cytosolic Ca^{2+} or Ca^{2+} spikes,[27] much like those previously described in a variety of cell types.[28] As in other classes of vascular smooth muscle cells, the Ca^{2+} spikes are modulated by extracellular Ca^{2+} as they are reversibly abolished, or their frequency decreased, following the removal of extracellular Ca^{2+} from the bathing medium.[27–30] The Ca^{2+} spikes in some conduit and resistance pulmonary myocytes are also modulated by changes in bathing Po_2, although in diametrically opposed manners.[27] In the majority of conduit myocytes, a reduction in bathing Po_2 induces a drop in basal cytosolic Ca^{2+} concentration ($[Ca^{2+}]_i$) and a decrease, or complete supression, of the Ca^{2+} spike frequency. These changes are generally associated with an increase in Ca^{2+} spike amplitude (Figure 2A, top). This response to hypoxia is also seen in some resistance myocytes. However, in more than 50% of the resistance myocytes, low Po_2 induces the opposite response: increase in basal $[Ca^{2+}]_i$ accompanied by a decrement in Ca^{2+} spike amplitude (Figure 2B, top). This latter hypoxic response, only observed in resistance myocytes, resembles the common effect of membrane depolarization on the Ca^{2+} spikes observed in all vascular myocytes classes thus far examined by the authors,[27,30] and probably arises as a consequence of voltage-dependent Ca^{2+} entry. In accord with this idea, the decrement in basal $[Ca^{2+}]_i$ observed in conduit myoyctes in response to a drop in Po_2 can be counteracted with elevated extracellular K^+, suggesting that low Po_2 is attenuating voltage-dependent Ca^{2+} entry (Figure 2A, bottom). However, the increment in basal $[Ca^{2+}]_i$ observed in resistance myocytes can be reversibly counteracted by selectively blocking the activity of L-type Ca^{2+} channels with nifedipine (0.5 μM) (Figure 2B, bottom). These results strongly suggest that low Po_2 modulates the activity of L-type Ca^{2+} channels in diametrically opposed manners in different regions of the pulmonary arterial tree, such that, hypoxia would inhibit Ca^{2+} channels in myocytes of conduit arteries, but potentiate Ca^{2+} channel activity in a subpopulation of resistance myocytes. These results also agree with previous work showing that the development of HPV in the distal regions of the pulmonary artery[31] can be either inhibited[32] or enhanced[33] with L-type Ca^{2+} channel antagonist or agonist, respectively.

Hypoxia appears to specifically modulate extracellular Ca^{2+} entry through voltage-gated Ca^{2+} channels since the liberation of sequestered Ca^{2+} from intracellular pools, seems to be unaffected by low Po_2. The effect of hypoxia on Ca^{2+} release has been studied in cells exposed to norepinephrine (NE) which is known to evoke release of Ca^{2+} from intracellular pools[28] as well as to promote the influx of extracellular Ca^{2+} through L-type Ca^{2+} channels.[17] Figure 2C (left) illustrates the typical response of a myocyte to NE demonstrating the component due to release from the internal stores (fast transient spike) and the one attributed to transmembrane Ca^{2+} entry (arrow). Figure 2C (right) shows that hypoxia reversibly attenuates the component of the response mediated by transmembrane Ca^{2+} entry (arrow) without influencing the liberation of Ca^{2+}

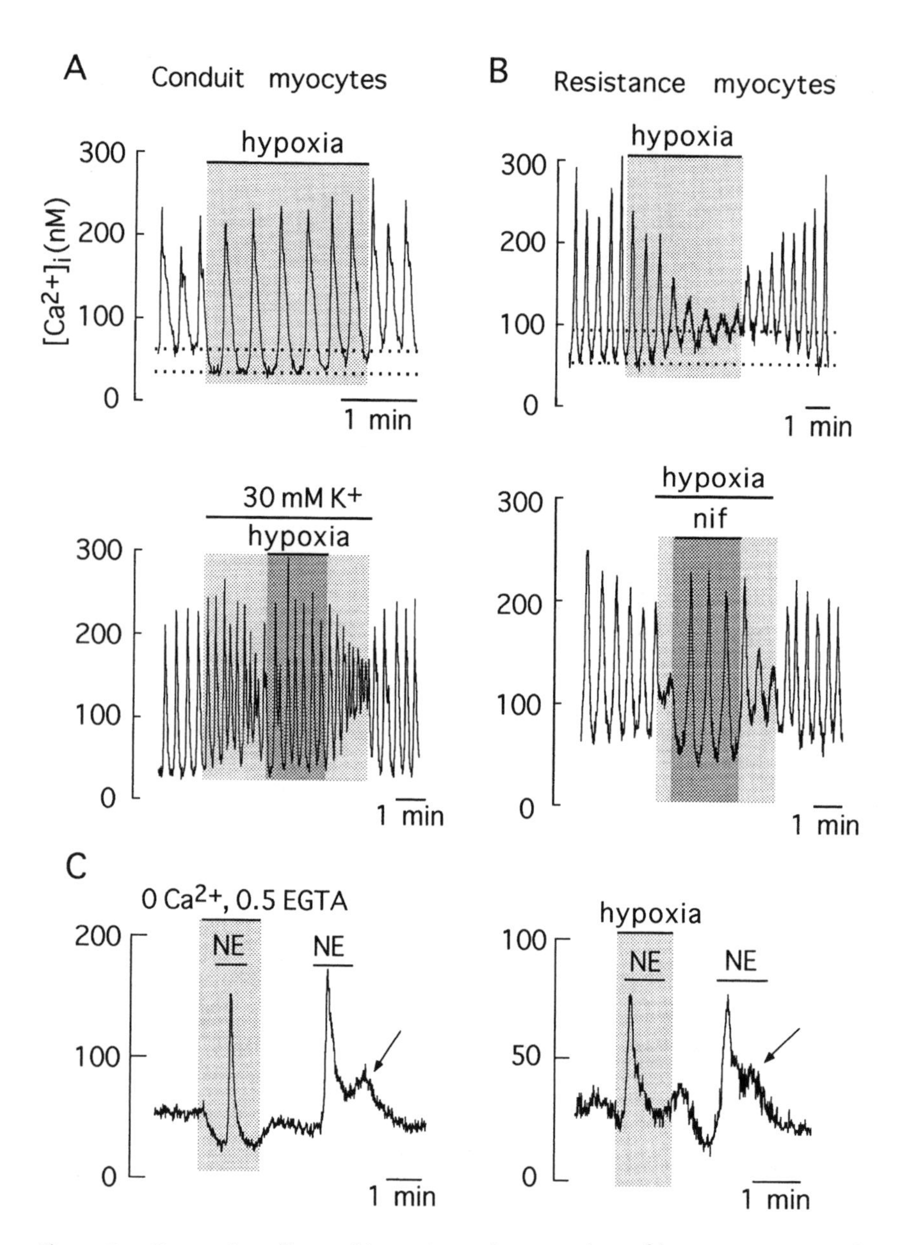

Figure 2. Contrasting effects of hypoxia on the cytosolic Ca^{2+} concentration and Ca^{2+} oscillations (Ca^{2+} spikes) in conduit and resistance pulmonary myocytes. **A.** Recordings from a representative conduit myocyte. **Top**. Reduction of basal Ca^{2+} levels (**dotted lines**) and the frequency of the oscillations by low Po_2 in a representative conduit myocyte. **Bottom**. Increase of basal Ca^{2+} and the frequency of the

from intracellular pools. The distinct effects of hypoxia on Ca^{2+} spike amplitude in conduit (amplitude increase) and resistance (amplitude decrease) pulmonary myocytes most likely reflect the bell-shaped dependence on $[Ca^{2+}]_i$ of the sarcoplasmic reticulum Ca^{2+} release channel.[28,34] Through such a mechanism, Ca^{2+} release would be potentiated at low basal $[Ca^{2+}]_i$ and inhibited at elevated basal $[Ca^{2+}]_i$. Therefore, it appears that low Po_2 is exerting its dual effect on $[Ca^{2+}]_i$ by selectively modulating extracellular Ca^{2+} influx without directly altering the release of Ca^{2+} from intracellular reservoirs. Reuptake of Ca^{2+} from previously depleted stores is also unaffected by low Po_2.[30]

Blockade of K_{ATP} Channels Does not Alter the Hypoxia-Induced Reduction of Cytosolic Ca^{2+} Concentration

Since K_{ATP} channels have also been broadly implicated in the control of arterial resistance,[16] we have studied whether blockade of this channel type can prevent the hypoxia-induced reduction of cytosolic Ca^{2+} concentration. We used glibenclamide (up to 10 μM) in these experiments as a potent blocker of K_{ATP} channels in vascular smooth muscle. Figure 3A shows that glibenclamide neither influenced spike generation nor precluded spike inhibition by low Po_2, indicating that these phenomena are independent of K_{ATP} channel activity. Furthermore, Figure 3B shows that low Po_2 could counteract the effects of membrane depolarization due to the exposure to high external K^+, even in the presence of glibenclamide.[35] Therefore, blocking the activity of K_{ATP} channels apparently has little influence over the hypoxic modulation of voltage-dependent Ca^{2+} channels in arterial myocytes. It is, therefore, likely that the activity of K_{ATP} and

Figure 2. *(continued)* oscillations by high external K^+. The effect of K^+ is counteracted by hypoxia. **B.** Recordings from a representative resistance myocyte. **Top**. Increase of basal Ca^{2+} (**dotted lines**) and reduction of the Ca^{2+} spikes amplitude during exposure to hypoxia. **Bottom**. The effect of hypoxia is counteracted by blockade of L-type Ca^{2+} channels with nifedipine (0.5 μM). **C.** Transmembrane Ca^{2+} influx and Ca^{2+} release induced by norepinephrine (NE, 3 μM) in a conduit pulmonary myocyte. Note on the **left panel** how the component due to Ca^{2+} entry (**arrow**) is abolished in the absence of external Ca^{2+} (0 mM Ca^{2+} and 0.5 mM EGTA added to the external solution). The **right panel** illustates the lack of effect of hypoxia on Ca^{2+} release from internal stores and the abolition of transmembrane Ca^{2+} influx in a celiac myocyte. The Po_2 of the solutions were approximately 150 (normoxia) and 20 to 30 (hypoxia) mm Hg. (Modified with permission from References 27, 30, 37.)

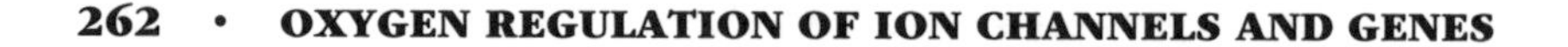

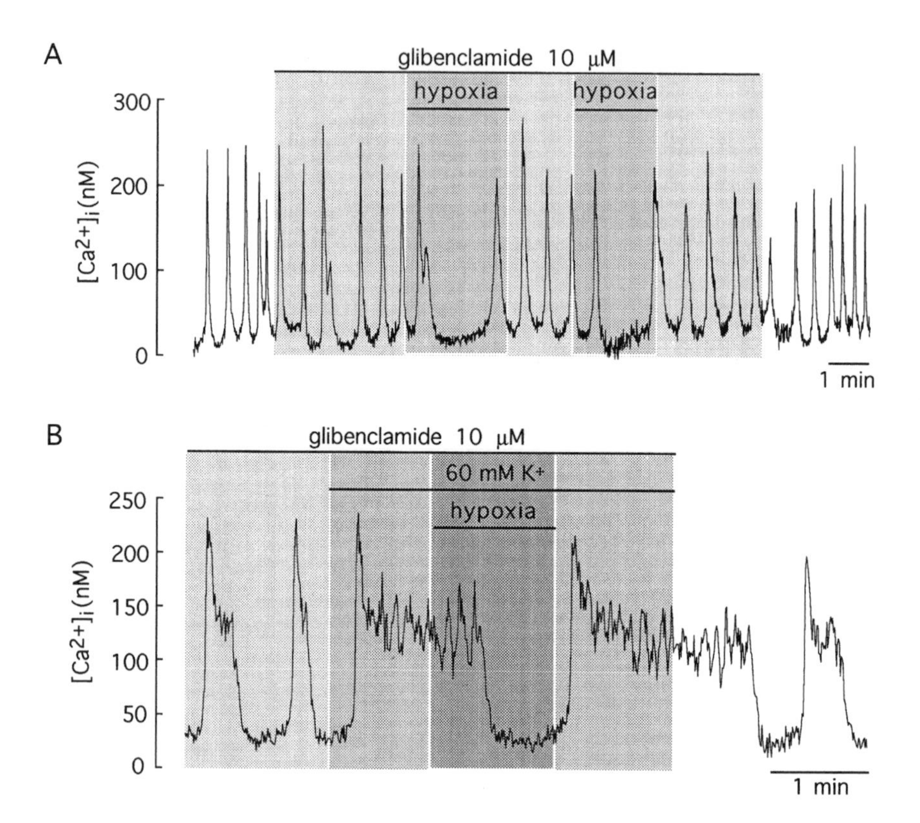

Figure 3. The activity of K_{ATP} channels does not appear to mediate the effect of hypoxia on the cytosolic Ca^{2+} concentration and Ca^{2+} spikes in conduit pulmonary myocytes. **A.** Typical responses to hypoxia (reduction in basal Ca^{2+} and in spike frequency) in a myocyte exposed to an external solution with glibenclamide added to block the activity of K_{ATP} channels. **B.** Hypoxia counteracts the effect of high external K^+ in the presence of glibenclamide. The application of the different test solutions is indicated by the **bars** and the **shaded regions**.

voltage-dependent Ca^{2+} channels are recruited into the hypoxic vasomotor response under distinct physiologic circumstances.

Differential Oxygen Sensitivity of Ca^{2+} Channels of Conduit and Resistance Pulmonary Myocytes

To ascertain whether the differential hypoxic modulation of $[Ca^{2+}]_i$ in pulmonary myocytes is mediated by distinct regulatory modes of L-type Ca^{2+} channels, we examined the macroscopic Ca^{2+} currents of conduit and resistance myocytes under conditions of normoxia and hypoxia. Figure 4A (top) shows a family of Ca^{2+} currents recorded from a conduit myocyte at the indicated membrane potentials. The current traces obtained in normoxia (before hypoxia [n], and following recovery [r]) are compared with those recorded during hypoxia (h). Consistent with the inhibitory effect of low Po_2 on $[Ca^{2+}]_i$, hypoxia strongly attenuates the whole-cell Ca^{2+} current at negative membrane potentials.[35] However, at membrane potentials more positive than +20 mV, hypoxia exhibited little effect. In direct opposition to this response characteristic of conduit myocytes, hypoxia reversibly potentiates the Ca^{2+} current at negative membrane potentials in many resistance myocytes (Figure 4A, bottom). At strongly depolarized membrane potentials, hypoxia inhibits the Ca^{2+} current of pulmonary resistance myocytes. A summary of the voltage dependence of the hypoxic modulation of the Ca^{2+} currents in the population of pulmonary myocytes studied is shown in Figure 4B. It thus appears that near the resting potential, hypoxia can have a dual effect either inhibiting or augmenting the influx of extracellular Ca^{2+} into conduit (solid diamonds) and resistance (solid circles) myocytes, respectively. The mechanism of the differential regulation of Ca^{2+} channels by low Po_2 is for the moment unknown, although it could be related to the dual redox modulation of L-type Ca^{2+} channels reported to occur in ventricular myocytes.[36] Conduit and resistance myocytes seem to express a pharmacologically homogeneous population of L-type Ca^{2+} channels, but the density of the channels in resistance myocytes is about two times higher than in conduit myocytes[37] (see below). Therefore, it seems that the properties of myocytes change along the pulmonary arterial tree, possibly to subserve different functional roles. The existence of smooth muscle cell diversity in the pulmonary artery has been reported in regards to their morphological phenotype,[38,39] as well as the type of K^+ channels present in their plasmalemma.[20]

Oxygen Sensing by Ca^{2+} Channels and the Systemic and Pulmonary Vasomotor Responses to Hypoxia

Generally speaking, both conduit pulmonary, as well as systemic, arteries vasodilate in response to regional hypoxia.[1] We have previously shown that in systemic myocytes, hypoxia modulates $[Ca^{2+}]_i$ in a manner that closely resembles that previously demonstrated in conduit myocytes.[30] In agreement with their equivalent vasomotor responses to hypoxia, the effect of low Po_2 on the Ca^{2+} current of systemic myocytes is

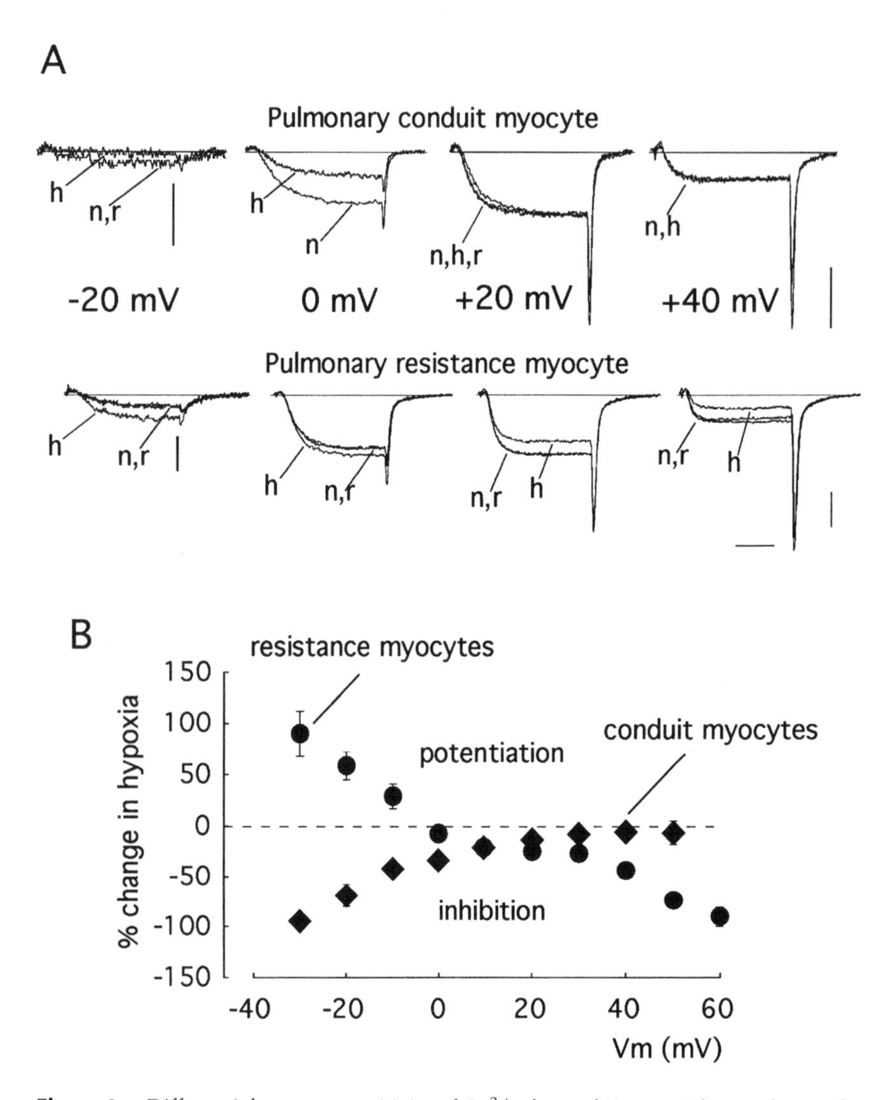

Figure 4. Differential oxygen sensitivity of Ca^{2+} channels in arterial smooth muscle cells isolated from conduit and resistance regions of the pulmonary arterial tree. **A.** Current traces demonstrating the differential effects of hypoxia (**h**) on the calcium currents elicited by voltage pulses to −20, 0, +20, and +40 mV (holding potential = −80 mV) in a conduit and resistance pulmonary arterial myocyte. Control (**n**) and recovery (**r**) traces are shown superimposed. **Vertical scale bars** represent 200 pA (trace at −20 mV) and 400 pA (traces at 0, +20, and +40 mV). **Horizontal scale bar** corresponds to 5 ms and applies to all traces. **B.** Summary of the voltage-dependent modulation of current amplitude by hypoxia. Percentage of the change in current amplitude in hypoxia (negative representing inhibition and positive poten-

similar to that of conduit pulmonary myocytes (Figure 5A).[30,35,37] The whole-cell Ca^{2+} current of systemic myocytes is reversibly attenuated by low P_{O_2} with a voltage dependence similar to that observed in pulmonary conduit myocytes. A summary of this voltage dependence is shown in Figure 5B, which is a plot made with the combined data obtained from celiac, femoral, cerebral, and coronary myocytes.[35] The effect of P_{O_2} appears to be selective for the L-type Ca^{2+} current, since the macroscopic Ca^{2+} current of vascular smooth muscle cells is almost completely blocked with low concentrations of nifedipine and is similar in magnitude to the current inhibition observed with hypoxia.[35] Interestingly, in all myocyte classes studied (systemic, conduit pulmonary, and resistance pulmonary), the position along the voltage axis of the current-voltage relationships are similar (Figure 5C). However, the average peak current amplitude is greater in resistance pulmonary myocytes than in conduit pulmonary or systemic myocytes (Figure 5C). Mean Ca^{2+} current density (in pA/pF) is also greatest in pulmonary myocytes of resistance branches (~21), when compared to either conduit (~13) or systemic myocytes (~5) (Figure 5D).[35,37] Archer et al[20] recently reported that pulmonary myocytes from resistance branches also possess a higher density of oxygen-sensitive delayed rectifier K^+ channels than conduit myocytes. Therefore, the potent hypoxic potentiation of the Ca^{2+} current in resistance myocytes may act in conjunction with the inhibition of the K^+ conductance in response to hypoxia to produce HPV.

The opposed voltage dependence of the Ca^{2+} current modulation by hypoxia in conduit and resistance pulmonary myocytes is consistent with the contrasting hypoxic-vasomotor responses of these same arterial segments. In this respect, the modulation of Ca^{2+} channel activity by P_{O_2} may represent a unifying mechanism contributing to both the hypoxic vasoconstriction and vasorelaxation of the distinct arterial segments. The effect of hypoxia is rapid and reversible, since both inhibition and recovery of the current are observed within seconds of changing P_{O_2}. Furthermore, the modulation of the Ca^{2+} current by P_{O_2} typically becomes appreciable at values below ~80 mm Hg,[35] near the range of P_{O_2} values previously described to cause vasodilation in intact perfused organs (~40 mm Hg).[1] The oxygen-regulated Ca^{2+} channels described here are, therefore, more sensitive to rapid changes in P_{O_2} than the K_{ATP} channels previously shown

Figure 4. *(continued)* tiation) expressed as a function of membrane potential. Data pooled from 8 pulmonary conduit (**solid diamonds**) and 19 pulmonary resistance (**solid circles**) myocytes. The data are represented as mean ± standard error. (Adapted with permission from References 35 and 37.)

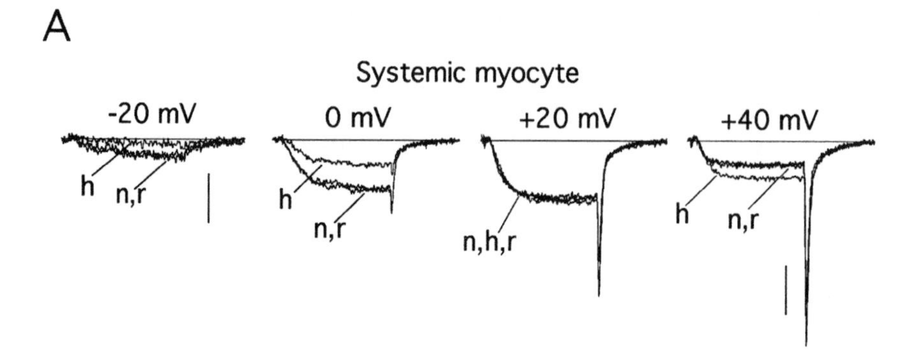

Figure 5. Oxygen sensitivity of Ca^{2+} channels in systemic arterial smooth muscle cells. **A.** Recordings demonstrating the effect of hypoxia (**h**) on the calcium currents elicited by voltage pulses to −20, 0, +20, and +40 mV (holding potential = −80 mV) in a celiac arterial myocyte. Control (**n**) and recovery (**r**) traces are shown superimposed. **Vertical scale bars** represent 100 pA (trace at −20 mV) and 200 pA (traces at 0, +20, and +40 mV). Pulse duration was 15 ms. (Adapted with permission from References 35 and 37.)

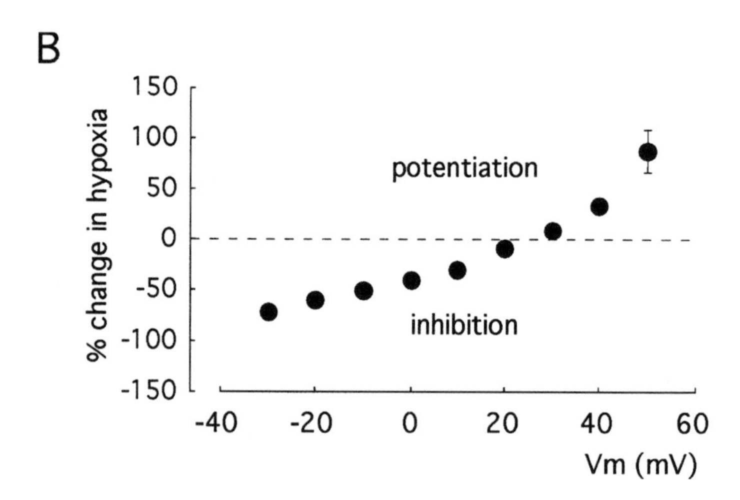

Figure 5. *(continued)* **B.** Summary of the voltage-dependent modulation of current amplitude by hypoxia. Percentage of the change in current amplitude in hypoxia (negative representing inhibition and positive potentiation) expressed as a function of membrane potential. Data pooled from 17 systemic myocytes. The data are represented as mean ± standard error. (Adapted with permission from References 35 and 37.)

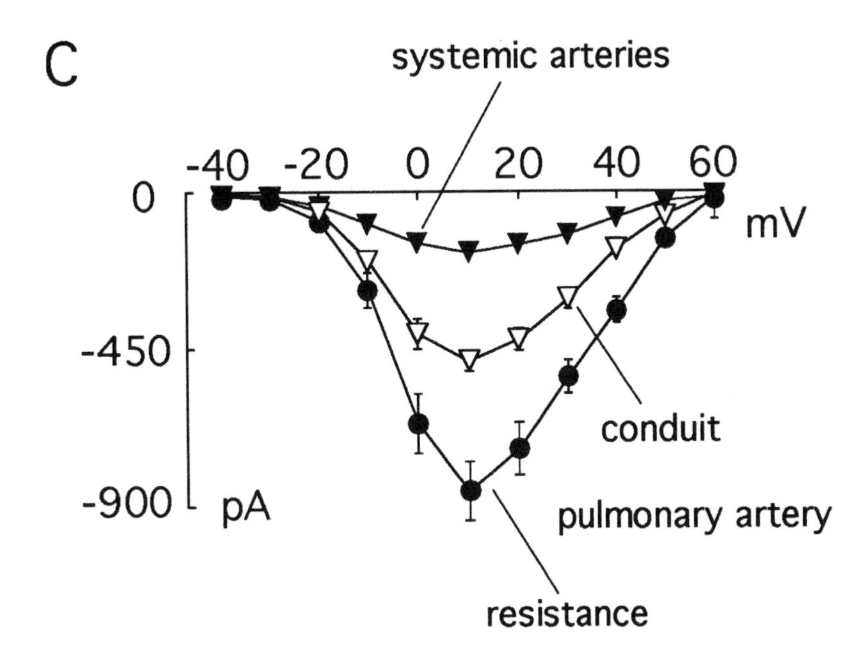

Figure 5. *(continued)* **C.** Mean current-voltage relationships for systemic, pulmonary conduit, and pulmonary resistance myocytes. (Adapted with permission from References 35 and 37.)

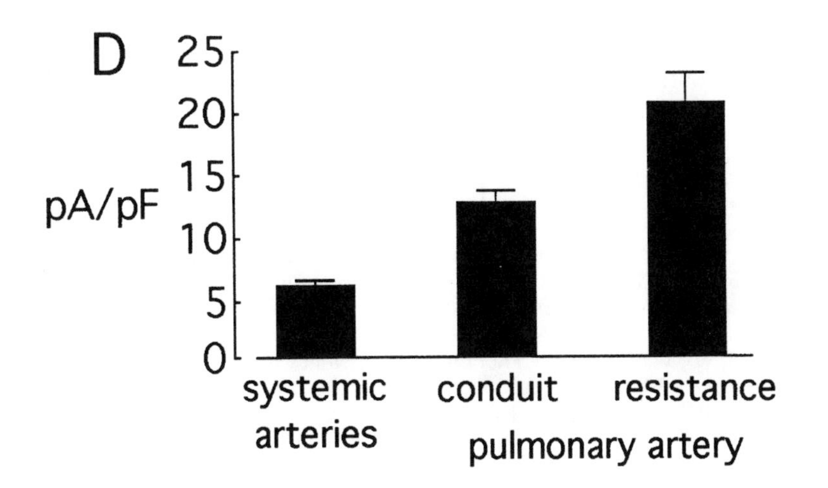

Figure 5. *(continued)* **D.** Mean current density in the different myocyte classes as indicated. (Adapted with permission from References 35 and 37.)

to be involved in the dilatation of the coronary circulation in response to hypoxia.[26] Since it is well established that cytosolic Ca^{2+} is the variable that determines smooth muscle contractility,[13] and that L-type Ca^{2+} channels are major regulators of smooth muscle tension, as well as the target of vasoactive agents,[15] it is reasonable to presume that oxygen-regulated Ca^{2+} channels, in conjunction with other channel types and cellular mechanisms, contribute directly to the regulation of cytosolic Ca^{2+} levels and, hence, arterial tone.

In conclusion, several experimental observations suggest that oxygen interacts directly with the channel moiety to confer oxygen sensitivity. Since the effect of oxygen on the Ca^{2+} channels is rapid and unaffected following intracellular dialysis with agents which irreversibly activate G-proteins,[37] it appears that hypoxia acts via a membrane delimited mechanism without the involvement of soluble cytosolic mediators.[14] The identification of the molecular domains conferring oxygen sensitivity to L-type Ca^{2+} channels would motivate the development of pharmacologic agents to be used in treatment of pulmonary and systemic hypertension.

Acknowledgments

This work was supported with grants from the Dirección General de Investigación Científica y Técnica (DGICYT) of the Spanish Ministry of Science and Education, the Andalusian Government, and the European Community (DGXII). During the tenure of this work Dr. Alfredo Franco-Obregón was funded by Postdoctoral Fellowships of the International Human Frontiers Science Program (1993–1995) and the National Science Foundation—North Atlantic Treaty Organization (1996).

References

1. Sparks H: Effect of local metabolic factors on vascular smooth muscle. In: Bohr DF, Somlyo AP, Sparks HV (eds): *Handbook of Physiology. The Cardiovascular System. II. Vascular Smooth Muscle.* Bethesda, MD: American Physiology Society; 475–513, 1980.
2. Schini VB, Vanhoutte PM: Endothelin-1: a potent vasoactive peptide. *Pharmacol Toxicol* 69:303–309, 1991.
3. Ward JPT, Robertson TP: The role of the endothelium in hypoxic pulmonary vasoconstriction. *Exp Physiol* 80:793–801, 1995.
4. Umans JG, Levi R: Nitric oxide in the regulation of blood flow and arterial pressure. *Annu Rev Physiol* 57:771–790, 1995.
5. Yanagisawa M, Kurihara H, Kimura S, et al: A novel potent vasoconstrictor peptide produced by vascular endothelial cells. *Nature* 332:411–415, 1988.
6. Yoshida M, Suzuki A, Itoh T: Mechanisms of vasoconstriction induced by endo-

thelin-1 in smooth muscle of rabbit mesenteric artery. *J Physiol* 477:253–265, 1994.
7. Huang PL, Huang Z, Mashimo H, et al: Hypertension in mice lacking the gene for endothelial nitric oxide synthase. *Nature* 377:239–242, 1995.
8. Kurihara Y, Kurihara H, Suzuki H, et al: Elevated blood pressure and craniofacial abnormalities in mice deficient in endothelin-1. *Nature* 368:703–710, 1994.
9. Wadsworth RM: Vasoconstriction and vasodilator effects of hypoxia. *Trends Pharmacol Sci* 15:47–53, 1994.
10. Leach RM, Robertson TP, Twort CHC, et al: Hypoxic vasoconstriction in rat pulmonary and mesenteric arteries. *Am J Physiol* 266:L223-L231, 1994.
11. Yuan X, Tod ML, Rubin LJ, et al: Contrasting effects of hypoxia on tension in rat pulmonary and mesenteric arteries. *Am J Physiol* 259:H281-H289, 1990.
12. Madden JA, Vadula MS, Kurup VP: Effects of hypoxia and other vasoactive agents on pulmonary and cerebral artery smooth muscle cells. *Am J Physiol* 263:L384-L393, 1992.
13. van Breemen C, Saida K: Cellular mechanisms regulating $[Ca^{2+}]_i$ in smooth muscle. *Annu Rev Physiol* 51:315–329, 1989.
14. López-Barneo J: Oxygen-sensing by ion channels and the regulation of cellular functions. *Trends Neurosci* 19:435–440, 1996.
15. Nelson MT, Patlak JB, Worley JF, et al: Calcium channels, potassium channels and voltage-dependence of arterial smooth muscle tone. *Am J Physiol* 259:C3-C18, 1990.
16. Nelson MT, Quayle JM: Physiological roles and properties of potassium channels in arterial smooth muscle. *Am J Physiol* 268:C799-C822, 1995.
17. Nelson MT, Standen NB, Brayden JE, et al: Noradrenaline contracts arteries by activating voltage-dependent calcium channels. *Nature* 336:382–385, 1988.
18. Langston PD, Standen NB: Calcium currents elicited by voltage steps and steady voltages in myocytes isolated from the rat basilar artery. *J Physiol* 469:535–548, 1993.
19. Nelson MT, Cheng H, Rubart M, et al: Relaxation of arterial smooth muscle by calcium sparks. *Science* 270:633–637, 1995.
20. Archer SL, Huang JMC, Reeve HL, et al: Differential distribution of electrophysiologically distinct myocytes in conduit and resistance arteries determines their response to nitric oxide and hypoxia. *Circ Res* 78:431–442, 1996.
21. Yuan X, Goldman WF, Tod ML, et al: Hypoxia reduces potassium currents in cultured rat pulmonary but not mesenteric arterial myocytes. *Am J Physiol* 264: L116-L123, 1993.
22. Post JM, Gelband CH, Hume JR: $[Ca^{2+}]_i$ inhibition of K^+ channels in canine pulmonary artery: novel mechanism for hypoxic-induced membrane depolarization. *Circ Res* 77:131–139, 1995.
23. Post JM, Hume JR, Archer SL, et al: Direct role for potassium channel inhibition in hypoxic pulmonary vasoconstriction. *Am J Physiol* 262:C882-C890, 1992.
24. Daut J, Maier-Rudolph W, von Beckerath N, et al: Hypoxic dilation of coronary arteries is mediated by ATP-sensitive potassium channels. *Science* 247: 1341–1344, 1990.
25. von Beckerath N, Sabine C, Dischner A, et al: Hypoxic vasodilatation in isolated, perfused Guinea-pig heart: an analysis of the underlying mechanisms. *J Physiol* 442:297–319, 1991.
26. Dart C, Standen NB: Activation of ATP-dependent K^+ channels by hypoxia in

smooth muscle cells isolated from the pig coronary artery. *J Physiol* 483:29–39, 1995.
27. Ureña J, Franco-Obregón A, López-Barneo J: Contrasting effects of hypoxia on cytosolic Ca^{2+} spikes in conduit and resistance myocytes of the rabbit pulmonary artery. *J Physiol* 496:103–109, 1996.
28. Berridge MJ: Inositol trisphosphate and calcium signalling. *Nature* 361:315–325, 1993.
29. Blatter LA, Wier WG: Agonist-induced $[Ca^{2+}]_i$ waves and Ca^{2+}-induced Ca^{2+} release in mammalian vascular smooth muscle cells. *Am J Physiol* 263:H576-H586, 1992.
30. Franco-Obregón A, Ureña J, López-Barneo J: Oxygen-sensitive calcium channels in vascular smooth muscle and their possible role in hypoxic arterial relaxation. *Proc Natl Acad Sci USA* 92:4715–4719, 1995.
31. Weir EK, Archer SL: The mechanism of acute hypoxic pulmonary vasoconstriction: the tale of two channels. *FASEB J* 9:183–189, 1995.
32. McMurtry I, Davidson B, Reeves J, et al: Inhibition of hypoxic pulmonary vasoconstriction by calcium antagonists in isolated rat lungs. *Circ Res* 38:99–104, 1976.
33. McMurtry I: Bay K8644 potentiates and A23187 inhibits hypoxic vasoconstriction in rat lungs. *Am J Physiol* 249:H741-H746, 1985.
34. Bezprozvanny I, Watras J, Ehrlich BE: Bell-shaped calcium-response curves of Ins(1,4,5)P_3- and calcium-gated channels from endoplasmic reticulum of cerebellum. *Nature* 351:751–754, 1991.
35. Franco-Obregón A, López-Barneo J: Low Po_2 inhibits calcium channel activity in arterial smooth muscle cells. *Am J Physiol* 271:H2290-H2299, 1996.
36. Campbell DL, Stamler JS, Strauss HC: Redox modulation of L-type calcium channels in ferret ventricular myocytes. *J Gen Physiol* 108:277–293, 1996.
37. Franco-Obregón A, López-Barneo J: Differential oxygen sensitivity of calcium channels in rabbit smooth muscle cells of conduit and resistance pulmonary arteries. *J Physiol* 491:511–518, 1996.
38. Frid MG, Moiseeva EP, Stenmark KR: Multiple phenotypically distinct smooth muscle cell populations exist in the adult and developing bovine pulmonary arterial media in vivo. *Circ Res* 75:669–681, 1994.
39. Whorley JD, Frid MG, Orton EC et al: Hypoxia selectively induces proliferation in a specific subpopulation of smooth muscle cells in the bovine neonatal pulmonary arterial media. *J Clin Invest* 96:273–281, 1995.

Chapter 20

Hypoxia, Adenosine, and K_{ATP} Channels of Coronary Arterial Smooth Muscle

Caroline Dart
Christina S. Davie
John M. Quayle
George C. Wellman
Nicholas B. Standen

Introduction

The mammalian heart has the highest oxygen consumption per unit weight of any organ in the body. The coronary circulation is characterized by the close correlation between the metabolic needs of the cardiac tissue and the supply of oxygen and metabolites by the coronary blood vessels. This is achieved by appropriate adjustments of the diameter of coronary blood vessels, so that a local fall in oxygen tension, for example, will cause dilation of coronary arteries and arterioles.[1] Blood vessel diameter depends on the contractile tone of smooth muscle cells in the vessel walls, and there are a number of possible mechanisms by which a reduction in oxygen tension could lead to relaxation of coronary arterial smooth muscle. First, the oxygen tension might act directly on the smooth muscle

From: López-Barneo, J and Weir, EK: *Oxygen Regulation of Ion Channels and Gene Expression*. Armonk, NY: Futura Publishing Company, Inc., ©1998.

cells. Second, hypoxia could lead to release of vasodilator substances from the endothelial cells lining the arteries. Third, cardiac myocytes could release metabolites which act on coronary smooth muscle to cause vasodilation, for example, adenosine, protons, and potassium (K^+). Adenosine, in particular, has been suggested to play a pivotal role in matching coronary blood flow to cardiac metabolism.[2] These mechanisms are clearly not mutually exclusive, and each could exert part of its dilator effect through the activation of K^+ channels.

Opening K^+ channels can provide a powerful mechanism for relaxation of vascular smooth muscle. K^+ channel activation is transduced into vasorelaxation by the membrane hyperpolarization that it causes. It has recently become clear that the membrane potential of arterial smooth muscle is a major determinant of contractile tone and, therefore, of vessel diameter, acting by way of its effect on intracellular $[Ca^{2+}]$.[3] Membrane potential controls the open probability of voltage-dependent Ca^{2+} channels which are active at voltages around the physiologic resting potential, and may also affect Ca^{2+} release from intracellular stores. The activity of K^+ channels plays a central role in the control of membrane potential, since its value depends on the balance between K^+ conductance and depolarizing conductances, comprising, for example, channels permeable to cations, Ca^{2+}, or Cl^-. Because the number of channels active in the membrane of arterial smooth muscle near to the resting membrane potential is very low, opening or closure of just a few K^+ channels can cause a significant change in this potential and, therefore, in contractile tone.[3]

One class of K^+ channel, the adenosine triphosphate (ATP)-sensitive K^+ (or K_{ATP}) channel seems particularly specialized to respond to changes in cellular metabolism. K_{ATP} channels have the characteristic property of being closed by intracellular ATP, and in the heart are expressed both in cardiac myocytes and in coronary smooth muscle cells.[4,5] The action of ATP to cause channel closure is antagonized by intracellular adenosine diphosphate (ADP), and in some tissues by hydrogen ions. K_{ATP} channels can also be activated by a number of endogenous transmitters; adenosine is known to activate the channels in both cardiac and smooth muscle, while activators of K_{ATP} channels of smooth muscle also include calcitonin gene-related peptide (CGRP), vasoactive intestinal peptide, nitric oxide, and prostacyclins.[6,7]

This chapter covers some of the evidence that K_{ATP} channels are involved in coronary vasodilation in response to hypoxia and ischemia, and describes experiments investigating the activation of K_{ATP} channels of isolated coronary smooth muscle cells by hypoxia, adenosine, and CGRP.

Hypoxic Coronary Vasodilation Involves K_{ATP} Channels

A number of recent studies using isolated hearts or coronary vessels have suggested that K_{ATP} channels provide an important mechanism for hypoxic vasodilation in the coronary circulation.[8–12] Such vasodilation is blocked or reduced by glibenclamide, a sulphonylurea blocker of K_{ATP} channels, in guinea pig, dog, rabbit, bovine, and pig coronary circulations. In the intact perfused guinea pig heart, vasodilation to either hypoxia or adenosine is glibenclamide sensitive, but early hypoxic vasodilation in this preparation is not blocked by adenosine receptor antagonists, so that this phase may be a direct consequence of decreased tissue P_{O_2}.[8] The later phase of hypoxic vasodilation in perfused guinea pig heart may involve both adenosine and prostaglandins, while adenosine release seems to play an important role in K_{ATP} channel activation in the rabbit heart.[10] Hypoxia or ischemia also lead to a fall in pH in the heart; the vasodilator response of porcine coronary arterioles to acidosis has also been found to be substantially blocked by glibenclamide, suggesting that K_{ATP} channel activation is also involved in this response.[13]

Hypoxia Activates K_{ATP} Channels in Cells Isolated from Coronary Arteries

We have obtained evidence that hypoxia can act directly on coronary smooth muscle to open K_{ATP} channels from experiments using smooth muscle cells isolated enzymatically from pig coronary arteries.[14] To minimize disruption of cytoplasmic composition by dialysis, we used the perforated patch technique with the pore-forming antibiotic amphotericin, and we usually measured currents at -60 mV in high K^+ external solution, so that K^+ channel activation would lead to an inward current. Hypoxic solutions were obtained by bubbling the solution used to superfuse the cell with N_2, giving a P_{O_2} of 25 to 40 mm Hg. This solution was applied directly onto the cell through gas-impermeable tubing, and a high flow rate was maintained throughout. Figure 1A shows the effect of applying hypoxic solution in a typical experiment, while mean results are shown in Figure 1B. Hypoxic solution activated an inward current and caused an increase in current noise, usually after a delay of 1 to 2 minutes. The properties of this hypoxia-activated current suggest that it flows through K_{ATP} channels. We used voltage ramps to measure the current-voltage

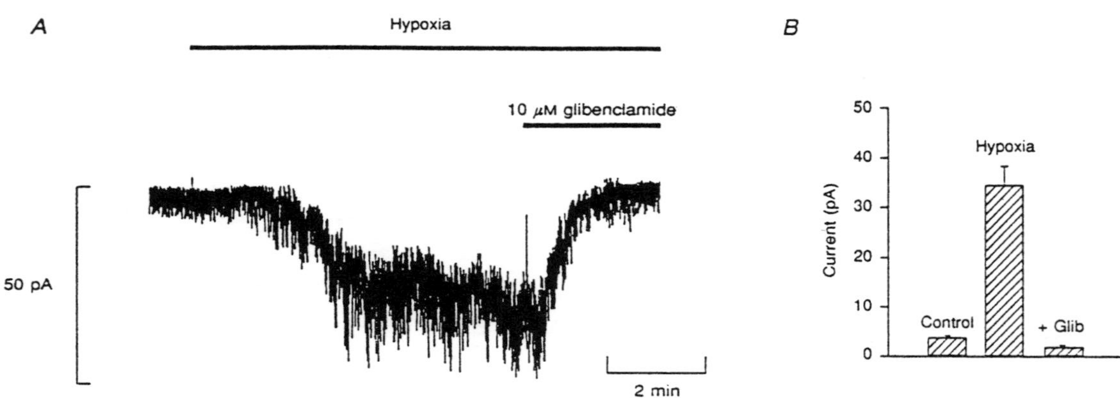

Figure 1. Activation of K_{ATP} current by hypoxia. **A.** The record shows whole-cell current measured using the perforated-patch technique from a smooth muscle cell isolated from a pig small diameter coronary artery. The cell was superfused with 143 mM K^+ solution and held at −60 mV throughout. Hypoxic solution (Po_2 25–40 mm Hg) and glibenclamide were applied as indicated. **B.** Mean currents from five cells under control (normoxic) conditions, in hypoxic solution, and in hypoxic solution with 10 μM glibenclamide. (Reproduced with permission from Reference 14.)

relation of the hypoxia-activated current. The reversal potential of the current shifted with a change in extracellular [K^+] as expected for a K^+ current, and the current-voltage relation was essentially linear in symmetrical high [K^+] solutions, as expected for channels whose gating shows little voltage dependence. In addition, the hypoxia-activated current was completely inhibited by the K_{ATP} channel blocker glibenclamide, but unaffected by the blocker of large conductance Ca^{2+}-activated K^+ channels, charybdotoxin[14]

K^+ channels activated by hypoxia can also be detected at the single-channel level. Because of the low channel open probability in arterial smooth muscle cells at physiologic membrane potentials, the noise in whole-cell recordings is low, and it is often possible to detect the activity of individual channels. Figure 2A shows recordings of whole-cell current made during the onset of the response to hypoxia. Using appropriate filtering, it is quite easy to resolve openings of a channel with a unitary current around −2 pA, and it is clear that increasing numbers of such channels become active as the response to hypoxia develops. Figure 2B shows a corresponding histogram of current amplitude, made at the beginning of the response to hypoxia, and shows peaks corresponding to current levels with zero, one, two, or three channels open simultaneously. The unitary current of about −2 pA at −60mV corresponds to a single-channel conductance of 34 pS. In some cells, we were also able to use cell-attached patches to demonstrate hypoxic activation of channels with the same conductance.

Activation of Coronary K_{ATP} Channels by Adenosine

As discussed above, adenosine released from cardiac myocytes may play an important role in the regulation of coronary blood flow, and adenosine can hyperpolarize coronary arteries.[1] We have used the same patch-clamp techniques as those described above to demonstrate the activation by adenosine of K_{ATP} channels in coronary arterial smooth muscle.[15] Like hypoxia, adenosine activated a whole-cell K^+ current in isolated pig coronary cells. Current-voltage relations were consistent, with channels showing little voltage dependence, and the current was blocked by glibenclamide (Figure 3A). Unitary currents of adenosine-activated channels measured in whole-cell recordings as described above were the same as those for the channels activated by hypoxia. Another way to estimate the unitary current of the channels activated by adenosine is to use noise analysis of the whole-cell current, and we found that this also gave values

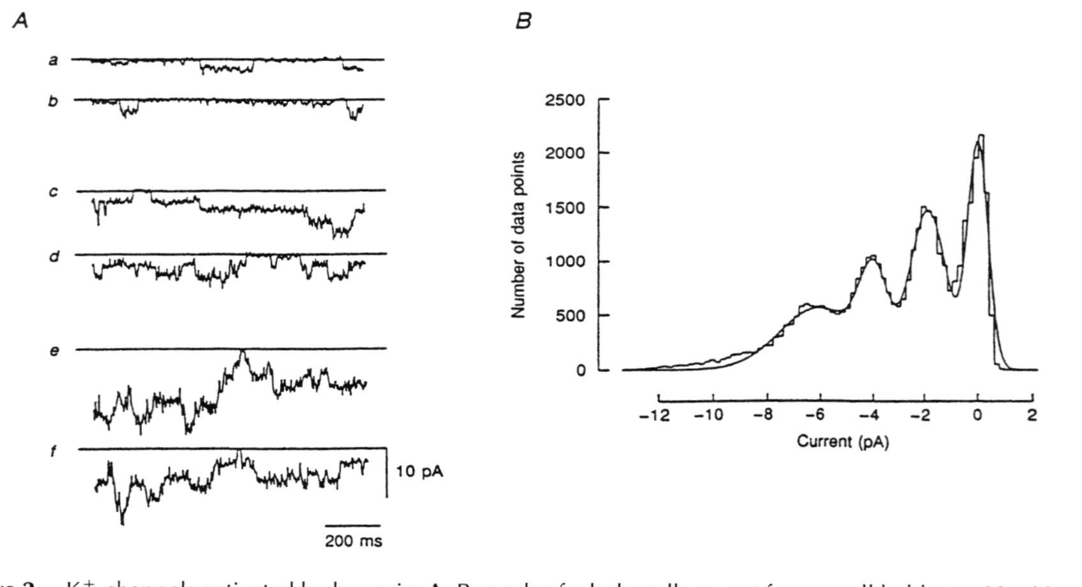

Figure 2. K^+ channels activated by hypoxia. **A.** Records of whole-cell current from a cell held at −60 mV and bathed in 143 mM $[K^+]$ solution. Records **a** and **b** were made while the cell was superfused with normoxic solution, and records **c**, **d**, **e**, and **f** progressively later during the response to hypoxic solution. The **straight line** indicates the zero current level in each case. **B.** Histogram of current amplitude formed from recordings made during the onset of the hypoxia-induced current. The histogram has been fitted with the sum of four Gaussian curves with means of 0, −1.87, −3.98 and −6.08 pA. (Reproduced with permission from Reference 14.)

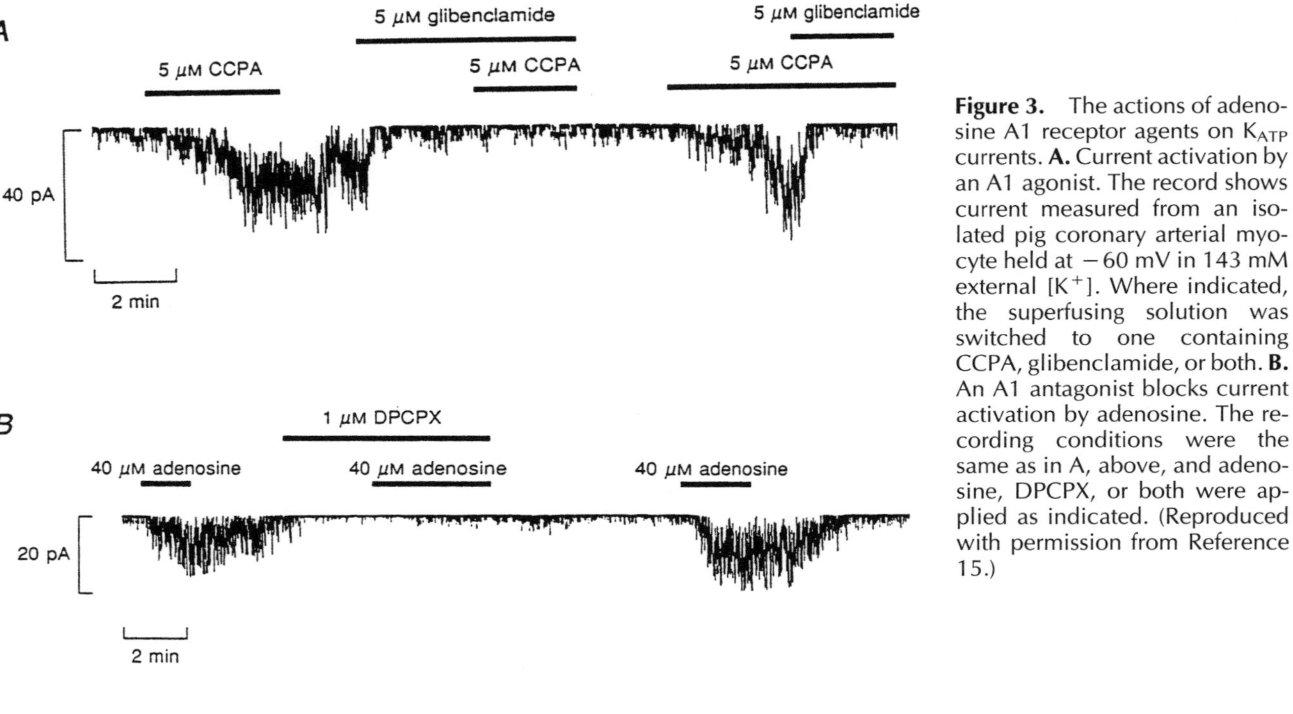

Figure 3. The actions of adenosine A1 receptor agents on K_{ATP} currents. **A.** Current activation by an A1 agonist. The record shows current measured from an isolated pig coronary arterial myocyte held at −60 mV in 143 mM external $[K^+]$. Where indicated, the superfusing solution was switched to one containing CCPA, glibenclamide, or both. **B.** An A1 antagonist blocks current activation by adenosine. The recording conditions were the same as in A, above, and adenosine, DPCPX, or both were applied as indicated. (Reproduced with permission from Reference 15.)

consistent with those measured from single channels. Thus, adenosine and hypoxia appear to activate the same type of K^+ channel in coronary smooth muscle.

We have also investigated the mechanism by which adenosine activates K_{ATP} current. Adenosine receptors can be divided into at least three subclasses, A1, A2, and A3. A2 receptors lead to activation of adenylyl cyclase and are most commonly associated with effects on vascular smooth muscle, although the glibenclamide relaxation of pig coronary arteries to adenosine has been proposed to occur through an A1 receptor.[16] Consistent with this suggestion, we found in isolated cells that A1 receptor agents mimicked or blocked the effects of adenosine in activating K_{ATP} current. Figure 3A shows that the highly selective A1 receptor agonist (2-chloro-N^6-cyclopentyladenosine) CCPA activated a K^+ current that was indistinguishable both in terms of block by glibenclamide and of the unitary conductance of the underlying channels, from that activated by adenosine itself. We also found that the selective A1 receptor antagonist DPCPX (8-cyclopentyl-1,3-dipropylxanthine) blocked current activation by adenosine, as shown in Figure 3B. The A2 receptor agents CGS 21680 and CGS 15943A, however, were ineffective in activating or blocking the adenosine-induced current, respectively. We conclude, therefore, that adenosine acts at an A1 receptor to activate K_{ATP} channels of pig coronary smooth muscle. Adenosine has also been reported to activate K_{ATP} current in smooth muscle from dog coronary arteries, although the receptor type involved was not investigated in this case.[17]

CGRP Activates K_{ATP} Channels Through Protein Kinase A

CGRP is a 37-amino acid peptide that occurs in autonomic sensory nerves innervating many tissues, including the heart and blood vessels.[18] CGRP is an extremely potent vasodilator, and in mesenteric arteries has been shown to act in part by activating K_{ATP} channels by way of adenylyl cyclase and protein kinase A.[19,20] Myocardial ischemia induces release of CGRP from nerves within the heart, providing another possible mechanism for ischemic vasodilation. We have, therefore, studied the effects of CGRP in isolated pig coronary arterial smooth muscle, using conventional whole-cell patch-clamp recording, rather than the permeabilized patch method.[21] Like hypoxia or adenosine, CGRP (50 nM) activated a substantial K^+ current that we attribute to K_{ATP} channels, since it was blocked by glibenclamide and was also substantially smaller when the intracellular solution contained 3 mM ATP rather than 0.1 mM ATP. The CGRP-activated current was reduced by the inhibitor of protein kinase A, H89 (1 μM), and we also found that activation of adenylyl cyclase with forskolin (10 μM) stimulated a glibenclamide-sensitive K^+ current in these cells. Our findings suggest that CGRP activates K_{ATP} channels in coronary arteries by causing stimulation of adenylyl cyclase to generate cyclic adenosine monophosphate (cAMP) and activate protein kinase A.

How Does Hypoxia Activate K_{ATP} Channels in Coronary Arteries?

The pathways by which the locally released vasodilators adenosine and CGRP can activate coronary K_{ATP} channels are at least partially understood. It is much less clear how hypoxia itself might lead to channel activation in isolated cells. Perhaps the most obvious mechanism by which a reduction in Po_2 could lead to channel activation would be by changing the energy metabolism of arterial myocytes, thus altering levels of nucleoside phosphates. Such a mechanism has been suggested to explain hypoxic vasodilation in the isolated heart, where metabolic inhibition with 2-deoxyglucose or dinitrophenol also produces vasodilation.[8] Such metabolic inhibition also activates glibenclamide-sensitive currents in our isolated coronary smooth muscle cells. However, it is not certain that the hypoxic solutions we used, which have a Po_2 in the range 25 to 40 mm Hg, would cause much change in intracellular nucleotide concentrations, since hypoxia has been reported to cause little change in intracellular [ATP] in aorta.[22] It is possible that the metabolism of small arteries differs from that of larger vessels, and also that submembrane nucleotide concentrations change differently from those in the bulk of the cytoplasm. Alternatively, it might be that K_{ATP} channels of coronary myocytes are activated by an oxygen-sensing mechanism similar to those proposed for cells of the carotid body or airway muscosal cells.

While the exact mechanism of hypoxic activation remains unclear, it is worth noting that the oxygen tensions we have used may not be very different from those found in small arteries and arterioles under physiologic conditions, since Po_2 may decrease to around 20 mm Hg in terminal arterioles.[23] This could contribute to a background level of K_{ATP} channel activity, and in line with this, several studies have reported that glibenclamide increases basal coronary tone in vivo.[24]

The Role of K_{ATP} Channels in the Ischemic Heart

Figure 4 summarizes a number of mechanisms that converge at the level of K_{ATP} channels to provide an integrated response in the ischemic

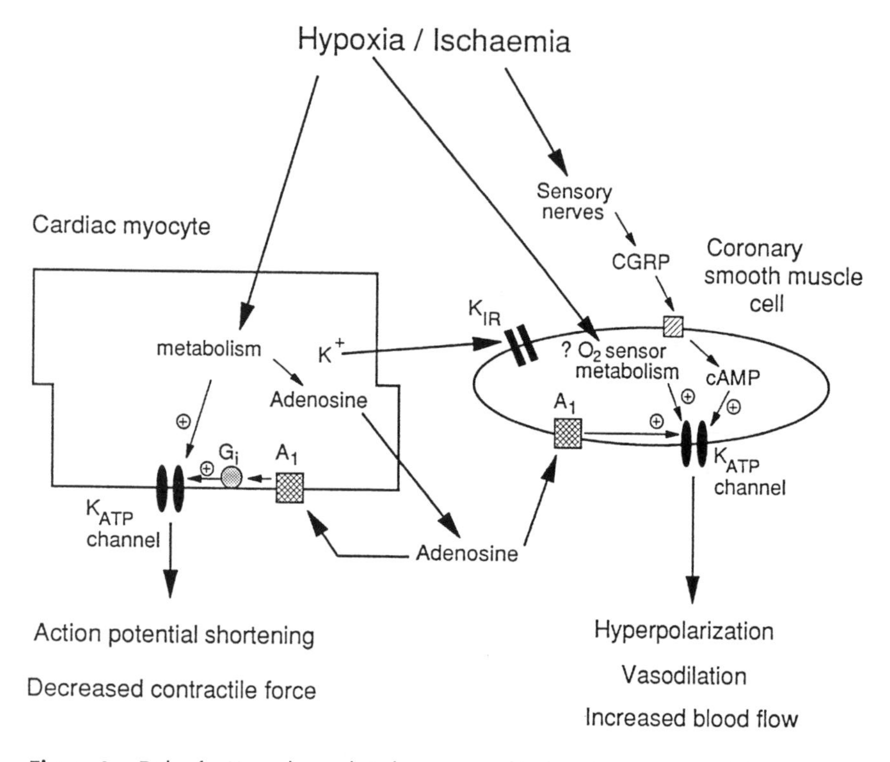

Figure 4. Roles for K_{ATP} channels in hypoxic and ischemic responses of the coronary circulation.

heart. In cardiac muscle cells, decreased oxygen delivery will compromise metabolism, leading to increases in intracellular ADP and lactate, decreased pH, possibly a small fall in ATP, and release of adenosine into the extracellular space. These metabolic changes will activate K_{ATP} channels in the cardiac muscle cells, and adenosine acting at A1 receptors on the cardiac myocytes will also contribute to their activation.[25] Channel activation will lead to action potential shortening, thus, decreasing calcium entry, contractile force, and so energy consumption. Opening of K_{ATP} channels will also lead to efflux of K^+, and probably also to the cardioprotective effects associated with preconditioning.[26]

In the smooth muscle cells of the coronary vasculature, K_{ATP} channels will be activated by hypoxia either directly or through consequent metabolic changes. Adenosine released from cardiac muscle will contribute to their activation, and CGRP released from sensory nerves as a consequence of ischemia may also play a role, as may a fall in tissue pH. K_{ATP} channel activation will cause hyperpolarization and vasodilation, increasing blood flow and thus delivery of oxygen and metabolites. The K^+ released from cardiac muscle, primarily through K_{ATP} channels, may also contribute to this vasodilation by activating another K^+ channel, the inward rectifier, which appears to be preferentially expressed in small coronary arteries.[27]

Thus, the final results of K_{ATP} activation in ischemia are to reduce cardiac energy consumption and to restore blood flow as far as possible, both of which counteract the ischemia and its effects.

Conclusions

K_{ATP} channels of coronary arterial smooth muscle are activated both by hypoxia itself and also by adenosine and CGRP which will be released as a consequence of hypoxia or ischemia in the intact heart. Together with K_{ATP} channels of cardiac myocytes themselves, these mechanisms form part of an integrated response of the coronary circulation to changes in metabolic demand of the cardiac tissue. It is clear that more work is needed to resolve the mechanism of K_{ATP} channel activation by hypoxia itself, and recent information on the molecular structure of these channels[28] will pave the way for further understanding of the mechanisms that control the activity of cardiovascular K_{ATP} channels at the molecular level.

References

1. Daut J, Standen NB, Nelson MT: The role of the membrane potential of endothelial and smooth muscle cells in the regulation of coronary blood flow. *J Cardiovasc Electrophysiol* 5:154–181, 1994.
2. Berne RM: The role of adenosine in the regulation of coronary bloodflow. *Circ Res* 47:807–813, 1980.
3. Nelson MT, Patlak JB, Worley JF, et al: Calcium channels, potassium channels, and voltage dependence of arterial smooth muscle cell tone. *Am J Physiol* 259: C3-C18, 1990.
4. Davies NW, Standen NB, Stanfield PR: ATP-dependent potassium channels of muscle cells: their properties, regulation, and possible functions. *J Bioenerg Biomembr* 23:509–535, 1991.
5. Nichols CG, Lederer WJ: Adenosine triphosphate-sensitive potassium channels in the cardiovascular system. *Am J Physiol* 261:H1675-H1686, 1991.
6. Quayle JM, Standen NB: K_{ATP} channels in vascular smooth muscle. *Cardiovasc Res* 28:797–804, 1994.
7. Nelson MT, Quayle JM: Physiological roles and properties of potassium channels in arterial smooth muscle. *Am J Physiol* 268:C799-C822, 1995.
8. von Beckerath N, Cyrys S, Dischner A, et al: Hypoxic vasodilatation in isolated, perfused guinea-pig heart: an analysis of the underlying mechanisms. *J Physiol* 442:297–319, 1991.

9. Clayton FC, Hess TA, Smith MA, et al: Coronary reactive hyperaemia and adenosine-induced vasodilation are mediated partially by a glyburide-sensitive mechanism. *Pharmacology* 44:92–100, 1992.
10. Nakhostine N, Lamontagne D: Adenosine contributes to hypoxia-induced vasodilatation through ATP-sensitive K^+ channel activation. *Am J Physiol* 265: H1289-H1293, 1993.
11. Mellemkjaer S, Nielsen-Kudsk JE: Glibenclamide inhibits hypoxic relaxation of isolated porcine coronary arteries under conditions of impaired glycolysis. *Eur J Pharmacol* 270:307–312, 1994.
12. Kalsner S: Hypoxic relaxation in functionally intact cattle coronary artery segments involves K^+_{ATP} channels. *J Pharmacol Exp Ther* 275:1219–1226, 1995.
13. Ishizaka H, Kuo L: Acidosis-induced coronary arteriolar dilation is mediated by ATP-sensitive potassium channels in vascular smooth muscle. *Circ Res* 78: 50–57, 1996.
14. Dart C, Standen NB: Activation of ATP-dependent K^+ channels by hypoxia in smooth muscle cells isolated from the pig coronary artery. *J Physiol* 483:29–39, 1995.
15. Dart C, Standen NB: Adenosine-activated potassium current in smooth muscle cells isolated from the pig coronary artery. *J Physiol* 471:767–786, 1993.
16. Merkel LA, Lappe RW, Rivera LM, et al: Demonstration of vasorelaxant activity with an A_1-selective adenosine agonist in porcine coronary artery: involvement of potassium channels. *J Pharmacol Exp Ther* 260:437–443, 1992.
17. Xu X, Lee KS: Characterization of the ATP-inhibited K^+ current in canine coronary smooth muscle cells. *Pflügers Arch* 427:110–120, 1994.
18. Bell D, McDermott BJ: Calcitonin gene-related peptide in the cardiovascular system: characterization of receptor populations and their (patho)physiological significance. *Pharmacol Rev* 48:253–288, 1996.
19. Nelson MT, Huang Y, Brayden JE, et al: Activation of K^+ channels is involved in arterial dilations to calcitonin gene-related peptide. *Nature* 344:770–773, 1990.
20. Quayle JM, Bonev AD, Brayden JE, et al: Calcitonin gene-related peptide activated ATP-sensitive K^+ currents in rabbit arterial smooth muscle via protein kinase A. *J Physiol* 475:9–13, 1994.
21. Wellman GC, Quayle JM, Everitt DE, et al: Calcitonin gene-related peptide (CGRP) activates an ATP-sensitive (K_{ATP}) potassium current in pig coronary vascular smooth muscle cells via cyclic AMP-dependent protein kinase (PKA). *J Physiol* 499P:11P, 1997.
22. Post JM, Jones AW: Stimulation of arterial K efflux by ATP depletion and cromakalim is antagonized by glyburide. *Am J Physiol* 260:H848-H854, 1991.
23. Duling B, Berne RM: Longitudinal gradients in periarteriolar oxygen tension: a possible mechanism for the participation of oxygen in local regulation of blood flow. *Circ Res* 27:669–678, 1970.
24. Samaha FF, Heineman FW, Ince C, et al: ATP-sensitive potassium channel is essential to maintain basal coronary vascular tone in vivo. *Am J Physiol* 262: C1220-C1227, 1992.
25. Kirsch GE, Codina J, Birnbaumer L, et al: Coupling of ATP-sensitive K^+ channels to A_1 receptors by G proteins in rat ventricular myocytes. *Am J Physiol* 259: H820-H826, 1990.
26. Yellon DM, Gross GJ: *Myocardial Protection and the K_{ATP} Channel.* Norwell, MA: Kluwer Academic Publishers; 1995.

27. Quayle JM, Dart C, Standen NB: The properties and distribution of inward rectifier potassium currents in pig coronary arterial smooth muscle. *J Physiol* 494: 715–726, 1996.
28. Inagaki N, Gonoi T, Clement IP, et al: A family of sulfonylurea receptors determines the pharmacological properties of ATP-sensitive K^+ channels. *Neuron* 16:1011–1017, 1996.

Section 5

OXYGEN SENSING IN NERVE CELLS

Chapter 21

Oxygen Sensing in Neurons:
Direct and Indirect Modulation of Ion Channels

Gabriel G. Haddad

Introduction

Since ion channels represent one of the most important effector systems responsible for neuronal activity and excitability in the central and peripheral nervous systems, it is no surprise that understanding of how ion channels function has become central in a number of conditions that seem to disturb or alter neuronal discharge. An increasing number of examples has been forthcoming in the past decade. Consider, for example, the importance of the glutamate receptor/channels in processes such as development, differentiation, and pathophysiologic conditions, such as excitotoxicity of ischemia and hypoxia.[1] Also, consider the role of voltage-gated sodium (Na) channels in congenital muscle diseases.[2] Other important examples have implicated mutations in potassium (K) channels in central neurological diseases.

Although oxygen deprivation can be severe and pathophysiologic, lack of oxygen can certainly occur as part of physiologic alterations in the microenvironment of neurons, either as a result of changes in blood flow to small regions, or as a result of intense neuronal activity in comparison to the level of oxygenation provided. Since hypoxia has been shown by

From: López-Barneo, J and Weir, EK: *Oxygen Regulation of Ion Channels and Gene Expression*. Armonk, NY: Futura Publishing Company, Inc., ©1998.

a number of investigators to affect neuronal excitability and discharge, ion channels have been examined for a better understanding of the cascade of events that occur with low oxygen.

There are at least two major reasons for the interest in how oxygen is sensed and the initial events that occur when nerve cells are challenged with low levels of oxygen. The first is that this initial cascade may be very important in steering the response of nerve cells toward adaptive or deleterious effects on nerve cell function. The thorough understanding of this initial response might lead us to design interventions that may lead to cell survival or prevention of cell injury. The second, is that understanding the mechanisms that are responsible for sensing the lack of oxygen is a fundamental question that might help in understanding certain natural processes that are dependent on oxygen, such as those that occur at birth or shortly after (changes in vessel caliber and change in blood flow, change in carotid body sensitivity with age, etc.). In addition, understanding these mechanisms will most likely prove to be important in trying to understand the interactions between the microenvironment of a cell and its genetic endowment; for example, how the changes in the environment of a nerve cell, including oxygen or lack thereof, interact with neuronal gene expression and its regulation.

This chapter focuses mostly on work from the author's laboratory to illustrate: 1) how hypoxia induces cytosolic changes that in turn influences the activity of ion channels and neuronal excitability; and 2) how hypoxia can directly alter the activity of ion channels without first affecting other cytosolic functions. The first example will be obtained from work performed on the voltage-activated Na channels and the second part will focus on certain species of K channels.

Hypoxic Modulation of the Voltage-Activated Na^+ Channels

At the beginning of our investigations, we subjected neurons, in the neocortical or hippocampal slice of rats, to hypoxia or anoxia, in order to examine the response of neurons to lack of oxygen while preserving their local connections. In addition, to the degree that the responses of neurons are altered by the presence of glial elements, these elements were present in the slice preparation and the glial-neuronal interactions are present in the slice. A typical response for these rat neurons is biphasic: first they hyperpolarize, 2 to 3 minutes after hypoxia, and then they depolarize. The hyperpolarization is small in general, but the depolarization gets larger in time and ends up with a depolarization blockade.[3] Typically in these studies, the input resistance drops and by the time neurons have depolarized in a major way, input resistance has become very small.[3]

One intriguing finding with CA1 or neocortical neurons in the rat is that these neurons decrease their excitability and increase their rheobase even before any changes in membrane potential or input resistance.[3] Although this decrease in excitability can certainly be explained by the hyperpolarization and by the decrease in input resistance, when they occur, the initial decrease in excitability does not seem to be related to the alterations in potential or conductance seen. We hypothesized, therefore, that the early decrease in excitability depends on another phenomenon, namely a mechanism that is related to firing threshold and Na^+ channel activation.

Neocortical nerve cells were obtained from rats (25–30 days old) by triturating thin slices after enzyme exposure. The peak whole cell Na^+ current (I_{Na}) was recorded with a step depolarization to −10 mV from a holding potential of −70 mV.[3] This peak current stabilized by 2 minutes after rupture of the membrane, and experiments were performed between minutes 2 and 10 of whole-cell recording. Control studies showed a slow rundown of I_{Na} over 3 minutes of recording to about 85% of the initial current. In addition, both the steady-state inactivation curve and the activation curve showed a slow drift of approximately −1.0 mV/min.[3,4]

When the extracellular bath was changed from control perfusate to the hypoxic solution, there was a rapid inhibition of peak I_{Na}, with no effect on the kinetics of activation or inactivation.[3] After 3 minutes of hypoxic exposure, I_{Na} was reduced to about 35% to 40% of baseline. In addition, steady state inactivation was shifted by approximately −10.0 mV, while the change in activation was not different from control.[3] This was the first demonstration that the Na current can be inhibited by hypoxia.

Prolonged periods of deprivation can lead to disturbance in ionic homeostasis and irreversible brain damage, not only in animals but also in humans. Because the majority of animal studies have focused on hippocampal and brain stem tissue, we focused on neocortical cells and their properties, not only in animals but also in human neocortical neurons.

To examine the effect of anoxia on human neocortical neurons and determine whether they have a similar response to that in animals, slices were first exposed to anoxia for 10 to 30 minutes.[5] As in rat neocortical slices, membrane potential of the human neurons (V_m) showed a biphasic response to anoxia in most neurons. The initial phase, occurring in the first few minutes of anoxic exposure, consisted of a relatively small hyperpolarization. V_m then started to become more positive, returning to baseline and becoming depolarized after 8 to 15 minutes of anoxic exposure.

Although R_m did not change in the first several minutes of anoxia, it subsequently decreased in all cells.[5]

Interestingly, as in rats, before there was any change in R_m and at a time when V_m was either still at, or had returned to baseline levels, rheobase was found to increase.[5] The hyperpolarization, decrease in R_m and elevation of $K^+{}_o$ during anoxia could be explained by an increase in potassium conductance, as has been shown in previous studies in rat hippocampal and brain stem neurons. However, since the anoxic depression of neuronal excitability could not be adequately explained by an increased potassium conductance alone, especially that, in some neurons, excitability was reduced before any changes in V_m or R_m we asked whether anoxia altered voltage-dependent inward currents. Using the whole-cell patch-clamp technique, pyramidal CA1 neurons were studied. Anoxia decreased I_{Na} in human neocortical neurons, but typically the response took two to three times longer to elicit than that elicited with CN. Although both CN and hypoxia depressed I_{Na}, recovery was much more complete after CN than anoxia. Both CN and oxygen deprivation had a major effect on the voltage dependence of steady-state inactivation. The midpoint of the steady-state inactivation curve [$H\infty(V)$] was shifted in the negative direction by about 20 mV for both CN and anoxia. This shift to the left was also present in control experiments (no hypoxia), but to a much lesser extent. Since dialysis might have occurred with whole-cell recording, nystatin patches were used and similar results were obtained during hypoxia.

Because adenosine triphosphate (ATP) might have been reduced with oxygen deprivation, we determined whether ATP played an important role in maintaining I_{Na}. Using whole-cell recordings with electrodes containing 2 to 10 mM K_2ATP, we examined I_{Na} during hypoxia or CN. When holding these cells at -70 mV and stepping to 0 mV, CN decreased the magnitude of I_{Na} by only 8%.[3] Further, the negative shift in the $H\infty(V)$ curve was 7 mV ($n = 10$), indicating that intracellular ATP levels are crucial in the modulation of I_{Na} when human neocortical neurons are deprived of oxygen.[5]

This study of membrane currents in adult human cortical neurons demonstrates that dissociation of neurons from adult human brains can be successfully performed and isolated neurons studied. Our voltage-clamp recordings of neocortical neurons also provide the first direct evidence that anoxic depression of human neocortical activity is largely mediated by modulations of I_{Na}. As has been described, rat and human neocortical neurons respond in a similar way to anoxia by inhibiting I_{Na}, and at least part of this inhibition is related to a steady state inhibition of the Na channels. The underlying mechanism(s) for this phenomenon is not yet known, but we have preliminary evidence that activation of protein kinases, in particular protein kinase C, is involved in the decrease of the Na current.

The functional implications of this phenomenon may be related to Na entry into a nerve cell during lack of oxygen. The inhibition of the Na channels is most likely an adaptive mechanism that tries to render cells less vulnerable to anoxia, since restricting Na entry will have beneficial effects on survival and the prevention of cell death. At a time when ATP and energy supplies may be dwindling, decreasing Na load on the cell will have major implications on maintaining ATP levels and minimizing the mismatch between supplies and demand. Clearly, if the stress is severe and prolonged enough, decreasing Na load in this fashion will not be enough to prevent Na load. This is consistent with our data which shows that Na gets into nerve cells when oxygen deprivation is severe enough.[6] It is also consistent with our observations that we can markedly blunt the probability for cell death if the extracellular space does not have Na.[7,8]

Modulation of K^+ Channels by Po_2

Another example that has been the subject of many recent investigations is a K^+ conductance that is sensitive to a number of cytosolic factors. K^+ conductances that are sensitive to ATP have been found in pancreatic, myocardial, and smooth muscle cells and in neurons. In relation to hypoxia in the central nervous system, we have recently presented the first direct evidence that this type of channel responds to low oxygen levels in the cellular microenvironment.[9,10] Since these channels are sensitive to ATP and Ca^{++} in nerve cells,[11] it is possible that channel activity is modulated during low oxygen conditions by alterations in ATP and Ca^{++}, alterations known to occur during hypoxia (Figure 1).[12,13] The importance of the opening of this K^+ channel is related to our previous data showing that blockade of this channel with glibenclamide during anoxia leads to further depolarization and all the cells that have been studied did not recover from anoxia, in sharp contrast to control cells (not exposed to glibenclamide), which all recovered after even as short a period as 10 to 15 minutes into reoxygenation.[14]

The new development in this area is related to recent findings from our laboratory showing that ion channels of neuronal plasma membranes respond to changes in molecular oxygen, not indirectly through cytosolic changes, but directly in a cytosol-independent and membrane delimited manner.[9–11] Qualitatively, this is not dissimilar to oxygen partial pressure (Po_2) modulation of K^+ channels in carotid glomus cells or pulmonary smooth muscle cells.[15–19] We have shown experimentally that certain spe-

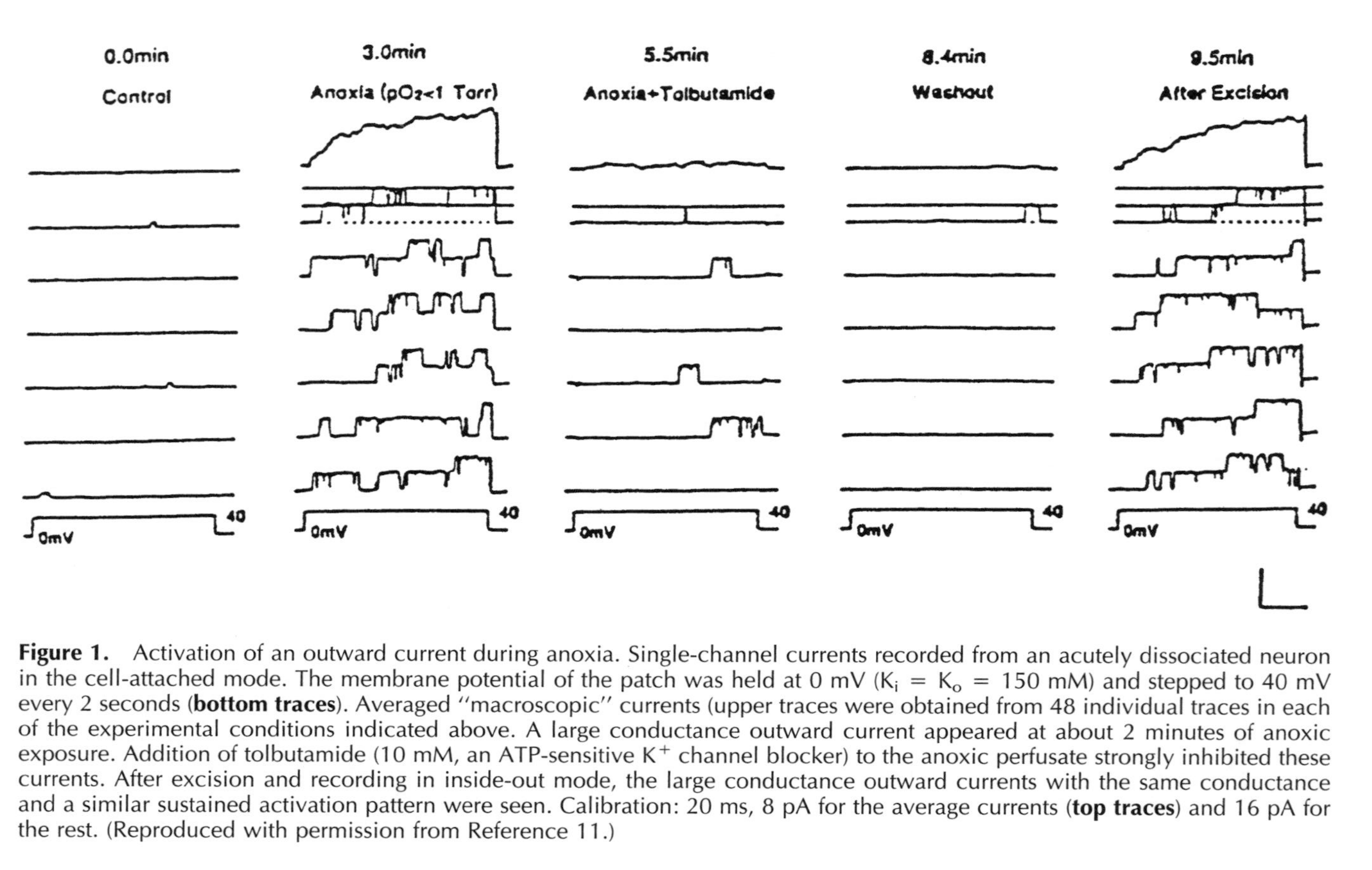

Figure 1. Activation of an outward current during anoxia. Single-channel currents recorded from an acutely dissociated neuron in the cell-attached mode. The membrane potential of the patch was held at 0 mV (K_i = K_o = 150 mM) and stepped to 40 mV every 2 seconds (**bottom traces**). Averaged "macroscopic" currents (upper traces were obtained from 48 individual traces in each of the experimental conditions indicated above. A large conductance outward current appeared at about 2 minutes of anoxic exposure. Addition of tolbutamide (10 mM, an ATP-sensitive K^+ channel blocker) to the anoxic perfusate strongly inhibited these currents. After excision and recording in inside-out mode, the large conductance outward currents with the same conductance and a similar sustained activation pattern were seen. Calibration: 20 ms, 8 pA for the average currents (**top traces**) and 16 pA for the rest. (Reproduced with permission from Reference 11.)

cies of K^+ channels in neocortical neurons decrease their activity when oxygen is depleted around the excised patch. This decrease in overall channel activity is mostly due to a decrease in open probability (Popen). The Po_2-Popen dose-response curve is relevant to the physiology of oxygen delivery and transport to the brain, since the channel response seems to be very consistent with the Po_2 that normally exists in the interstitium.[9,10] These K^+ channels start responding to Po_2 at or just below 20 Torr, with 50% reduction of activity at about 10 Torr (Figure 2). Although the exact molecular mechanism underlying the change in activity as a function of Po_2 is not completely understood, these K^+ channels seem to be directly sensitive to oxygen. We have recently named these channels oxygen-sensing K^+ channels or "OK" channels. We have, in addition, performed experiments that bear on potential mechanisms underlying K^+-sensing mechanisms.

We have performed experiments and gathered data that suggest that a change in the redox state of the OK channel itself during oxygen deprivation alters its own activity.[9,10] Indeed, when we have used reducing agents such as reduced glutathione (GSH) or dithiothreitol on excised patches, K^+ channel Popen decreased markedly. Oxidized GSH did not significantly affect ion channel activity in neuronal excised patches.[10] The basis for such modulation could be similar to the reduction of thiol groups of cysteine residues on the N-terminal portion of a shaker-type channel molecule, found to be critical in fast inactivation kinetics.[20] Indeed, K^+ channels with fast inactivation kinetics, such as the A current, have been shown to be modulated by intracellular substances that can reduce or oxidize cysteine residues.[20]

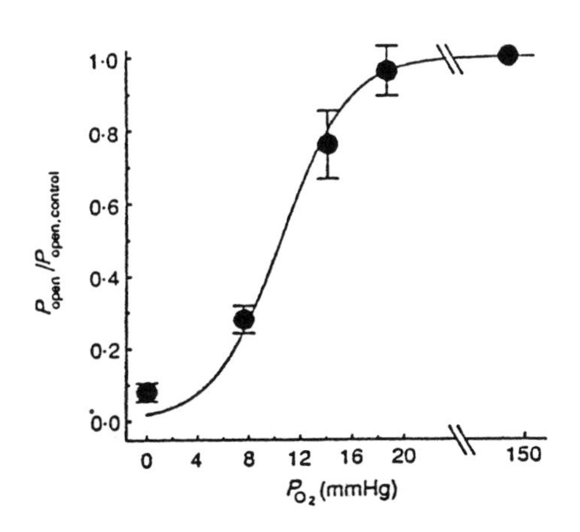

Figure 2. Dose-dependent inhibition of P_{open} by graded hypoxia. Inside-out patches were recorded with an equal concentration of K^+ (150 mM) on both sides of the membrane. Po_2 was measured with polarographic electrodes. Graded hypoxia was induced by perfusing patches with one of the solutions bubbled for at least 2 hours with either 2% (balanced with N_2), 1% or 0% oxygen, or 0% oxygen plus 2 mM $Na_2S_2O_4$. The measured Po_2 from these solutions was 18:7, 14:1, 7:6, and 0 mm Hg, respectively. (Reproduced with permission from Reference 9.)

It is possible that molecules such as plasma membrane metal-containing proteins are associated with these specific K^+ channels that, by a so far unknown mechanism, affect channel activity when oxygen is depleted.[9,10] This idea of a link between a membrane protein and the OK channel is based on recent data from our laboratory showing that metal center blockers or chelators, such as 1 to 10 phenanthroline, deferoxamine, or cyanide, suppress K^+ channel activity in a similar fashion as hypoxia.[9,10] Oxidant species and radicals such as hydrogen peroxide and nitric oxide are probably not important modulators of this K^+ channel in neurons, since superoxide dismutase and hemoglobin were not effective in altering channel activity.[9,10] Clearly, this does not totally eliminate their role in vivo or in whole-cell situations, since enzyme systems (e.g., oxidases) that are not membrane bound can generate oxidant species and affect K^+ channel activity.

In conclusion, there are a number of processes that get triggered with hypoxia in nerve cells. It is possible, actually likely, that these processes are parallel and that they interact. What constitutes an oxygen "sensor" and the mechanisms of oxygen sensing are not well understood at present. Whether there are a number of them in each cell type, whether each cell type has a different sensor, and whether the same sensor is present in all cells is not clear. However, we favor the idea that the sensors will vary, depending on function and the level of oxygen sensing. We should also recognize that chronic hypoxia may be totally different from acute hypoxia in terms of oxygen sensing. Since oxygen tolerant and oxygen nontolerant animals sense oxygen, but do not respond to it in the same way, oxygen sensors in these two different types of animals might be very different.

References

1. Haddad GG, Jiang C: O_2 deprivation in the central nervous system: on mechanisms of neuronal response, differential sensitivity, and injury. *Prog Neurobiol* 40:277–318, 1993.
2. Barchi RL: Molecular pathology of the skeletal muscle sodium channel. *Annu Rev Physiol* 57:355–385, 1995.
3. Cummins TR, Donnelly DF, Haddad GG: Effect of metabolic inhibition on the excitability of isolated hippocampal CA1 neurons: developmental aspects. *Neurophysiol* 66:1471–1482, 1991.
4. O'Reilly JP, Haddad GG: Hypoxia reduces Na^+ current in hippocampal neurons via a kinase mediated pathway (abstr). *Soc for Neurosci* 22(3):2151, 1996.
5. Cummins TR, Jiang C, Haddad GG: Human neocortical excitability is decreased during anoxia via sodium channel modulation. *J Clin Invest* 91:608–615, 1993.
6. Friedman JE, Haddad GG: Anoxia induces an increase in intracellular sodium in rat central neurons in vitro. *Brain Res* 663:329–334, 1994.

7. Friedman JE, Haddad GG: Removal of extracellular sodium prevents anoxia-induced injury in freshly dissociated rat CA1 hippocampal neurons. *Brain Res* 641:57–64, 1994.
8. Chidekel AS, Friedman JE, Haddad GG: The role of extracellular sodium in anoxia-induced injury in rat neocortical neuronal culture (abstr). *Soc for Neurosci* 21:218, 1995.
9. Jiang C, Haddad GG: Oxygen deprivation inhibits a K^+ channel independently of cytosolic factors in central neurons. *J Physiol (Lond)* 481:15–26, 1994.
10. Jiang C, Haddad GG: A direct mechanism for sensing low oxygen levels by central neurons. *Proc Natl Acad Sci USA* 91:7198–7201, 1994.
11. Jiang C, Sigworth FJ, Haddad GG: O_2 deprivation activates an ATP-inhibitable K^+ channels in substantia nigra neurons. *J Neurosci* 14:5590–5602, 1994.
12. Friedman JE, Haddad GG: Major differences in $Ca^{2+}{}_i$ between neonatal and adult rat CA1 neurons in response to anoxia: role of $Ca^{2+}{}_o$ and $Na_o{}^+$. *J Neurosci* 13(1):63–72, 1993.
13. Kass IS, Lipton P: Protection of hippocampal slices from young rats against anoxic transmission damage is due to better maintenance of ATP. *J Physiol* 413:1–11, 1989.
14. Jiang C, Haddad GG: The effect of anoxia on intracellular and extracellular potassium activity in hypoglossal neurons in vitro. *J Neurophysiol* 66:103–111, 1991.
15. Archer SL, Huang J, Henry TD, et al: A redox-based O_2 sensor in rat pulmonary vasculature. *Circ Res* 73:1100–1112, 1993.
16. Lopez-Barneo J, Lopez-Lopez JR, Urena J, et al: Chemotransduction in the carotid body: K^+ current modulated by Po_2 in type I chemoreceptor cells. *Science* 241: 580–582, 1988.
17. Peers C: Hypoxic suppression of K^+ currents in type I carotid body cells: selective effect on the Ca^{2+} activated K^+ current. *Neurosci Lett* 119:253–256, 1990.
18. Post J, Hume J, Weir E: Direct role of potassium channel inhibition in hypoxic pulmonary vasoconstriction. *Am J Physiol* 262:C882-C890, 1992.
19. Post J, Weir EK, Archer SL, et al: Redox regulation of K^+ channels and hypoxic pulmonary vasoconstriction. In: Weir EK, Hume J (eds). *Ion Flux in Pulmonary Vascular Control.* New York: Plenum Press; 189–204, 1993.
20. Ruppersberg JP, Stocker M, Pongs O, et al: Regulation of fast inactivation of cloned mammalian IK(A) channels by cysteine oxidation. *Nature* 352:711–714, 1991.

Chapter 22

Ischemia and Oxidative Regulation of Neuronal Calcium-Permeable AMPA Receptors

Laura L. Dugan
Dorothy M. Turetsky
Chung Y. Hsu
Dennis W. Choi

Introduction

Glutamate, which represents the major excitatory neurotransmitter in mammalian brain, acts through three types of ionotropic receptors: N-methyl-D-aspartate (NMDA); -amino-3-hydroxy-5-methyl-4-isoxazole-propionic acid (AMPA); and kainate receptors. Overactivation of glutamate receptors —"excitotoxicity"— has been implicated as an important injury process in central nervous system (CNS) hypoxia-ischemia. Such excitotoxic neuronal damage has been attributed in part to receptor-gated calcium (Ca^{2+}) influx,[1] and although initial attention was focused on the role of the highly Ca^{2+}-permeable NMDA receptor in excitotoxic neuronal injury,[2–4] more recent studies have reported that activation of AMPA or kainate receptors can also lead to neuronal loss.[5–7]

Most AMPA or kainate-type glutamate receptor channels are permeable only to monovalent cations. This relative impermeability to Ca^{2+} demonstrated by most AMPA receptors (compared to NMDA receptors) corre-

From: López-Barneo, J and Weir, EK: *Oxygen Regulation of Ion Channels and Gene Expression*. Armonk, NY: Futura Publishing Company, Inc., ©1998.

lates well with the longer exposure times necessary for AMPA or kainate to cause neuronal death.[8] For example, 5-minute exposure to NMDA will result in death of nearly half of all neurons over the next few hours, while 5-minute exposure to AMPA is essentially nontoxic. Over the past few years, however, subpopulations of neurons bearing Ca^{2+}-permeable AMPA or kainate receptors have been identified in hippocampus,[9] cerebellum,[0–11] cortex,[12–13] and spinal cord.[14] Such Ca^{2+}-permeable AMPA/kainate receptors allow rates of $^{45}Ca^{2+}$ influx similar to NMDA[16] and increased vulnerability to kainate receptor-mediated neuronal death.[12,17] Expression studies have demonstrated that AMPA receptor Ca^{2+}-permeability depends on the subunit composition of the receptor, with the inclusion of an edited GluR 2/GluR B subunit dominantly conferring Ca^{2+}-impermeability to the AMPA receptor channel (Figure 1).[18–19]

Since AMPA receptor subunit expression and resultant cation permeability would likely have important functional consequences, considerable attention has been focused on changes in the relative abundance of AMPA receptor subunits during development and after various neurological insults. Subsequent to an initial report by Pellegrini-Giampietro and col-

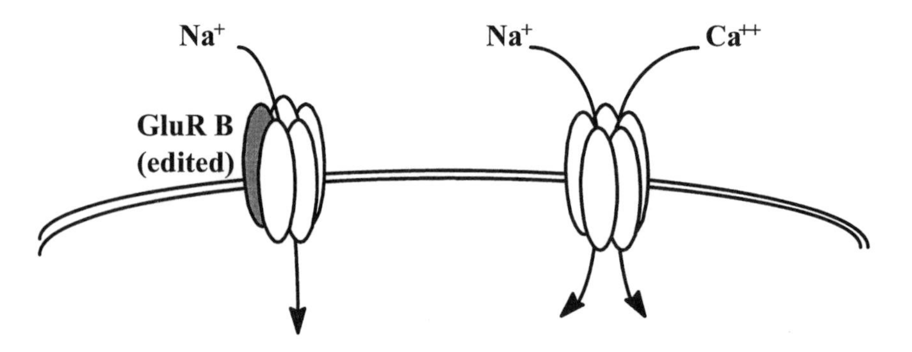

Figure 1. The presence of a GluR B subunit (in its edited Q → R form) determines cation selectivity of AMPA receptor channels. Channels which lack GluR B are highly permeable to Ca^{2+} as well as Na^{+}. Editing of GluR B occurs via a specific adenosine deaminase, which converts an adenosine in the GluR B mRNA to an inosine, resulting in substitution of arginine for glutamine in the protein product.

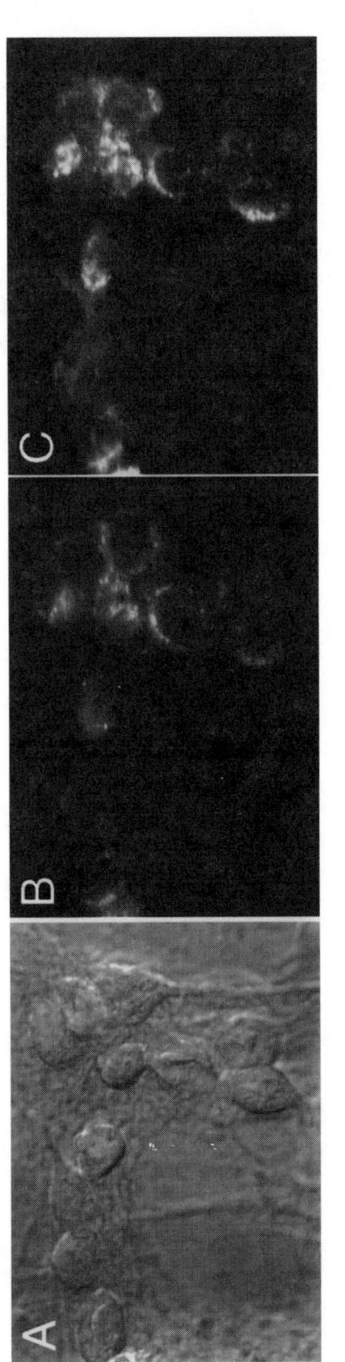

Figure 2. Confocal images of cortical neurons generating ROS following NMDA receptor stimulation. **A.** Differential interference contrast image of a field of cultured neurons using Nomarski optics. **B.** Fluorescence photomicrograph of same field showing low basal fluoresence intensity due to oxidation of dihydrorhodamine 123 to its fluorescent product, rhodamine 123. **C.** Increased fluorescence 15 minutes after application of 100 mm NMDA for 5 minutes. Sham washed controls had no fluorescence increase over the same period (not shown).

leagues[20] that selective decreases in GluR B messenger ribonucleic acid (mRNA) occurred in the hippocampal CA1 region after global ischemia, decreased GluR B mRNA or protein has been reported in kainate induced-seizures[21–22] and in a model of amygdaloid kindling.[23] Although the mechanism by which these insults decrease GluR B expression remains unclear, we noted that one possibility might be enhanced free radical generation. Production of reactive oxygen species (ROS) has been documented to occur during excitotoxicity[24–26] (Figure 2), as well as in CNS hypoxia-ischemia[27–29] (Figure 3). We set out to test the hypothesis that

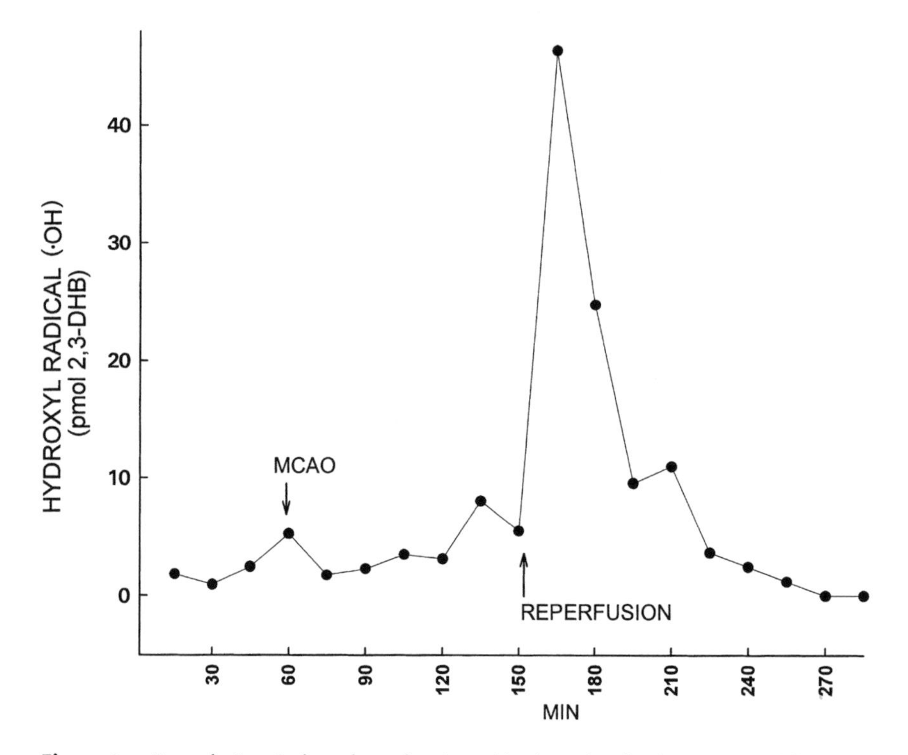

Figure 3. Reperfusion-induced production of hydroxyl radical in a rat middle cerebral artery occlusion (MCAO) model of focal ischemia. Salicylate was included in artificial cerebrospinal fluid which was dialyzed through a microprobe implanted 2 mm deep in the ipsilateral cortex prior to onset of ischemia. After equilibration, the dialysate was collected every 15 minutes during ischemia (90 minutes), and following reperfusion (120 minutes). The hydroxyl radical metabolite of salicylate (2,3-dihydroxybenzoic acid; DHB) was analyzed by HPLC in line with an electrochemical detector. A several-fold increase in ·OH was observed within 15 minutes after the reintroduction of oxygen. (From Reference 30.)

brief, nonlethal oxidative stress could alter AMPA receptor subunit expression. An abstract of this work has appeared.[30]

Experimental Procedures

Cell Culture

Cortical neuronal cultures, containing neurons only, or neurons and glia, were prepared as previously described.[31] Briefly, dissociated neocortices obtained from fetal mice at 14 to 16 days gestation were plated onto culture plates coated with poly-D-lysine:laminin (pure neuronal), or onto a previously established glial monolayer (mixed cultures). Medium was changed biweekly. Neurons for imaging experiments were prepared similarly, on 35 mm culture dishes possessing an oval cutout sealed by a glass cover slip.[25] Experiments were performed between days 14 and 18 in vitro.

Confocal Microscopy for Neuronal Reactive Oxygen Species

Confocal microscopy and detection of ROS formation were performed as described.[25] Cultures were washed into hydroxyethylpiperazine-N′-2-ethane sulfonic acid (HEPES), bicarbonate-buffered balanced salt solution (HBBSS, containing, in mM, 116 NaCl, 5.4 KCl, 0.8 $MgSO_4$, 1.8 $NaPO_4$, 12 HEPES, 25 $NaHCO_3$, 5.5 D-glucose, pH 7.40). Dihydrorhodamine 123 (Molecular Probes, Eugene, OR) stock (10 mM) made in dimethyl sulfoxide (DMSO) was stored at $-20°$ C, and used for only 3 to 4 days of experiments. Stock solutions have been shown to contain a small amount of contaminating rhodamine 123, as measured using a Perkin-Elmer LB50 Fluorescence Spectrometer. Cells loaded with 5 μM dihydrorhodamine were incubated at 37° C in a 5% carbon dioxide (CO_2) incubator for 30 minutes prior to microscopy.

In cells loaded with dihydrorhodamine, cellular fluorescence was imaged using a laser scanning confocal microscope (Noran Odyssey), with an argon-ion laser coupled to an inverted microscope (Nikon Diaphot) equipped with a 60× oil-immersion objective (Nikon Plan Apo, N.A. 1.4). For dihydrorhodamine, excitation $\lambda = 488$ nm and fluorescence is monitored at > 515 nm. The laser beam was attenuated to less than 5% of maximum illumination, and laser exposure limited to brief image acquisition intervals (2 sec every 4 min) using a computer-controlled shutter. Laser settings and exposure duration were held constant for all experiments. Frame-averaged confocal images were digitized at 512 × 480 or 640 × 480 pixels using microcomputer-based imaging software (MetaMorph, Universal Imaging). Exposure to NMDA was carried out by application of 100 μM NMDA (added as an aliquot of a 20 mM stock) to 1 mL medium in the culture dish, and was terminated by addition of the receptor antagonist, MK-801 (10 μM, also as an aliquot from a 5 mM stock). Combined oxygen, glucose deprivation was performed as described. Cultures were placed in an anoxic chamber ($O_2 < 2$ mm Hg), and the media was exchanged three times with a balanced salt solution (BSS_0) lacking glucose and oxygen. After 60 minutes, the cells were washed back into oxygen, glucose-containing medium containing dihydrorhodamine, and returned to the aerobic culture incubator for 20 minutes.

Microdialysis and Analysis of Reactive Oxygen Species in Ischemia-Reperfusion In Vivo

Artificial cerebrospinal fluid (ACSF) containing salicylic acid (1 mM) was dialyzed through a probe implanted in the region of the cortex which typically encompasses the ischemic penumbra, and rats were then subjected to ischemia for 90 minutes, followed by reperfusion. Samples were collected every 15 minutes, and analyzed by High Performance Liquid Chromatography (HPLC) for production of the ·OH metabolite of salycylate, 2,3-dihydroxybenzoic acid.[29]

Pretreatment with Hydrogen Peroxide and Reactive Oxygen Species Generating Systems

Cells were washed into a HEPES-bicarbonate buffered salt solution (HBBSS: 116 mM NaCl, 5.4 mM KCl, 0.8 mM MgSO4 , 1.8 mM NaPO4, 1.8 mM CaCl2, 5.5 mM glucose, 12 mM HEPES acid, 25 mM NaHCO3, pH 7.4). Cultures were then treated with hydrogen peroxide (H_2O_2) (60 μM + 10 μM MK-801) and placed into the 5% CO_2 incubator for 30 minutes. The culture medium was then replaced three times to remove H_2O_2, and the cultures returned to the incubator for 24 hours.

Kainate-Activated Cobalt Uptake

Cobalt uptake was performed as described.[10] Cells were exposed to 100 μM kainate, plus 5 mM $CoCl_2$ in uptake buffer (139 mM sucrose,

57.5 mM NaCl, 5 mM KCl, 2 mM $MgCl_2$, 1 mM $CaCl_2$, 12 mM glucose, 10 mM Hepes, pH 7.6) for 25 minutes at room temperature. Cultures were then washed in uptake buffer plus 3 mM ethylenediaminetetraacetic acid (EDTA) to remove extracellular Co^{2+}, and incubated in 0.12% $(NH_4)_2S$ for 5 minutes to precipitate intracellular Co^{2+}. After three washes in uptake buffer, cells were fixed in 4% paraformaldehyde for 30 minutes.

For silver enhancement, cultures were washed three times in development buffer (292 mM sucrose, 15.5 mM hydroquinone, 42 mM citric acid), and incubated in 0.1% silver nitrate ($AgNO_3$) in development buffer at 50° C on a slide warmer. This solution was changed at 15-minute intervals until complete, and the reaction was terminated by triple exchange of the medium with warm development buffer.

The number of Co^{2+}-positive cells was determined by direct counts under bright field optics. Eight adjacent 200× fields running along a radius of the well were counted in each culture to ensure a representative sample of neuronal density. In each experiment, the number of Co^{2+}-positive cells in treated conditions was normalized to the number in sham-washed cultures to determine percent change in the Co^{2+}-positive population.

^{45}Calcium Influx Assay

Twenty-four hours after H_2O_2 pretreatment, cultures were washed into HBBSS and exposed to excitatory amino acids in the presence of 2 μCi/mL $^{45}Ca^{2+}$ (New England Nuclear) for 15 minutes.[8] After exposure, cells were washed thoroughly to remove all traces of $^{45}Ca^{2+}$, and the cell layer extracted in 0.2% SDS. Cell lysates then underwent β-counting.

Exposure to N-Methyl-D-Aspartate Leads to Production of Oxygen Radicals

Neurons exposed to NMDA rapidly increase production of ROS, detectable as increased fluorescence from oxidation of the nonfluorescent compound, dihydrorhodamine 123, to its fluorescent product, rhodamine 123.[25] This increase in fluorescence was not blocked by a nitric oxide synthase inhibitor (N^G-L-Arginine, 1 mM, 15 minute pretreatment), or an inhibitor of arachidonic acid metabolism (Meclofenamate, 100 μM), but was attenuated by two inhibitors of the mitochondrial electron transport chain, rotenone 10 μM (with MK-801) or Antimycin A (1 μg/mL with MK-801), and by removal of oxygen. Application of kainate failed to cause enhanced radical formation. Similar results were obtained by electron paramagnetic resonance spectroscopy using a spin-trapping agent.[25]

Production of ROS can be observed in vivo in ischemia-reperfusion, as well (Figure 3). Within minutes after reintroduction of oxygen, a substantial increase in salicylate oxidation was observed.[29] Similarly, preliminary data in vitro suggest that there is enhanced formation of ROS following oxygen-glucose deprivation, and that this increase can be blocked, in part, by NMDA receptor antagonists.

Overactivation of NMDA and AMPA/ Kainate Receptors Differentially Affects Reactive Oxygen Species Production

Overactivation of glutamate receptors, as either a primary or secondary event, is believed to occur in many types of CNS injury. One consequence of overactivation of NMDA receptors appears to be enhanced production of ROS, with the mitochondrial electron transport chain likely to be an important (but not the only) source. While our data suggest that NMDA and AMPA/kainate receptors may differ in their ability to recruit downstream pathways which generate ROS during insults such as ischemia-repersion injury, there may be many different pathological processes contributing to the substantial production of ROS observed both in vivo and in vitro. While reactive oxygen species generated in the setting of CNS trauma, ischemia, and other disease states may produce direct injury to CNS cells, it is also likely that ROS may have more delayed effects on gene regulation. We explored the ability of ROS to affect the GluR B subunit because of its important role in determining Ca^{2+}-permeability of AMPA receptors, and the fact that lack of this subunit may confer enhanced vulnerability on selected neuronal populations.

Sublethal Exposure to H_2O_2 Increases the Expression of Ca^{2+}-Permeable AMPA/Kainate Receptors in Neurons

Approximately 13% of cultured cortical neurons exhibit kainate-activated cobalt uptake, a marker for cells bearing Ca^{2+}-permeable AMPA/ kainate receptors.[12] Cultures exposed to a nontoxic concentration of H_2O_2 (60 μM H_2O_2 + 10 μM MK-801)[32] had a 25% increase in the number of neurons with Ca^{2+}-permeable AMPA/kainate receptors over the subsequent 24 hours (Figure 4A). Coapplication of 30 μM NBQX *during* Co^{2+}

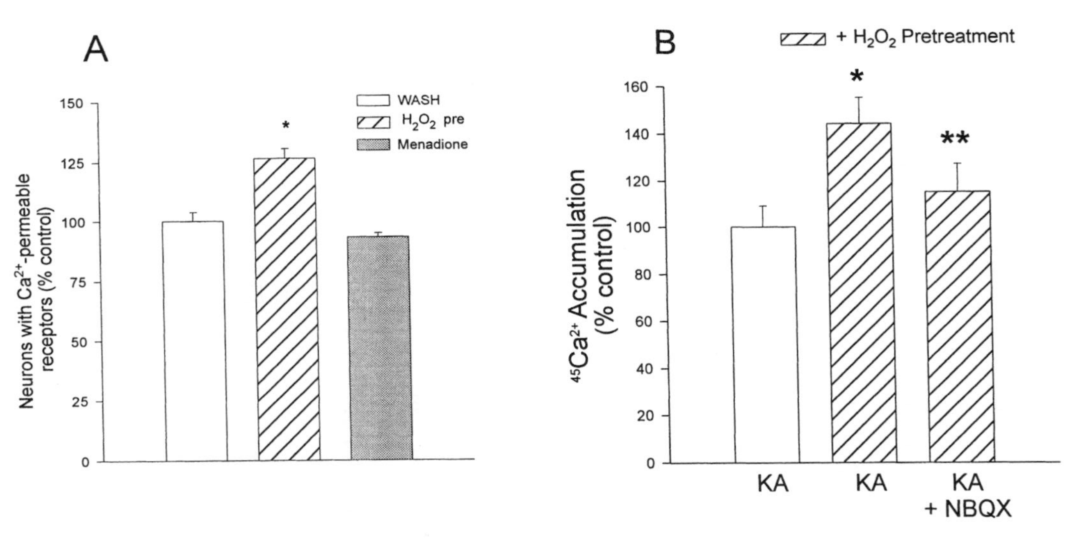

Figure 4. Exposure of cortical neuronal cultures to a sublethal concentration of H_2O_2 results in a delayed increase (25% at 24 hours) in the number of neurons (**A**) with Ca^{2+}-permeable AMPA/kainate receptors, as detected by a histochemical stain for kainate-stimulated Co^{2+} uptake which is specific for Ca^{2+}-permeable AMPA/kainate receptors. Menadione, which generates superoxide anion, failed to mimic the effect of H_2O_2 (**A**), indicating that the phenomenon might be specific for H_2O_2. H_2O_2 pretreatment not only increased the number of neurons with Ca^{2+}-permeable AMPA/kainate receptors, but increased the amount of kainate-stimulated Ca^{2+} entry (**B**), as detected by kainate-stimulated tracer $^{45}Ca^{2+}$ uptake.

staining eliminated all kainate-stimulated Co^{2+} uptake in both control and H_2O_2-treated cultures (not shown), indicating that Co^{2+} entry continued to be through Ca^{2+}-permeable AMPA/kainate receptors (and not due to nonspecific membrane damage). The effect appears to be specific for hydroxyl radical, since neither 30-minute pretreatment with menadione (1 μM), a superoxide generator (Figure 4A), nor DEA/NO (1 mM), a nitric oxide generator (not shown) altered the number of cobalt-positive neurons.

Cultures exposed to H_2O_2 24 hours previously also showed enhanced uptake of tracer $^{45}Ca^{2+}$ during a 15-minute stimulation with 100 μM kainate + 10 μM MK-801 (Figure 4B). Again, inclusion of 30 μM NBQX in the stimulation solution reduced $^{45}Ca^{2+}$ accumulation to baseline levels, suggesting that the increased $^{45}Ca^{2+}$ influx was via AMPA/kainate receptors.

The increase in percentage of neurons with Ca^{2+}-permeable AMPA/kainate receptors required several hours to appear; preliminary data indicates that there is a delayed, selective decrease in newly synthesized GluR B protein. Twenty-four-hour ^{35}S-methionine labeling of pure neuronal cultures and subsequent immunoprecipitation showed GluR B levels to be reduced by approximately one third. Levels of GluR A were only slightly reduced in H_2O_2 treated cultures, and GluR D levels were generally nondetectable. GluR C, which is either less abundant, or detected with less efficiency by the antibody, may also have somewhat decreased levels after H_2O_2 treatment. Overall levels of protein synthesis, as assessed by TCA precipitation of ^{35}S-methionine labeled pure neuronal cultures, were unaffected by H_2O_2 pretreatment (not shown).

The pattern of decreased GluR B expression seen after H_2O_2 pretreatment is similar to the changes observed after global ischemia[20] and kainate-induced seizures.[22] Both of these injury paradigms caused alterations in AMPA receptor subunit mRNA by 12 hours after the insult. Although the decrease in GluR B expression seen 24 hours after H_2O_2 treatment is not as large as that reported after global ischemia[20] or kainate-induced seizures,[22] it should be noted that both of the later studies were measuring mRNA levels in cells destined to die. In a study examining AMPA receptor subunit protein levels in piriform cortex/amygdala after amygdaloid kindling, Prince and colleagues[23] found a 25% reduction in total GluR B protein 24 hours after the last severe seizure, a change more in line with changes we observed. It should also be noted that the decreases in GluR B expression reported after global ischemia or kainate-induced seizures have been assayed in subfields of the hippocampal pyramidal cell layer, a layer where all cells exhibit kainate-activated cobalt uptake. Our measurements were made in a system where only a minority of the cells are cobalt positive, and it is possible that cells already expressing Ca^{2+}-permeable AMPA receptors regulate GluR B differently.

References

1. Choi DW: Calcium: still center-stage in hypoxic-ischemic neuronal death. *Trends Neurosci* 18:58–60, 1995.
2. Meldrum B: Possible therapeutic applications of antagonists of excitatory amino acid transmitters. *Clin Sci* 68:113–122, 1985.
3. Rothman SM, Olney JW: Glutamate and the pathophysiology of hypoxic-ischemic brain damage. *Ann Neurol* 19:105–111, 1986.
4. Choi DW: Glutamate neurotoxicity and diseases of the nervous system. *Neuron* 1:623–634, 1988.
5. Spencer P, Lynch MA, Bliss TV: In-vitro release of [14C]glutamate from dentate gyrus is modulated by GABA. *J Pharm Pharmacol* 38:393–395, 1986.
6. Teitelbaum JS, Zatorre RJ, Carpenter S, et al: Neurologic sequelae of domoic acid intoxication due to the ingestion of contaminated mussels. *N Engl J Med* 322:1781–1787, 1990.
7. Sheardown MJ, Nielsen EO, Hansen AJ, et al: 2,3-ihydroxy-6-nitro-7-sulfamoyl-benzo(F)quinoxaline: a neuroprotectant for cerebral ischemia. *Science* 247: 571–574, 1990.
8. Hartley DM, Kurth MC, Bjerkness L, et al: Glutamate receptor-induced $^{45}Ca^{2+}$ accumulation in cortical cell culture correlates with subsequent neuronal degeneration. *J Neurosci* 13:1993–2000, 1993.
9. Iino M, Ozawa S, Tsuzuki K: Permeation of calcium through excitatory amino acid receptor channels in cultured rat hippocampal neurons. J Physiol 424: 151–165, 1990.
10. Pruss RM, Akeson RL, Racke MM, et al: Agonist-activated cobalt uptake identifies divalent cation-permeable kainate receptors on neurons and glial cells. *Neuron* 7:509–518, 1991.
11. Brorson JR, Bleakman D, Chard PS: Calcium directly permeates kainate/alpha-amino-3-hydroxy-5-methyl-4-isoxazolepropionic acid receptors in cultured cerebellar Purkinje neurons. *Mol Pharmacol* 41:603–608, 1992.
12. Turetsky DM, Canzoniero LMT, Sensi SL, et al: Cortical neurons exhibiting kainate-activated Co^{2+} uptake are selectively vulnerable to AMPA/kainate receptor-mediated toxicity. *Neurobiol Dis* 3:101–110, 1994.
13. Jonas P, Spruston N: Mechanisms shaping glutamate-mediated excitatory postsynaptic currents in the CNS. *Curr Opin Neurobiol* 4:366–372, 1994.
14. Carriedo SG, Yin HZ, Lamberta R, et al: In vitro kainate injury to large, SMI-32(+) spinal neurons is Ca^{2+} dependent. *Neuroreport* 6:945–948, 1995.
15. Lu YM, Yin HZ, Weiss JH: Ca^{2+} permeable AMPA/kainate channels permit rapid injurious Ca^{2+} entry. *Neuroreport* 6:1089–1092, 1995.
16. Gu JG, Albuquerque C, Lee CJ, et al: Synaptic strengthening through activation of Ca^{2+}-permeable AMPA receptors. *Nature* 381:793–796, 1996.
17. Brorson JR, Manzolillo PA, Miller RJ: Ca^{2+} entry via AMPA/KA receptors and excitotoxicity in cultured cerebellar Purkinje cells. *J Neurosci* 14:187–197, 1994.
18. Hollmann M, Hartley M, Heinemann S: Ca^{2+} permeability of KA-AMPA—gated glutamate receptor channels depends on subunit composition. *Science* 252: 851–853, 1991.
19. Verdoorn TA, Burnashev N, Monyer H, et al: Structural determinants of ion flow through recombinant glutamate receptor channels. *Science* 252:1715–1718, 1991.

20. Pellegrini-Giampietro DE, Zukin RS, Bennett MV, et al: Switch in glutamate receptor subunit gene expression in CA1 subfield of hippocampus following global ischemia in rats. *Proc Natl Acad Sci USA* 89:10499–10503, 1992. (published erratum appears in *Proc Natl Acad Sci USA* 90:780, 1993.)
21. Pollard H, Heron A, Moreau J, et al: Alterations of the GluR-B AMPA receptor subunit flip/flop expression in kainate-induced epilepsy and ischemia. *Neuroscience* 57:545–554, 1993.
22. Friedman LK, Pellegrini-Giampietro DE, Sperber EF, et al: Kainate-induced status epilepticus alters glutamate and GABAA receptor gene expression in adult rat hippocampus: an in situ hybridization study. *J Neurosci* 14:2697–1707, 1994.
23. Prince HK, Conn PJ, Blackstone CD, et al: Down-regulation of AMPA receptor subunit GluR2 in amygdaloid kindling. *J Neurochem* 64:462–465, 1995.
24. Lafon-Cazal M, Pietri S, Culcasi M, et al: NMDA-dependent superoxide production and neurotoxicity. *Nature* 364:535–537, 1993.
25. Dugan, LL, Sensi, SL, Canzoniero, LMT, et al: Mitochondrial production of reactive oxygen species in cortical neurons following exposure to N-methyl-D-aspartate. *J Neurosci* 15:6377–6388, 1995.
26. Reynolds IJ, Hastings TG: Glutamate induces the production of reactive oxygen species in cultured forebrain neurons following NMDA receptor activation. *J Neurosci* 15:3318–3327, 1995.
27. Cao, W, Carney, JM, Duchon, A, et al: Oxygen free radical involvement in ischemia and reperfusion injury to brain. *Neurosci Lett* 88:233–238, 1988.
28. Zini I, Tomasi A, Grimaldi, et al: Detections of free radicals during brain ischemia and reperfusion by spin trapping and microdialysis. *Neurosci Lett* 138:279–282, 1992.
29. Dugan LL, Lin TT, He YY, et al: Detection of free radicals by microdialysis/spin trapping EPR following focal cerebral ischemia-reperfusion and a cautionary note on the stability of 5,5-dimethyl-1-pyrroline N-oxide (DMPO). *Free Rad Res* 23:27–32, 1995.
30. Dugan LL, Turetsky DM, Snider BJ, et al: H_2O_2 induces a delayed increase in the number of cortical neurons with Ca^{2+}-permeable AMPA/kainate receptors, and enhances kainate-induced Ca^{2+} entry. *Soc Neurosci Abs* 353, 1995.
31. Dugan LL, Bruno VMG, Amagasu SM, et al: Glia modulate the response of murine cortical neurons to excitotoxicity: glia exacerbate AMPA neurotoxicity. *J Neurosci* 15:4545–4555, 1995.
32. Dugan LL, Choi DW: Exposure to oxygen free radicals potentiates injury in cortical cultures. *Soc Neurosci Abs* 1993.

Section 6

SENSITIVITY TO HYPOXIA

Chapter 23

Short- and Long-Term Modulation of Oxygen Sensitivity:
Lessons from the Carotid Body

Prem Kumar
David R. Pepper

Introduction

Given the pivotal role of molecular oxygen in not only the production of metabolic energy, but also in gene expression and bioelectric phenomena, it is perhaps not surprising that the ability to sense oxygen appears to be a ubiquitous feature of cell physiology.[1] Such a sensing mechanism may have evolved initially to enable single-celled organisms to combat the potential production of the high, lethal amounts of reactive oxygen species generated during aerobic metabolism. With the evolution of multicellular organisms, many cells would no longer be in direct contact with the atmosphere and the establishment of an essentially energy-conserving and protective response to oxygen lack (hypoxia) may, thus, have also proved beneficial to these cells. This ability for self-preservation at the level of the individual cell would not, however, be absolute and if the state of hypoxia were not relieved, the cell would eventually fail and die. The sensing of low oxygen partial pressure (Po_2), at a systemic level, coupled to appropriate, coordinated, cardiorespiratory reflexes, would then have conferred an adaptive potential to the whole organism allowing

From: López-Barneo, J and Weir, EK: *Oxygen Regulation of Ion Channels and Gene Expression.* Armonk, NY: Futura Publishing Company, Inc., ©1998.

the delivery of oxygen at an appropriately high tension (Po_2) in the face of varying metabolic, environmental, or pathologic demands. Many cell types appear to have become specialized in the sensing of low Po_2; these include systemic and pulmonary arterial smooth muscle, certain central neurones, and adrenal chromaffin cells (as described by others in Chapters 11 and 19), as well as neuroepithelial bodies in the airways,[2] although perhaps the most studied and archetypal oxygen sensor remains the mammalian carotid body. The distinction between oxygen sensing per se and an oxygen sensor may, therefore, be quite subtle and may lie in the range of Po_2 over which the system is maximally sensitive. It could, thus, be argued that the physiologic role of any putative systemic oxygen sensor can only be assessed fully when a quantitative assessment of its oxygen sensitivity is determined. The full definition of any such sensor should, therefore, contain such a measurement. This obviously requires a comparison to be made between measurements made from at least two different levels of Po_2. Unfortunately, this minimum two levels is also commonly the maximum number of levels studied which, assuming the system under investigation is nonlinear (an assumption that should be made until proven otherwise), makes it quite apparent why the oxygen sensitivity of a system is rarely quoted.

In this chapter, we wish to make the case (using the carotid body as our example) that oxygen sensitivity, even within a single system, is so crucially dependent upon a number of contributory factors, that its quantification is only meaningful under the conditions at which it was derived. Specifically, once the stimulus and the response have been satisfactorily defined, mammalian oxygen sensitivity can depend upon (in no particular order): 1) the level of Po_2 around which it is measured; 2) the steady state level of Pco_2/pH; 3) the postnatal age of the cells; 4) the environmental temperature; and 5) the history of arterial oxygenation. Additionally, the effects of these variables upon oxygen sensitivity are not always mutually exclusive.

Stimulus and Response

The stimulus must always be measured at some fixed site which, in most cases, is invariably not the site at which oxygen is being sensed by the cell. The farther away the gas tension is measured from the site of chemoreception, the greater the degree of uncertainty as to the actual stimulus intensity. It is, therefore, important to state how the level of oxygen at the site of measurement might differ from that at the site of the sensor and, if possible, to offer some quantitative assessment of this difference. In the whole animal, arterial chemoreceptor discharge is most often related to arterial blood gas tensions. This is perhaps the best that one can do in this situation and it is certainly preferable to relating discharge to end-tidal gas tensions or, even worse, to inspired tensions where the difference between the recorded stimulus and that reaching the carotid body artery, never mind the carotid body tissue, cannot be known with any certainty.

Chemoreceptors respond to a fall in Po_2 by an increase in the mean level of their steady state discharge frequency.[3] The relation between arterial Po_2 and discharge is nonlinear, increases substantially only at levels of arterial Po_2 below $\approx$ 90 mm Hg (at normal arterial levels of Pco_2). At high levels of stimulation ($<\approx$ 30 mm Hg Po_2), discharge frequency tends to plateau or may even fall. The responses obtained in vivo and those obtained using an in vitro superfused preparation are qualitatively similar; the few differences in the positions of the response curves observed between the two approaches could be explained by differences in the site of measurement of the stimulus intensity. The level of stimulus at the site of transduction, in an in vitro preparation, will clearly be greater than that measured in the superfusate and greater, at any given Po_2, in larger organs due to the increased mass of metabolizing tissue through which gases would need to diffuse. In our preparation, the Po_2 of the superfusate is measured continuously at the surface of the carotid body and is ramped down while discharge is recorded. The resultant in vitro Po_2 stimulus response curve must, therefore, be shifted rightward from that which would be recorded in vivo. The actual rightward shift cannot be determined accurately in our preparation and this is its major limitation. It is, however, possible to calculate (given published measurements of gas solubilities and carotid body metabolic rates[4,5]) that for a sphere of carotid body cells with a radius of 100 μm, a maximum Po_2 difference of $\approx$ 80 mm Hg would exist between the surface and the center of the sphere. Thus, in the worst case, the Po_2 stimulus response curves generated in vitro are shifted to the right by $\approx$ 80 mm Hg Po_2 when compared to similar curves generated in vivo. The depth, within the carotid body, of the cell recorded from would determine the actual Po_2 difference, and some of the variability in the position of the response curves found between preparations may reflect a variability in cell location. Alternatively, of course, there is no reason to exclude the possibility that such variability observed in the whole organ may simply reflect the affinity range of the oxygen sensor(s).

In isolated type I carotid body cells, the Po_2 of the bathing superfusate is assumed to be equivalent to the tissue Po_2 in vivo. Unfortunately, a determination of this tissue Po_2 of the carotid body remains a key issue in chemoreceptor physiology, and knowledge of the position and shape of the tissue stimulus afferent neural response curves is required. The first step in achieving this ideal situation comes from noninvasive, phosphorescence quenching studies which have revealed a strong correlation between microvascular Po_2 and arterial Po_2 and hence with afferent discharge.[6,7] These studies provide a value of microvascular Po_2 of ≈ 50 mm Hg during arterial normoxaemia and, therefore, equate reasonably well with earlier microelectrode measurements of mean tissue Po_2 levels of around 20 to 40 mm Hg.[3] Clearly then, one might not expect to observe a response in single cells until the bath Po_2 falls below ≈ 40 mm Hg. While an exponential response curve must be generated at some point between stimulus transduction and afferent fiber discharge, there is no reason to believe that the shape of the response at a single cell level should mimic that of the response of the whole organ. It is certainly, however, beneficial to any hypothesis based at the single cell level if the response measured is at least positively correlated with the response of the whole organ.

The Level of Po_2

Chemoreceptor discharge increases alinearly with reduced Po_2. This response is well fitted by a single exponential with offset, although hyperbolic functions can and have also been used. If, however, the arterial Po_2 is reduced to below ≈ 20 to 30 mm Hg (in vivo), the discharge increase per unit drop in Po_2 gradually reduces and may even decrease or fail, if the Po_2 is allowed to fall too far. The best fit over the entire range of Po_2 is, thus, sigmoidal and its similarity in shape (although inverted) and position to that of the hemoglobin saturation curve gave rise to the idea that the carotid body could act via desaturation of a sensor with hemoglobin-like properties. Given the alinearity, the sensitivity to oxygen, i.e., the change in response between two defined levels of Po_2, will depend upon the actual levels of Po_2 examined. It is possible, of course, simply to measure the response in the absence of stimulus and then in the presence of a maximal stimulus, i.e., anoxia. This approach has been employed on many occasions and can provide a valuable start in the search for potential chemotransducing mechanisms. Such an approach can also be employed to guarantee a reproducible stimulus between preparations and, thus, avoid the complications outlined in the section above.[8] At its best, however, such a two-point determination of oxygen sensitivity can only provide a mean sensitivity over the entire operational range of the transducer. The generation of a true response curve, therefore, requires the determination of many more stimulus response coordinates, but such an approach can take time during which the system under study may alter its characteristics, more especially in the artificial in vitro situation. A significant return of the response to control levels should, therefore, be determined whenever possible to separate pathology from physiology. In common with many other biological transducer systems, the carotid body chemoreceptor exhibits its highest sensitivity over a stimulus range appropriate for the initiation of corrective reflexes. On either side of this range, the sensitivity is reduced. The range of maximal or near maximal sensitivity can, however, be altered by other variables (as described below) to ensure the optimum response in most situations.

Intracellular pH

As well as transducing arterial Po_2 into afferent neural discharge, the carotid body also responds to elevations in Pco_2 or H^+. Over the physiologic range, the relation between partial pressure of carbon dioxide (Pco_2) or H^+ and discharge is linear. In adult rat carotid bodies, an interdependent interaction between Po_2 and Pco_2 is observed both in vivo[9] and in vitro,[10] such that a unit increase in the intensity of one stimulus has a greater effect upon afferent discharge at more intense levels of the other stimulus. This is best described by a consideration of Pco_2 stimulus response curves generated at different, steady levels of Po_2. This shows that, as Po_2 is decreased, the sensitivity of the receptor to Pco_2 is increased, thus generating a characteristic "fan" of Pco_2 chemoreceptor response curves that is maintained in the whole animal, including humans[11,12] at the level of reflex respiratory responses to these stimuli. The two stimuli clearly do not interact in a simple additive way. Alternatively, this interaction can be observed as an upward and rightward shift in the position of the Po_2 response curve by increasing Pco_2. The responses of chemoreceptors to their stimuli are also quantified by their thresholds. In the case of Po_2, at normal levels of arterial Pco_2, there appears to be no high level of Po_2 at which discharge is silenced, with single fibers, in vitro, exhibiting mean discharge frequencies of $\approx$ 0.5 to 2 Hz at Po_2s in excess of 400 mm Hg and of $\approx$ 2 to 5 Hz at an arterial Po_2 of $\approx$ 100 mm Hg in vivo. There is also no high level of Po_2 at which an increase in Pco_2 fails to excite the receptor. Chemoreceptor discharge is, however, silenced at levels of Pco_2 below $\approx$ 18 mm Hg, with the threshold being lower, at lower values of Po_2, such that the fan of Pco_2 response curves appears to originate from below the Pco_2 abscissa.

Perhaps then, given the relatively ubiquitous nature of oxygen sensing, a more characteristic feature of the carotid body chemoreceptor is the ability of each of its afferent nerve fibers to be able to signal both P_{O_2} and P_{CO_2} and in an interdependent manner. The transduction mechanisms for these two stimuli must, therefore, converge at some point between stimulus detection and the generation of an action potential in the afferent nerve. The basic question as to how and where this interaction occurs has been relatively ignored in recent years, but must be addressed by any unifying hypothesis of chemotransduction. Alterations in intracellular pH (pHi) can affect a number of cellular functions in many different cell types,[13] including ion channel conductances in neural tissue. The carotid body is no exception and the outward potassium (K^+) current in type I cells from different species and at different ages is inhibited by hypercapnia and/or acid.[14,15] It is now apparent that the final common stimulus to an extracellular respiratory or metabolic acidosis is a decrease in pHi; the action of carbon dioxide being mediated via an intracellular acidification subsequent to its carbonic anhydrase-catalyzed hydrolysis to H^+. Isohydric hypercapnia (increasing P_{CO_2} without change in $[H^+]$) is without sustained effect upon pHi,[16] lending further support to the notion of arterial pH rather than P_{CO_2} as the preeminent carotid body chemostimulant as had been previously suggested.[17] A number of transmembrane acid (or acid equivalent) transport mechanisms, whereby carotid body type I cells can regulate their pHi, have now been characterized[18] and these show similarities to other cell types. Thus, at an external pH of 7.4 (in carbon dioxide-bicarbonate buffered media), the type I cell pHi is ca. 7.28 in 10-day-old, neonatal rat cells.[18] (Note that at an external pH of 7.4, but this time in hydroxyethylpiperazine-N'-2-ethane sulfonic acid [HEPES]-buffered saline, the pHi was measured as 7.77,[18] indicating the considerable impact that the choice of buffer may have upon the experimental outcome). Unlike many other cells, however, steady state pHi in the type I cell is extremely sensitive to external pH with a slope coefficient of 0.63 relating pHi to external pH.[16] This is about twice that found in many other cell types.[19,20] The intrinsic (non-carbon dioxide) buffering power of type I cells is low and does not appear different from many other cell types.[18] The carotid body's uniqueness for acid transduction appears, therefore, to lie not in the nature of its proton extrusion mechanisms, but in the tight coupling between type I cell pHi and extracellular acidification by hypercapnia. We have recently shown (Figure), using our in vitro carotid body preparation, that an intracellular acidification of ca. 0.15 pH units caused by the addition of 10 mM of the weak organic acid, sodium propionate, to the extracellular superfusate has similar, multiplicative effects upon the P_{O_2} stimulus response curve in the adult as an

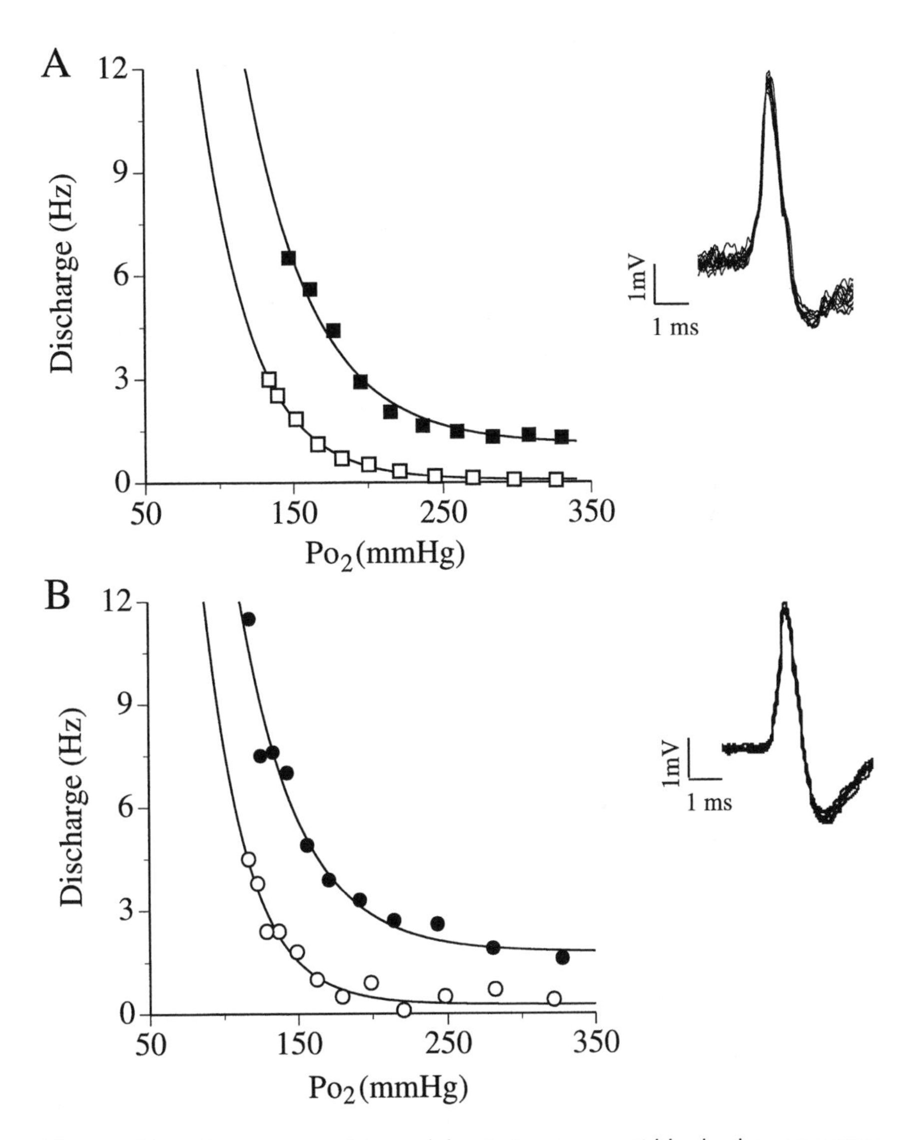

Figure. Hypoxic responses of two adult rats in vitro carotid body chemoreceptor preparations. **A.** The effect of P_{CO_2} (□, 35; ■, 60 mm Hg) and **B.** The effect of sodium propionate (○, 0 mM (control); ●, 10 mM propionate) upon the position of the P_{O_2}-response curve. All data has been fit by single exponentials with offset (**continuous lines**). Vertical distances between the pairs of response curves in both A and B are proportional to CO_2 and propionate sensitivity, respectively, and show a clear P_{O_2} dependence. Superimposed action potentials (**16 traces**) confirm both recordings as single fiber.

elevation of P_{CO_2} to ≈ 60 mm Hg which itself causes an extracellular acidification in bicarbonate-buffered medium of ≈ 0.20 units, i.e., a similar slope coefficient between extra- and intracellular pH as described in single cells.

Postnatal Maturation of Carbon Dioxide-Oxygen Interaction

Fetal chemoreceptors are spontaneously active in utero and show their greatest sensitivity to hypoxia at an arterial P_{O_2} below ≈ 25 mm Hg,[21] i.e., at a considerably lower tension than in the adult, but at a level more commensurate with fetal levels of P_{O_2}. It is now established that with increasing postnatal age after birth, an increase, or resetting, occurs in chemoreceptor afferent sensitivity in vivo and consequently in the reflex respiratory response to an acute hypoxic challenge.[22] Resetting, as described by an increase in hypoxic chemosensitivity, also occurs in vitro and is, therefore, a process intrinsic to carotid body tissue. Perhaps more interestingly, between birth and 5 weeks of age in the rat, a postnatal increase in the degree of interaction between carbon dioxide and hypoxia also occurs, whereby the afferent response to an asphyxial stimulus (i.e., carbon dioxide plus hypoxia) becomes increasingly greater than the sum of the two stimuli given separately.[10] This is seen as a progressively greater rightward shift in the position of the hypoxic response curves with increasing levels of P_{CO_2} in older animals; however, it is most clearly demonstrated as an age-dependent increase in the carbon dioxide sensitivity of the peripheral chemoreceptors with decreasing P_{O_2}, giving rise to the characteristic fan of carbon dioxide response curves in the adult, but producing a set of essentially parallel carbon dioxide response curves in the neonate. It may be suggested, therefore, that resetting, rather than being a development of hypoxic chemosensitivity per se, could be due to an increase in the degree of interaction between the hypoxic and hypercapnic/acidic chemotransduction mechanisms. Designing an experimental protocol to distinguish between these two possibilities remains a challenge. In the context of resetting as an increase in carbon dioxide-oxygen interaction, it is interesting that in adult rat type I cells, pHi in bicarbonate-buffered medium at an external pH of 7.4 is 7.17,[23] i.e., lower than that found in neonatal cells and the slope coefficient relating the two pH levels is even greater at 0.85. Thus, the pHi of the adult may be lower than that of the neonate, and its dependence upon extracellular pH greater, but it should be noted that contamination with nigericin may have affected, adversely, the results from adult cells.[23a].

While the full chemotransduction pathway in the carotid body remains undetermined, there appears a consensus for a stimulus-induced modification of ion channel open probability in the neural crest-derived type I cell as a seminal feature of chemotransduction.[24] It is evident that a variety of calcium (Ca^{2+}), sodium (Na^{+}), chloride (Cl^{-}), and K^{+} currents are present in the membrane of type I cells, and the stimulus-induced, Ca^{2+}-dependent release of putative transmitter(s)[3] lends further support to the idea of the primary transducer residing within this cell type. The specific details of the various ion channels described in these cells differ between groups, but a consistency exists regarding a role for a stimulus-induced inhibition of outward K^{+} currents[25,14,15,2] leading to cell depolarization or an increased electrical activity with concomitant Ca^{2+} entry[27,28] and neurosecretion.[29,30] The controversy revolves around the contribution that these various K^{+} channels make toward the resting membrane potential and the effect of K^{+} channel blockers upon sinus nerve discharge. Thus, patch-clamp studies have demonstrated that hypoxia can depolarize neonatal rat type I cells by reversibly and specifically inhibiting a Ca^{2+}-dependent, high conductance K^{+} current (K^{+}_{ca}),[15,31] while in adult rabbit the K^{+} current inhibited by hypoxia appears Ca^{2+}-independent and of lower conductance.[32] In collaboration with Dr. Chris Peers and colleagues at the University of Leeds, United Kingdom, we have recently described a specific maturational increase in the density of the hypoxia-sensitive, K^{+}_{ca} channels in type I cells of rats between birth and adult.[33] More recently, however, evidence has been forwarded which demonstrates a novel, small conductance, voltage-insensitive K^{+} current in the rat carotid body type I cell that is inhibited by hypoxia, and it has been proposed that this is the sole current responsible for stimulus-induced depolarization.[34] This channel is insensitive to pharmacologic blockers of other K^{+} channels and, thus, appears to fit with findings in adult rat carotid bodies, superfused in vitro, where the addition of charybdotoxin to block K^{+}_{ca} channels fails to increase chemoreceptor discharge in hyperoxia.[35] This does not, however, discount the importance of the voltage-sensitive channels previously described, as upon depolarization, these would become activated, increasing their contribution to the membrane potential and they may, thus, play an important role in the shaping of the hypoxia-response curve of this receptor system. The relative importance of these voltage-sensitive channels is, thus, determined by the membrane potential and perhaps more importantly by the resting membrane potential. No maturational measurements of this important variable have yet been reported.

Temperature

Chemoreceptors are sensitive also to temperature,[36] increasing and decreasing their discharge with increasing and decreasing temperature above and below 37° C, respectively. Experiments in vitro show this thermal sensitivity to be high. Thus, an elevation of temperature by just 2° C can ≈ double resting discharge, while a similar decrease can significantly reduce spontaneous discharge. We find no spontaneous discharge at room temperature in vitro (unpublished observations), a finding that may have some impact on the interpretation of experiments performed on single cells at that temperature. This effect of temperature has reflex consequences, but these are so slight (at least in normoxia) as to make it unlikely that the carotid body acts also as a functional thermosensor. More important, however, is the potential for this thermal sensitivity to act as a modifier of the chemotransduction process. A particularly interesting finding here is that when the superfused carotid body is made mildly hypoxic, increases in temperature now act to decrease discharge.[36] Such an effect, if observed in vivo, could have a profound impact on respiratory control in the overheated, chronically hypoxic neonate. A further effect of increasing temperature is to increase the sensitivity of the chemoreceptors to carbon dioxide,[37] i.e., acting not unlike hypoxia in this respect. Given the interaction between carbon dioxide and hypoxia, these findings may have important consequences during exercise in the adult or in the developing oxygen and carbon dioxide sensitivities seen during the postnatal period, although other consequences of temperature changes in vivo may attenuate the effect observed in vitro.

Chronic Hypoxia

Resetting appears contingent upon the elevation in arterial Po_2 that occurs as a consequence of the postnatal establishment of pulmonary ventilation and of cardiovascular readjustment. While not affecting in any qualitative way, the ability of the carotid body to transduce either hypoxia or hypercapnia, chronic hypoxemia from birth does prevent the natural development of a multiplicative carbon dioxide-oxygen interaction.[38] Thus, at 5 weeks of age, animals reared in a low oxygen environment (≈ 12% inspired oxygen) maintain the responses characteristic of a 5-day-old normoxic neonate. This blunting of hypoxic chemosensitivity in animals and humans who are chronically hypoxic from birth, while similar to the blunting observed in high altitude natives, is in marked contrast to the increased hypoxic sensitivity or acclimatization reported in adult sojourners to altitude. The importance of the carotid bodies in the ventilatory acclimatization to altitude is clear[39] and the intriguing possibility arises, therefore, that there exists a postnatal period where chemoreceptors are particularly vulnerable to blunting by chronic hypoxemia. This appears to be the case as this effect of chronic hypoxia upon carbon dioxide-oxygen interaction is indeed labile.[40] Thus, the blunting effect of chronic hypoxia in newborns was reversible and could be abolished after a 3-week return to room air and adult rats, born into normal, sea level room air and only placed into a hypoxic environmental chamber for 3 to 5 weeks at 3 weeks of age, maintained a significant carbon dioxide-oxygen interaction at the level of the carotid body chemodischarge. Thus, as stated previously,[41] chronic hypoxia should indeed be considered in terms both of the severity of stimulus and the duration of exposure and with a suitable weighting given to the early period of postnatal life. A reduction in the density of the hypoxia-sensitive, K^{+}_{ca} channels in type I cells from rats exposed to chronic hypoxia for $\approx$ 10 days from birth[42] provides further, albeit more circumstantial, evidence that this channel plays a role in resetting, although other differences between the effects of resetting and chronic hypoxia make it almost certain that different mechanisms are operative under these two conditions (see Chapter 13).

Conclusion

This chapter illustrates the importance of a number of factors in determining carotid body oxygen sensitivity and, therefore, also highlights the impact of experimental conditions upon the final response. The electrophysiologic and microfluorometric findings from single cell studies, as well as the new findings from more molecular approaches, will eventually need to explain the often much older and established findings from the whole organ and indeed from the whole animal. Similarly, innovative new experiments on these larger systems will have to be designed to test the physiologic significance of the findings at the more microscopic level as the mechanism of action of this receptor may turn out to be greater than the sum of its component parts.

Acknowledgments

We gratefully acknowledge the financial support of the Medical Research Council and The Wellcome Trust. P. Kumar is a Lister Institute Research Fellow.

References

1. Bunn HF, Poyton RO: Oxygen sensing and molecular adaptation to hypoxia. *Physiol Rev* 76:839–885, 1996.
2. Youngson C, Nurse C, Yeger H, et al: Oxygen sensing in airway chemoreceptors. *Nature* 365:153–155, 1993.
3. Gonzalez C, Almaraz L, Obeso A, et al: Carotid body chemoreceptors — from natural stimuli to sensory discharges. *Physiol Rev* 74:829–898, 1994.
4. Daly M, Lambertson CJ, Schweitzer A: Observations on the volume of blood flow and oxygen utilization of the carotid body in the cat. *J Physiol* 125:67–89, 1954.
5. Forster RE: The diffusion of gases in the carotid body. In: Torrance RW (ed): *Arterial Chemoreceptors*. Oxford: Blackwell Scientific Publications; 115–132, 1968.
6. Rumsey WL, Iturriaga R, Spergel D, et al: Optical measurements of the dependence of chemoreception on oxygen pressure in the cat carotid body. *Am J Physiol* 261:C614-C622, 1991.
7. Lahiri S, Rumsey WL, Wilson DF, et al: Contribution of in vivo microvascular Po_2 in the cat carotid body chemotransduction. *J Appl Physiol* 75:1035–1043, 1993.
8. Kholwadwala D, Donnelly DF: Maturation of carotid chemoreceptor sensitivity to hypoxia: in vitro studies in the newborn rat. *J Physiol* 453:461–473, 1992.
9. Lahiri S, DeLaney RG: Stimulus interaction in the responses of carotid body chemoreceptor single afferent fibers. *Respir Physiol* 24:249–266, 1975.
10. Pepper DR, Landauer RC, Kumar P: Postnatal development of CO_2-O_2 interaction in the rat carotid body in vitro. *J Physiol* 485:531–541, 1995.
11. Nielson M, Smith H: Studies on the regulation of respiration in acute hypoxia. *Acta Physiol Scand* 24:293–313, 1952.
12. Lloyd BB, Jukes MGM, Cunningham DJC: The relation between alveolar oxygen pressure and the respiratory response to carbon dioxide in man. *Q J Exp Physiol* 43:214–227, 1958.
13. Roos A, Boron WF: Intracellular pH. *Physiol Rev* 61:296–434, 1981.
14. Lopez-Lopez J, Gonzalez C, Urena J, et al: Low Po_2 selectively inhibits K channel activity in chemoreceptor cells of the mammalian carotid body. *J Gen Physiol* 93:1001–1015, 1989.
15. Peers C: Hypoxic suppression of K^+ currents in type I carotid body cells — selective effect on the Ca^+-activated K^+ current. *Neurosci Lett* 119:253–256, 1990.
16. Buckler KJ, Vaughan-Jones RD, Peers C, et al: Effects of extracellular pH, Pco_2, and HCO_3 on intracellular pH in isolated type I cells of the neonatal rat carotid body. *J Physiol* 444:703–721, 1991.
17. Hornbein TF, Roos A: Specificity of H ion concentration as a carotid chemoreceptor stimulus. *J Appl Physiol* 18:580–584, 1963.
18. Buckler KJ, Vaughan-Jones RD, Peers C, et al: Intracellular pH and its regulation in isolated type I carotid body cells of the neonatal rat. *J Physiol* 436:107–129, 1991.
19. Ellis D, Thomas RC: Microelectrode measurement of the intracellular pH of mammalian heart cells. *Nature* 262:224–225, 1976.
20. Aickin CC, Thomas RC: Microelectrode measurement of the intracellular pH

and buffering power of mouse soleus muscle fibres. *J Physiol* 267:571–585, 1977.
21. Blanco CE, Dawes GS, Hanson MA, et al: The response to hypoxia of arterial chemoreceptors in fetal sheep and newborn lambs. *J Physiol* 351:25–37, 1984.
22. Hanson MA, Kumar P: Chemoreceptor function in the fetus and neonate. In: O Regan RG, Nolan P, McQueen DS, Paterson DJ (eds): *Advances in Experimental Medicine and Biology*. Vol. 360, Arterial Chemoreceptors. Cell to System. New York: Plenum Publishing; 99–108, 1994.
23. Wilding TJ, Cheng B, Roos A: pH regulation in adult rat carotid body glomus cells — importance of extracellular pH, sodium, and potassium. *J Gen Physiol* 100:593–608, 1992.
23a. Richmond PH, Vaughan-Jones RD: Assessment of evidence for K^+-H^+ exchange in isolated type I cells of neonatal rat carotid body. *Pflugers Archiv* 434: 429–437, 1997.
24. Peers C, Buckler KJ: Transduction of chemostimuli by the type I carotid body cell. *J Membr Biol* 144:1–9, 1995.
25. Delpiano MA, Hescheler J: Evidence for a Po_2-sensitive K + channel in the type I cell of the rabbit carotid body. *FEBS Let* 249:195–198, 1989.
26. Stea A, Nurse CA: Whole-cell and perforated-patch recordings from O_2-sensitive rat carotid body cells grown in short-term and long-term culture. *Pflugers Arch* 418:93–101, 1991.
27. Buckler KJ, Vaughan-Jones RD: Effects of hypoxia on membrane potential and intracellular calcium in rat neonatal carotid body type I cells. *J Physiol* 476: 423–428, 1994.
28. Buckler KJ, Vaughan-Jones RD: Effects of hypercapnia on membrane potential and intracellular calcium in rat neonatal carotid body type I cells. *J Physiol* 478: 157–171, 1994.
29. Gonzalez C, Almaraz L, Obeso A, et al: Oxygen and acid chemoreception in the carotid body chemoreceptors. *Trends Neurosci* 15:146–153, 1992.
30. Montoro RJ, Urena J, Fernandez-Chacon R, et al: Oxygen sensing by ion channels and chemotransduction in single glomus cells. *J Gen Physiol* 107:133–143, 1996.
31. Wyatt CN, Peers C: Ca^{2+}-activated K^+ channels in isolated type I cells of the neonatal rat carotid body. *J Physiol* 483:559–565, 1995.
32. Ganfornina MD, López-Barneo J: Potassium channel types in arterial chemoreceptor cells and their selective modulation by oxygen. *J Gen Physiol* 100: 401–426, 1992.
33. Carpenter E, Hatton CJ, Pepper DR, et al: Developmental changes in isolated rat type I carotid body cell K^+ currents and their responses to hypoxia. *J Physiol* 497P:P26, 1996.
34. Buckler KJ: A novel oxygen sensitive potassium current in rat carotid body type I cells. *J Physiol* 1997. (In press.)
35. Pepper DR, Landauer RC, Kumar P: Effect of charybdotoxin on hypoxic chemosensitivity in the adult rat carotidbody, in vitro. J Physiol 487P:177P-178P, 1995.
36. Alcayaga J, Sanhueza Y, Zapata P: Thermal-dependence of chemosensory activity in the carotid body superfused in vitro. *Brain Res* 600:103–111, 1993.
37. Landauer RC, Pepper DR, Kumar P: Interaction of temperature and CO_2 in the adult rat carotid body, in-vitro. *J Physiol* 489P:162P-163P, 1995.
38. Landauer RC, Pepper DR, Kumar P: Effect of chronic hypoxaemia from birth

upon chemosensitivity in the adult rat carotid body in vitro. J Physiol 485: 543–550, 1995.
39. Smith CA, Bisgard GE, Nielsen AM, et al: Carotid bodies are required for ventilatory acclimatization to chronic hypoxia. J Appl Physiol 60:1003–1010, 1986.
40. Landauer RC, Conway AF, Pepper DR, et al: Age-dependent and reversible effects of chronic hypoxia upon carotid body CO_2-O_2 interaction. *J Physiol* 479P: 25P-26P, 1996.
41. Okuba S, Mortola JP: Long-term respiratory effects of neonatal hypoxia in the rat. *J Appl Physiol* 64:952–958, 1986.
42. Wyatt CN, Wright C, Bee D, et al: O_2-sensitive K^+ currents in carotid body chemoreceptor cells from normoxic and chronically hypoxic rats and their roles in hypoxic chemotransduction. *Proc Natl Acad Sci USA* 92:295–299, 1995.

Chapter 24

Sensitivity to Physiologic Hypoxia

Constancio González

Introduction

Cannon, the discoverer of the fight and flight reaction and, in conjunction with Rosenblueth, the creator of the concept of homeostasis, states in his autobiographical book, *The Way of a Researcher*, that the spirit that guides scientists in their enquiries into the secrets of nature is similar to the one that guided geographical explorers from the sixteenth to the eighteenth centuries to reach every place on our planet. In the physiology of hypoxia, which is the physiology of high altitude, there is a perfect blend of the geographical and the scientific spirit of adventure, as high altitude physiology has been developed in hazardous expeditions to the highest mountains on earth. There are, however, some instances in which important contributions to the understanding of high altitude physiology and medicine have been made with a different guiding spirit. Thus, the first account of mountain sickness in the occidental literature was given by a Jesuit, Father José de Acosta in 1590 in his *Historia Natural y Moral de las Indias* after crossing the Peruvian Andes at an estimated altitude of 4800 meters. In 1624, Jesuit Father Andrade, who was the first European to enter Tibet, thought that the cause of death of many people on the expedition at ≈5500 m was not the emanation of noxious vapors from earth, but the extreme cold and the reduction of the heat of the body. In 1661, another Jesuit, the German Father Grüber, in his crossing from Pe-

From: López-Barneo, J and Weir, EK: *Oxygen Regulation of Ion Channels and Gene Expression.* Armonk, NY: Futura Publishing Company, Inc., ©1998.

king to Kathmandu, wrote that in the mountains men cannot breathe because of the subtlety of the air. Aside from these pioneer observations, it was Paul Bert in the last quarter of the nineteenth century who dissociated cold from hypoxia with the use of decompression chambers. He demonstrated that breathing air at low barometric pressures, like those encountered at high altitudes, was dangerous, and that breathing oxygen even at those low pressures can restore the body functions.[1]

In 1890, Viault described the increase in the number of red blood cells as a response that develops in a short period of time. In 1906, Carnot and Deflandre suggested the presence of an erythropoietic factor in the blood of anemic animals. However, it was only in 1950 when Reissman showed that both partners of parabiotic pairs of rats exhibited normoblastic hypertrophy of the bone marrow, even though only one was subjected to hypoxic breathing, that interest for the erythropoietic factor was revived and the link between hypoxia and erythropoiesis was established. Experiments of nephrectomy in laboratory animals, and clinical observations in patients with chronic renal failure, identified the kidney as the main source for erythropoietin production in adult animals.[2]

Although Pflüger had reported the hyperpneic effect of breathing pure nitrogen (1868), it was only in 1908 that Boycott and Haldane described in detail the ventilatory effects of hypoxic hypoxia. In 1926 and 1928, Fernando de Castro, a disciple of Cajal, described the sensory nature of the carotid body and, in 1930, Heymans demonstrated that perfusion of isolated dogs' head with hypoxic blood produced hyperventilation that disappeared after sectioning the carotid sinus nerve.[3]

Liljestrand and von Euler, in 1946, observed for the first time a rise in pulmonary arterial pressure when cats were given a hypoxic gas mixture to breathe. An increase in pulmonary arterial blood pressure in response to acute hypoxia has been observed in many experimental models and in humans, as well as in subjects adapted to hypoxia and in some populations of native highlanders. Today, it is well established that hypoxia, mainly a decrease in alveolar oxygen partial pressure (Po_2) below 70 mm Hg, produces vasoconstriction of pulmonary arterial vessels, with a preference for the distal segments of the arterial tree. However, there is no consensus on the physiologic significance or the mechanisms of hypoxic pulmonary vasoconstriction.[1,4]

Physiologic Hypoxia:

The Adaptive Responses

Physiologic hypoxia is hypoxic hypoxia produced by ambient factors, i.e., by a decrease in ambient Po_2 as it happens naturally at high altitude due to a decrease in barometric pressure. It is physiologic because it proceeds without any pathology for the entire lifespan of individuals and from generation to generation. A reasonable limit to physiologic hypoxia is an altitude of ≈4,000 m above sea level, corresponding to a barometric pressure of 460 mm Hg, an inspired Po_2 of 87 mm Hg and, before hyperventilation, an alveolar Po_2 of ≈40 mm Hg. Nearly 15 million people live at this altitude, and when adequate corrections are made for racial and nutritional factors, they exhibit no differences from sea level inhabitants in reproduction, growth, or physical performance.[1]

I have mentioned the description of increased red cell mass and hyperventilation, and more recently hypoxic pulmonary vasoconstriction, as the adaptative physiologic responses observed upon short-term exposures to hypoxia, as well as in lowlanders residing at high altitude and in native highlanders. These responses are adaptative in the sense that they tend to reduce the physiologic strain produced by environmental hypoxia. Probably, every author would not agree with the adaptative nature of the forementioned responses, but I shall try to justify it.

The adaptative significance of hyperventilation is universally accepted. Hyperventilation washes the alveoli of carbon dioxide, and since $P_AO_2 \approx FIO_2(BP\text{-}P_{H_2O})\text{-}1.2 \times P_ACo_2$, it follows that a decrease in P_ACo_2 produces an increase in PAO_2. As it is discussed by West,[5] hyperventilation by decreasing P_ACo_2 allows P_AO_2 to approach to the inspired PO_2 (Table 1). The adaptative significance of polycythemia and hypoxic pulmonary vasoconstriction is less clear. There is no doubt that an increase in Hb concentration (for the present discussion, I shall assume a parallel increase in red cell number and Hb concentration) with altitude can com-

Table 1
Respiratory Gases at Different Barometric Pressures

Barometric Pressure/ Altitude (m)	$P_{At}O_2$	$P_{Ins}O_2$	$P_ACO_2/\Delta P_ACO_2$	$P_ACO_2/\Delta P_AO_2$	$C_AO_2/\Delta C_aO_2$ *(mL/100 mL)*
760/Sea level	159	149	40/0	101/0	19.2/0
600/2,000	125	116	34/−6	75/+7	18.4/+0.5
474/4,000	99	89	29/−11	54/+13	16.3/+3.4
370/6,000	77	68	23/−17	40/+20	12.6/+10.5

All pressures are expressed in mm Hg. For the calculation of the arterial O_2-content (C_aO_2) an alveolar-arterial Po_2 difference of 8 mm Hg, a hemoglobin (Hb) content of 14.5 g/100 mL of blood, and an O_2 transporting capacity of 1.34 mL/g of Hb have been assumed. It should be noted that the ventilatory responses are installed within minutes, before any compensatory polycythemia appears.

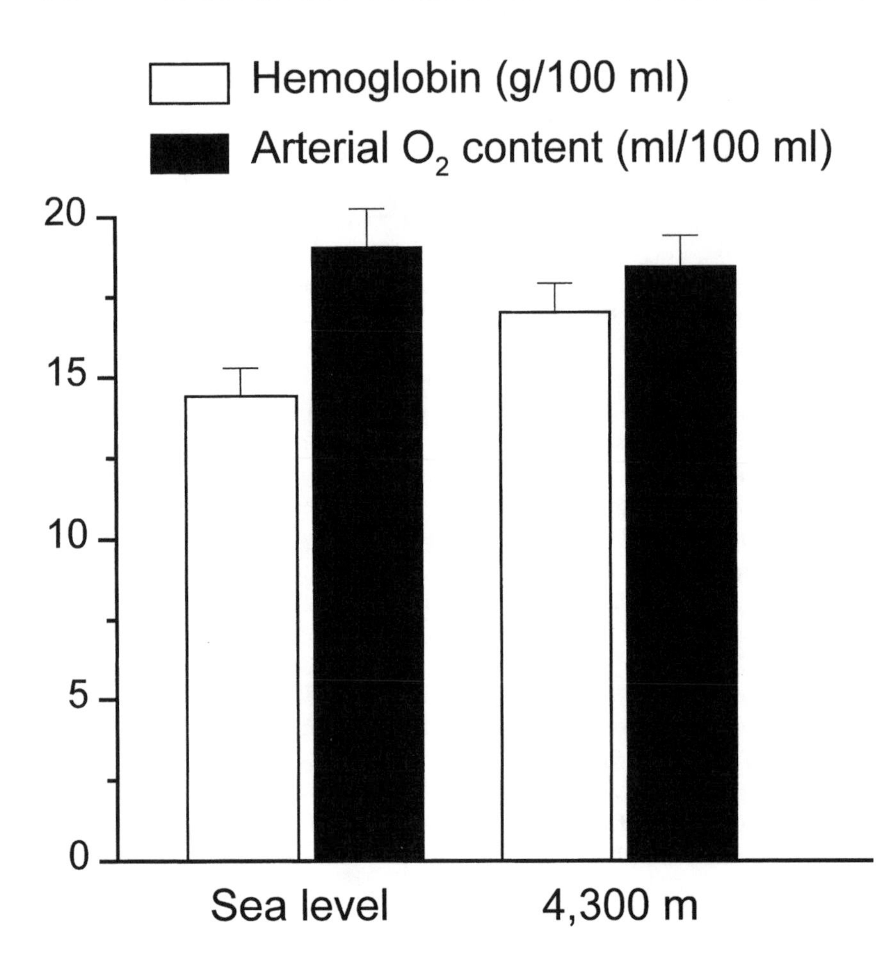

Figure 1. Adaptative polycythemia at high altitude. Hemoglobin concentrations have been taken from Reference 5a. Oxygen content has been calculated with arterial Po_2 of 93 (hemoglobin-O_2 = 97.25%) and 43 mm Hg (hemoglobin-O_2 = 80.36%) at sea level and 4,300 m of altitude, respectively.

pensate for a decrease in Pao_2 and a decrease in the saturation of Hb. It is also well documented that at altitudes well above 4000 m, this compensation results in an arterial oxygen content equal to that at sea level (Figure 1). However, the increase in the viscosity of the blood could offset the beneficial effect of polycythemia causing an increase in the peripheral resistance and, thereby, a decrease in cardiac output. In well acclimatized subjects and in highlanders, this is not the case. Their resting cardiac output, as well as their cardiac output in relation to work, are comparable to those seen at sea level, thereby physiologic polycythemias found at altitudes even higher than 4000 m are beneficial adaptative responses. It should be mentioned that the "loss of adaptation," to use Monge's words, can in fact produce a pathological polycythemia with hypertension and decreased cardiac output in some subjects, that is known as Monge's disease. According to Monge and León-Valverde,[6] a reduced hyperventilatory response to hypoxia (seen more frequently after 50 years of age) may be involved in the pathogenesis of Monge's disease.

The adaptative significance of hypoxic pulmonary vasoconstriction is also in debate. It is universally accepted that hypoxic pulmonary vasoconstriction plays a significant role in diverting the blood from the pulmonary circulation to the placenta in the fetus; it is also accepted that, in local lung pathology, hypoxic pulmonary vasoconstriction ameliorates blood oxygenation by reducing the circulation in nonaereated or poorly aereated alveoli. In fact, the improvement in blood oxygenation produced by almitrine in many types of lung diseases is due in part to the potentiation of hypoxic pulmonary vasoconstriction (almitrine also stimulates ventilation acting on carotid body chemoreceptors). But the real question is whether in generalized lung hypoxia, as it happens at low barometric pressure, pulmonary hypoxic vasoconstriction constitutes a beneficial adaptative response. The consideration of a beneficial effect for this response is frequently dominated, as it is the case with the polycythemic response, by the potential pathology associated with an increase in pulmonary arterial pressure, i.e., lung edema and right ventricular hypertrophy. In a healthy human, a moderate hypoxic pulmonary vasoconstriction should be beneficial, because it would divert blood from the lung bases with lower P_AO_2 (and then with more intense vasoconstriction) to the lung apices with higher P_AO_2. The apices have a relatively poor blood flow at normal pulmonary arterial pressure. A recent study[7] would agree with this notion, since it was found that hypoxia (4559 m, or breathing 10% oxygen at sea level) in control subjects moderately increased pulmonary arterial pressure, and inhalation of nitric oxide, which reduced the pulmonary arterial pressure, and worsened arterial oxygen saturation. On the contrary, in subjects prone to pulmonary edema, the same level of hypoxia produced a more intense pulmonary hypertension and a certain degree of lung edema that ameliorated together with arterial oxygen saturation upon nitric oxide inhalation. These findings lead the authors to conclude that the hyper-reactivity of pulmonary circulation to hypoxia, and the ensuing "loss of adaptation," is the result of a deficit in nitric oxide synthesis. Marshall et al[8] state this notion in a different manner: "the activities of hypoxic pulmonary vasoconstriction span the range from homeostasis to pathophysiology."

Physiologic Sensitivity to Hypoxia

From the above discussion, it is obvious that the adaptative responses generated by the chemoreceptor cells of the carotid body, the erythropoietin producing cells of the kidney, and the smooth muscle cells of the pulmonary artery are directed to the benefit of the entire organism, aiming to prevent hypoxia in body cells, and to maintain their metabolic rate and function. The significance of these responses is best appreciated when the relationship between arterial PO_2 and activation for these three cell types is considered. Figure 2 shows that this relationship is hyperbolic for the three cell types, and that the threshold of the response is around a PO_2 of 70 mm Hg, when the arterial oxygen content is ≈94% of that found at sea level. As a consequence of this threshold, hyperventilation, production of erythropoietin/increase in red cell mass and pulmonary hypoxic vasoconstriction start well before there is a significant drop in the availability of oxygen in the tissues; as a consequence of the shape of the curves, they proceed at progressively increasing intensity as arterial PO_2 continues to decrease.

The relationship between arterial PO_2 and the physiologic responses under consideration should imply that these three cell types must have metabolic machinery capable of supporting their progressively increasing activity as hypoxia increases. It is well documented in a great variety of tissues that sustained increased functional activity requires an increased energetic metabolic rate. In excitable cells, most of the extra energetic demand is used to maintain the ionic balance across cell membranes as a prerequisite for continuous cell spiking, and reflects the activation of the sodium/potassium (Na^+/K^+) pump.[9,10] The available experimental data indicate that this is in fact the situation in chemoreceptor cells of the carotid body during hypoxic stimulation. Thus, in rabbit carotid body, the rate of glucose consumption increased by around 45% under moderate hypoxic stimulation and ouabain completely suppressed this metabolic response.[11] On the contrary, in the nodose ganglion, used as control tissue, the same level of hypoxia did not alter the metabolic rate. Additionally, Verna et al[12] have shown that even more intense levels of hypoxia, capable of markedly increasing the level of discharge in the carotid sinus nerve, did not significantly alter the ATP content of the rabbit carotid body, but as expected[13] produced a significant change in the [ATP]/[ADP][AMP] quotient. In nonexcitable protein-secreting cells, such as erythropoietin producing cells, it is conceivable that activation would be associated with an increase in metabolism aimed to maintain an adequate rate of synthesis of hormone and its secretion, although secretion would require only a small percentage of the total cellular energy expenditure.[9,11]

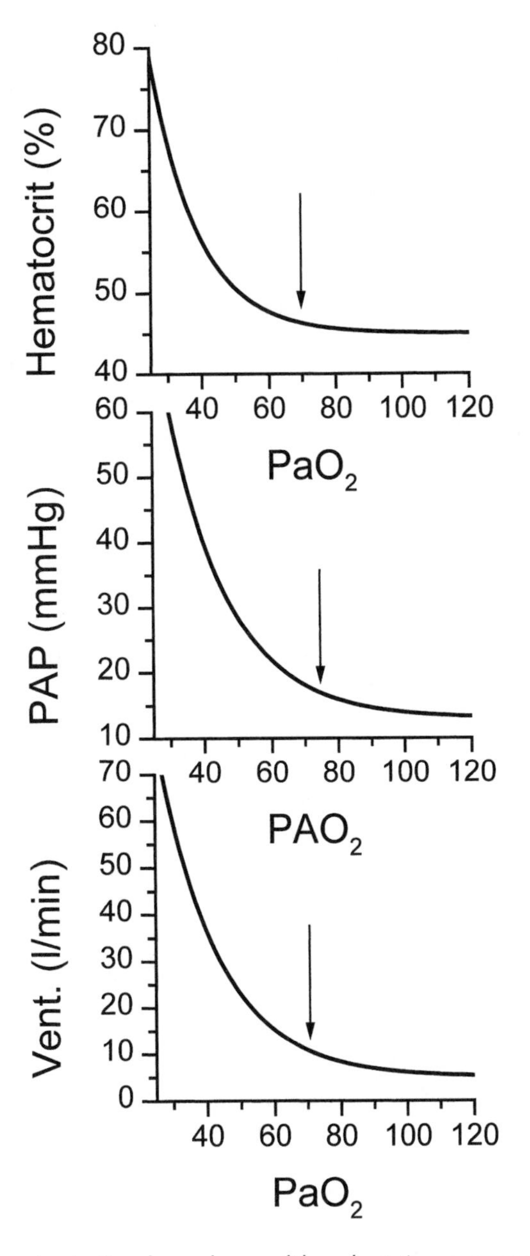

Figure 2. Approximate Po_2 dependence of the adaptative responses to physiologic hypoxia. Pao_2 = arterial blood oxygen pressure; PAo_2 = alveolar oxygen pressure; PAP = pulmonary arterial pressure; Vent = ventilation. The **arrows** indicate the threshold of the responses which, in all cases, is near 70 to 75 mm Hg.

The low threshold for hypoxia implies that chemoreceptor cells of the carotid body, erythropoietin producing cells, and smooth muscle cells of the pulmonary arteries must possess molecular oxygen-sensing mechanisms with low affinity for oxygen.

The three properties discussed here, i.e., the genesis of responses directed to prevent hypoxia in the entire organism and thus homeostasis, the required increased functional and metabolic activity during hypoxia, and the low threshold to hypoxia, define the physiologic sensitivity to hypoxia. It is the conjunction of these three properties that distinguishes the physiologic sensitivity to hypoxia, expressed only by chemoreceptor cells of the carotid body, erythropoietin-producing cells of the kidney and smooth muscle cells of the pulmonary arteries, from the general sensitivity to hypoxia shared by all cells in higher animals. All cell types in higher organisms exhibit a general sensitivity to hypoxia, if it is intense enough. The responses observed in most cells are directed to their own survival, and include shifts in metabolic routes, induction of glycolytic and oxidative enzymes, a general reduction of biosynthetic functions, and at the same time, an increase in the rate of synthesis of stress proteins acting as molecular chaperons or helping to repair possible mutations induced by hypoxia. These general responses of the cells mimic those encountered in lower organisms,[14] and are found at intense hypoxic levels.

Oxygen Sensing and Transduction of Physiologic Hypoxia

There are excellent reviews on oxygen sensing in general,[14] as well as on oxygen sensing in each of the cell types endowed with physiologic sensitivity to hypoxia (see Reference 15, for carotid body chemoreceptors; Reference 16, for erythropoietin producing cells, and; Reference 17, for pulmonary artery smooth muscle cells). In these reviews, as well as in the chapters of this book, each author defends a particular hypothesis of oxygen sensing and transduction according to personal research preferences.

I would agree with Bunn and Poyton[14] in stating that oxygen sensors are hemoproteins, whose identity in higher animal cells remains unknown. I refer to oxygen sensors because it is conceivable that different members of a family of hemoproteins are responsible for the general and for the physiologic sensitivity to hypoxia. In the same manner that punctual mutations and substitutions (normal hemoglobin vs. San Diego or Kansas hemoglobins) or oligomerization (myoglobin vs. hemoglobin) can generate well-characterized oxygen-transporting proteins with different

P_{50} for oxygen, evolution might have achieved oxygen sensors with very different oxygen affinities.

The strongest experimental support for the involvement of hemoproteins in oxygen sensing comes from the observation that carbon monoxide can inhibit low PO_2-triggered responses. As discussed in detail in References 14 and 18, carbon monoxide is so inert that in biological systems it is difficult to explain its actions by a mechanism different from its interactions with hemoproteins. In the carotid body chemoreceptors, the first evidence supporting a role for a hemoprotein in oxygen sensing was obtained by Lloyd et al[19]; these authors observed that a bolus of carbon monoxide inspired while breathing a hypoxic mixture significantly reduced ventilation. A few years later, Lahiri,[20] based in the analysis of hypoxic chemoreceptor discharges and the interactions between hypoxia and acidic stimuli, postulated that oxygen detection in the carotid body would be satisfactorily explained by a hemoglobin-like pigment with a P_{50} of 40 mm Hg and a particular Bohr effect. The discovery of oxygen-sensitive K^+ currents in the chemoreceptor cells of the carotid body[21] provided the possibility to test the effect of carbon monoxide on these K^+ currents, and as shown in Table 2, it was found that the presence of carbon monoxide in the hypoxic superfusing solution (10% carbon monoxide + 5% oxygen; i.e., carbon monoxide/oxygen = 2) reduced by nearly 70%, and in a readily reversible manner, the inhibition of the K^+ current produced by hypoxia in isolated chemoreceptor cells.[22] Lahiri et al[23] found that carbon monoxide/oxygen mixtures, in proportions similar to those used in isolated cells, inhibited the carotid sinus nerve chemoreceptor discharges elicited by hypoxia, while gas mixtures with higher carbon monoxide/oxygen proportions stimulated chemoreceptor discharges in a light-sensitive manner, indicating that this last effect was due to the interaction of carbon monoxide with cytochrome a_3. In fact the stimulatory effect of high proportions of carbon monoxide/oxygen was associated with a 30% to 40% decrease in the rate oxygen consumption. Intermediate carbon monoxide/oxygen proportions had dual effects. In the pulmonary circulation, we have recently observed that carbon monoxide also inhibits hypoxic pulmonary vasoconstriction[24] (Table 2), and Marshall et al[25] showed that higher concentrations of carbon monoxide produced pulmonary vasoconstriction. Goldberg et al,[26] in 1988, showed, and several authors have confirmed since, that carbon monoxide inhibited the production of erithropoietin produced by hypoxia. These, and some other pieces of experimental evidence, can only be interpreted on the basis of carbon monoxide interaction with hemoproteins, and since carbon monoxide also inhibits hypoxic responses in cell types with general sensitivity to hypoxia, the conclusion should be that oxygen sensors are indeed hemoproteins.

Table 2
Carbon Monoxide Prevents Hypoxic Inhibition of K^+ Currents in Chemoreceptor Cells of the Carotid Body and Hypoxic Pulmonary Vasoconstriction

Parameter Measured	*Control*	*Hypoxia*	*Hypoxia + CO*	*CO Inhibition of Hypoxia (%)*
K^+ current amplitude in the carotid body chemoreceptor cells (nA)	3.4 ± 0.9	2.2 ± 0.5	3.1 ± 0.7	68.4 ± 6.3[a]
Pulmonary arterial pressure (mm Hg)	15.2 ± 1.8	21.5 ± 1.3	16.0 ± 1.1	88.3 ± 2.7[b]

[a] Currents were recorded in short-term cultured rabbit carotid body chemoreceptor cells superfused with solutions equilibrated with 21% O_2 (control), 5% O_2 (hypoxia), and 5% O_2 + 10% CO (hypoxia + CO).
[b] Pulmonary arterial pressure was recorded in an isolated, blood perfused *in situ* preparation of rat lungs ventilated with 20% O_2/5% CO_2 (control), 2% O_2/5% CO_2 (hypoxia), and 2% O_2/5% CO_2/8% CO; in all cases N_2 was the balance gas.

The cellular location of the unknown hemoprotein acting as a putative oxygen sensor is not known. However, data obtained in isolated membrane patches of rabbit carotid body chemoreceptor cells strongly support the concept that the oxygen sensor is confined to the cellular plasma membrane. Thus, Ganfornina and Lopez-Barneo[27] found in isolated chemoreceptor cell membrane patches in the inside-out configuration that decreasing Po_2 in the bathing solution decreased the opening probabiliy of a K^+ channel with a unitary conductance of ≈20 pS. It should be mentioned, however, that cytoplasmic factors seem to be required for hypoxia to reduce the opening probalitity of the oxygen-sensitive $K^+{}_{Ca}$ in the rat carotid body chemoreceptor cells.[28]

Another hemoprotein that has been postulated as the oxygen sensor, triggering carotid body chemoreception, erythropoietin production, and hypoxic pulmonary vasoconstriction, is an NAD(P)H oxidase like that of neutrophils and macrophages. This oxidase is a multimeric complex in which an heme(Fe^{2+})-containing cytochrome β uses molecular oxygen to generate superoxide (O_2^-) becoming oxidized to cytochrome β heme(Fe^{3+}), which is back reduced in an NAD(P)H dependent manner. The O_2^- or the hydrogen peroxide (H_2O_2) formed by the superoxide dismutase, would be the nexus between the sensor and the transduction cascade. In the case of the carotid body chemoreceptor cells, the proposal is that hypoxia would reduce the rate of production of the peroxides, and these in turn would alter the ratio of oxidized/reduced glutathione, and thereby the ratio of -S-S-/SH in channel proteins. This would result in K^+ channel closure, cell depolarization, Ca^{2+} entry, and the release of neurotransmitters.[29] In pulmonary arteries, a dual proposal has been put forward: first, a decrease in peroxides produced by hypoxia would lead to a reduction in guanylate cyclase activity, cyclic guanosine monophosphate (cGMP) levels, and vasoconstriction[30]; second, hypoxia would trigger the closure of K^+ channels by increasing the ratios of GSH/GSSG, NADH/NAD, and probably other redox pairs.[17] In the case of erythropoietin-producing cells, support for the NAD(P)H oxidase comes from the observation that hydrogen peroxide can inhibit hypoxia-triggered erythropoietin production (see below).

The role of NAD(P)H oxidase as the primary oxygen sensor is not supported by experimental data. The oxidase does not react with carbon monoxide[31] and, therefore, cannot accommodate the forementioned observations; more importantly, a deficit in erythropoietin production is not an analytical or clinical feature of patients with chronic granulomatous disease, who lack functional oxidase. In fact, cells of patients with this disease exhibit a normal response to hypoxia.[32] I also question the significance of oxygen and H_2O_2 as key mediators of the physiologic sensitivity to hypoxia. My argument is based on the following points: 1) cells with physiologic sensitivity to hypoxia exhibit a higher metabolic rate during hypoxia than in normoxia (see above), and since there is a direct relation between oxygen consumption and peroxide generation[33] (see also Reference 35), one can question the assumed reduction in peroxides during hypoxia in these metabolically activated cells; 2) measurements made in the entire lung tissue under hypoxia only show very modest reductions (3% in a series of experiments) in activated oxygen species and, yet, in the same preparations, there was a marked increase in pulmonary arterial pressure[34]; 3) rotenone and antimycin A reduced activated oxygen species and produced an increase in pulmonary arterial pressure, but cyanide increased them and also produced an increase in pulmonary arterial pressure[34]; 4) to accept that the reduction of activated oxygen species produced by rotenone and antimycin A are the link for the reduction of K^+ currents, a minimal requirement should be the demonstration that these metabolic poisons do not inhibit K^+ channels by themselves, and; 5) the estimated steady-state concentrations of H_2O_2 in hepatocytes are in the range of 10^{-9} to 10^{-7} moles per liter,[35] and the first concentration of H_2O_2 inhibiting erythropoietin production in HepG2 cells was 300 mM, 100 mM being ineffective,[36] i.e., concentrations of H_2O_2 over 10^4 times higher than the physiologic one were needed, and even higher concentrations ($0.5–0.8 \times 10^{-3}$ M) of H_2O_2 were used to prevent the inactivation of voltage dependent K^+ channels.[37]

I also have some reservations regarding the redox state of the cells as a signal triggering the corresponding activities in the cells endowed with physiologic sensitivity to hypoxia. First, it should indeed be expected that during hypoxia, the three cell types with physiologic sensitivity to hypoxia have increased NAD(P)H/NAD(P) ratios as a regulatory mechanism to activate their metabolism[13,38] (in fact, Duchen and Biscoe[39] have measured such increase in isolated chemoreceptor cells at Po_2 below 60 mm Hg, while in the control adrenomedullary cells not sensitive to physiologic hypoxia the increase in NAD(P)H/NA(DP) was only evident at Po_2 below 10 mm Hg), and it should also be expected that rotenone, antimycin A, and cyanide produce an increase in the reduced species of all redox pairs located upstream of the inhibited step. Yet, cyanide did not inhibit K^+ currents (see Reference 40) while hypoxia, rotenone, and antimycin A did.[34] Finally, 2-deoxyglucose also inhibited K^+ currents in spite of the presence of a high ATP concentration in the recording pipettes, and it was assumed that an increase in NAD(P)H/NAD(P) ratio would be the effector of 2-deoxyglucose on K^+ currents.[17,41] However, it seems unlikely that the inhibition of glycolysis with 2-deoxyglucose can increase the NAD(P)H/NAD(P) ratio, since 2-deoxyglucose is not a substrate for glucose-6-phosphate dehydrogenase (i.e., the NADPH generating pentose shunt is inhibited),[42] and by definition 2-deoxyglucose inhibits the NADPH generating glycolitic pathway. Therefore, it is hard to accept an increase in the NAD(P)H/NAD(P) ratio as the primary regulator of the K^+ channel gating.

Another suggested link between physiologic hypoxia and cell responses is the energy charge of the cells, commonly studied by measuring ATP levels. As already mentioned, ATP levels in the carotid body are maintained in hypoxia, but it should be expected that rotenone, antimycin A, and cyanide reduce them. In the carotid body, cyanide produced a dose-dependent (10^{-5} to 2.5×10^{-4} M; 5 min) increase in the release of dopamine in chemoreceptor cells and in action potential frequency in the carotid sinus nerve; at the highest concentration, the nerve response was not sustained, suggesting a metabolic failure of the preparation; at a concentration of 10^{-4} M, cyanide reduced ATP levels in the carotid body by 45%.[43] In biopsies of the edges of ventilated and perfused lungs of the pig, which have received bolus injections of cyanide to yield final concentrations of 5×10^{-5}, 10^{-4}, and 10^{-3} M, the two lower concentrations produced a sustained increase in pulmonary arterial pressure and did not alter ATP levels; the highest dose injected reduced in an $\approx$40% the ATP levels, and produced a nonsustained increase in pulmonary arterial pressure.[44] However, the doses are uncertain because cyanide is very volatile and would pass to the ventilating gas, and on the other hand, it is not known how much pulmonary arteries have contributed to the actual ATP levels measured. In the carotid body, 2-deoxyglucose reduced ATP levels in a dose-dependent manner, but only in the absence of glucose in the bathing solution.[45] In other cell systems (e.g., platelets) at normal Po_2, even in the absence of glucose in the bathing solution, endogenous substrates are capable of maintaining ATP levels in spite of very high levels (up to 20 mM) of the glucose analog (unpublished observation). In addition, the inhibition of K^+ currents in pulmonary artery smooth muscle cells was observed with 5 mM ATP in the recording pipette.[41] Therefore, a decrease in the ATP levels does not seem to be the *universal* trigger for the transduction cascade.

Then, how do cells transduce the decrease in Po_2? If the oxygen sensor is indeed in the plasma membrane (see above), I envision the initiation of the transduction cascade in chemoreceptor cells and pulmonary artery smooth muscle cells as a change in the conformational state of the sensor upon oxygen saturation-desaturation, like that occurring in hemoglobin, which directly affects the gating of K^+ channels. The inmediate response generated in these cell types advocates a direct coupling between the oxygen sensor and the first element in the transduction cascade, the K^+ channels. At the present moment, there are no experimental data either to support or to deny this proposal. Long-term effects of hypoxia involving protein synthesis in these cells (e.g., induction of tyrosin hydroxylase) would be activated via second and third messenger systems, cAMP/cAMP inducible factor/CRE site, and Ca^{2+}-cAMP/*c-fos c-jun*/AP1 site. In erythropoietin producing cells, oxygen-sensor desaturation must generate a signal triggering the synthesis of transcription factors (e.g., hypoxia inducible factor 1 [HIF-1]) leading to an increase in erythropoietin production. This proposal has two drawbacks: first, it is speculative because there are no experimental data to support it; and second, it leaves unexplained the mechanisms of action of the forementioned metabolic poisons. Regarding the first point, it would appear that only when its chemical identity is known, will be possible to test it, and regarding the second point, a prerequisite to search for the mechanism of action of the metabolic poisons is to exclude a direct action of the poisons on isolated K^+ channels and on the effector machinery (contractile in smooth muscle cells, or secretory in chemoreceptor cells); nonetheless, there are some hints that might direct searches in different directions. For example, it is known that carbon monoxide excitation of carotid body chemoreceptors is accompanied by a reduction of the oxygen consumption at least in a 30% to 40% (see above), cyanide, rotenone, and antimycin A would also reduce oxygen consumption, and all of them would reduce ATP levels in parallel (see above). On the other hand it is also known that active Na^+ transport drops in parallel to the fall in oxygen consumption and ATP levels.[46] Therefore, at submaximal doses of cyanide, depolarization of chemoreceptor and pulmonary artery smooth muscle cells could be expected; at higher doses, a complete disruption of the energetic state of the cells would result in permanent depolarization of the cells and their incapacity to respond to any stimulus.[34,44] Regarding uncouplers and 2-deoxyglucose, it is known that in addition to their activity as metabolic inhibitors, both of them produce intracellular acidification in lymphocytes and polymorphonuclear leukocytes.[47,48] The sensitivity of $K^{+}{}_{ca}$ channels to hydrogen ions, as well as the sensitivity of chemoreceptor cells to intracellular acidification and the potentiation of pulmonary hypoxic vasoconstriction by acidosis, are well documented.

Acknowledgements

I want to thank Profs. B. Herreros, Sanchez-Crespo, Almaraz, and Obeso for critical reading of the manuscript. Supported by Spanish DGICYT Grant PB92–0267.

References

1. Ward MP, Milledge JS, West JB: *High Altitude Medicine and Physiology*. 2nd ed. London, UK: Chapman and Hall Medical; 1995.
2. Wintrobe MM: *Clinical Hematology*. Philadelphia: Lea and Febiger; 135–194, 1974.
3. Fidone SJ, Gonzalez C: Initiation and control of chemoreceptor activity in the carotid body. In: Fishman AP (ed). *Handbook of Physiology. The Respiratoy System*. Bethesda, MD: American Physiology Society; 247–312, 1986.
4. Reeves JT, Wagner WW, McMurtry IF, Grover RF: Physiological effects of high altitude on the pulmonary circulation. In: Guyton AC (ed): *Environmental Physiology III*. Boston, MD: University Park Press; 253–289, 1979
5. West JB: Human physiology at extreme altitudes on Mount Everest. *Science* 233: 784–788, 1984.

5a. Reynafarje B: Myoglobin content and enzymatic activity of muscle and altitude adaptation. *J Appl Physiol* 17:301–305, 1962.

6. Monge C, León-Valverde F: Physiological adaptation to high altitude: oxygen transport in mammals and birds. *Physiol Rev* 71:1135–1172, 1992.
7. Scherrer U, Vollenweider L, Delabays A, et al: Inhaled nitric oxide for high altitude pulmonary edema. *N Engl J Med* 334:624–629, 1996.
8. Marshall BE, Marshall C, Frasch F, Hanson CW: Role of hypoxic pulmonary vasoconstriction in pulmonary gas exchange and blood flow distribution. *Intensive Care Med* 20:291–297, 1994.
9. Mata M, Fink DJ, Gainer H, et al: Activity-dependent energy metabolism in rat posterior pituitary reflects sodium pump activity. *J Neurochem* 34:213–215, 1980.

10. Erecinska M, Dagani F: Relationships between the neuronal sodium/potassium pump and energy metabolism. *J Gen Physiol* 95:591–616, 1990.
11. Obeso A, Gonzalez C, Rigual R, et al: Effect of low O_2 on glucose uptake in rabbit carotid body. *J Appl Physiol* 74:2387–2393, 1993.
12. Verna A, Talib N, Roumy M, Pradet A: Effects of metabolic inhibitors and hypoxia on the ATP, ADP, and AMP content of the rabbit carotid body in vitro: the metabolic hypothesis in question. *Neurosci Lett* 116:156–161, 1990.
13. Erecinska M, Silver IA: ATP and brain function. *J Cereb Blood Flow Metab* 9: 2–19, 1989.
14. Bunn HF, Poyton RO: Oxygen sensing and molecular adaptation to hypoxia. *Physiol Rev* 76:839–885, 1996.
15. Gonzalez C, Almaraz L, Obeso A, Rigual R: Carotid body chemoreceptors: from natural stimuli to sensory discharges. *Physiol Rev* 74:829–898, 1994.
16. Ratcliffe PJ, Ebert BL, Ferguson DJP, et al: Regulation of the erythropoietin gene. *Nephrol Dial Transplant* 10:18–27, 1995.
17. Weir EK, Archer SL: The mechanism of acute hypoxic pulmonary vasoconstriction: the tale of two channels. *Faseb J* 9:183–189, 1995.
18. Coburn RF, Forman HJ: Carbon monoxide toxicity. In: Fishman AP, ed. *The Respiratory System.* Bethesda, MD: American Physiology Society; 439–456, 1987.
19. Lloyd BB, Cunningham DJC, Goode RC: Depression of hypoxic hyperventilation in man by sudden inspiration of carbon monoxide. In Torrance RW (ed). *Arterial Chemoreceptors.* Oxford, UK: Blackwell Scientific Publications; 145–148, 1968.
20. Lahiri S: Introductory remarks: oxygen linked response of carotid chemoreceptors. *Adv Exp Med Biol* 78:185–202, 1977.
21. López-Barneo J, López-Lopez JR, Ureña J, Gonzalez C: Chemotransduction in the carotid body: K^+ current modulated by Po_2 in type I chemoreceptor cells. *Science* 241:580–582, 1988.
22. Lopez-Lopez JR, Gonzalez C: Time course of K^+ current inhibition by low oxygen in chemoreceptor cells of adult rabbit carotid body: effects of carbon monoxide. *FEBS Lett* 299:251–254, 1992.
23. Lahiri S, Iturriaga R, Mokashi A, Ray DK, Chugh D: CO reveals dual mechanisms of chemoreception in the cat carotid body. *Res Physiol* 94:227–240, 1993.
24. Tamayo L, López-López JR, Castañeda J, Gonzalez C: Carbon monoxide inhibits hypoxic pulmonary vasoconstriction by a cGMP-independent mechanism. *Pflügers Arch-Evr J Physiol* 434:698–704, 1997.
25. Marshall C, Cooper DY, Marshall BE: Reduced availability of energy initiates pulmonary vasoconstriction. *Proc Soc Exp Biol Med* 187:282–286, 1988.
26. Goldberg M, Dunning SP, Bunn HF: Regulation of the erythropoietin gene: evidence that the oxygen sensor is a heme protein. *Science* 242:1412–1415, 1988.
27. Ganfornina MD, López-Barneo J: Single K^+ channels in membrane patches of arterial chemoreceptor cells are modulated by O_2 tension. *Proc Natl Acad Sci USA* 88:2927–2930, 1991.
28. Wyatt CN, Peers C: $Ca(^{2+})$-activated K^+ channels in isolated type I cells of the neonatal rat carotid body. *J Physiol Lond* 483:559–65, 1995.
29. Acker H, Xue D: Mechanisms of O_2 sensing in the carotid body in comparison with other O_2-sensing cells. *News Physiol Sci* 10:211–215, 1995.
30. Omar H, Wolin M: Endothelium-dependent and independent cGMP mechanisms appear to mediate O_2 responses in calf pulmonary resistance arteries. *Am J Physiol* 262:L560-L565, 1992.

31. Iizuka T, Kanegasaki S, Makino R, et al: Studies on neutrophyl β-type cytochrome in situ by low temperature absorption spectroscopy. *J Biol Chem* 260: 12049–12053, 1985.
32. Wenger RH, Marti HH, Schuerer-Maly CC, et al: Hypoxic induction of gene expression in chronic granulomatous disease-derived B-cell line: oxygen sensing is independent of the cytochrome b558-containing nicotinamide adenine dinucleotide phosphate oxidase. *Blood* 87:756–761, 1996.
33. Sohal RS, Weindruch R: Oxidative stress, caloric restriction, and aging. *Science* 273:59–63, 1996.
34. Archer SL, Huang J, Henry T, et al: A redox-based O_2 sensor in rat pulmonary vasculature. *Circ Res* 73:1100–1112, 1993.
35. Chance B, Sies H, Boveris A: Hydrogen peroxide metabolism in mammalian organs. *Physiol Rev* 59:527–605, 1979.
36. Fandrey J, Frede S, Jelkmann W: Oxygen sensing by H_2O_2-generating heme proteins. *Ann N Y Acad Sci* 718:341–343, 1994.
37. Vega-Saenz de Miera E, Rudy B: Modulation of K^+ channels by hydrogen peroxide. *Biochem Biophys Res Commun* 186:1681–1687, 1992.
38. Erecinska M, Wilson DF: Regulation of cellular energy metabolism. *J Memb Biol* 70:1–14, 1982.
39. Duchen MR, Biscoe TJ: Mitochondrial function in type I cells isolated from rabbit arterial chemoreceptors. *J Physiol Lond* 450:13–31, 1992.
40. Peers C, O'Donnell J: Potassium currents recorded in type I carotid body cells from the neontal rat and their modulation by chemoexcitatory agents. *Brain Res* 522:259–266, 1990.
41. Yuang X-J, Tod M, Rubin L, Blaustein M: Deoxyglucose and reduced glutathione mimic effects of hypoxia on K^+ and Ca^{2+} conductances in pulmonary artery cells. *Amer J Physiol* 267:L52-L63, 1994.
42. Horton RW, Meldrum BS, Bachelard HS: Enzymatic and cerebral metabolic effects of 2-deoxy-D-glucose. *J Neurochem* 21:507–520, 1973.
43. Obeso A, Almaraz L, Gonzalez C: Effects of cyanide and uncouplers on chemoreceptor activity and ATP content of the cat carotid body. *Brain Res* 481:250–257, 1989.
44. Buescher PC, Pearse DB, Pillai RP, et al: Energy state and vasomotor tone in hypoxic pig lungs. *J Appl Physiol* 70:1874–1881, 1991.
45. Obeso A, Almaraz L, Gonzalez C: Effects of 2-deoxy-D-glucose on in vitro cat carotid body. *Brain Res* 371:25–36, 1986.
46. Danisi G, Lacaz Vieira F: Nonequilibrium thermodynamic analysis of the coupling between active sodium transport and oxygen consumption. *J Gen Physiol* 64:372–391, 1974.
47. Grinstein S, Cohen S: Cytoplasmic (Ca^{2+}) and intracellular pH in lymphocytes. Role of membrane potential and volume-activated Na^+/H^+ exchange. *J Gen Physiol* 89:185–213, 1987.
48. Grinstein S, Furuya W: Characterization of the amiloride-sensitive Na^+-H^+ antiport of human neutrophils. *Am J Physiol* 250:C283-C291, 1986.

Index